International Classification of Procedures in Medicine

Volume 1

1. Procedures for Medical Diagnosis
2. Laboratory Procedures
4. Preventive Procedures
5. Surgical Procedures
8. Other Therapeutic Procedures
9. Ancillary Procedures

Published for trial purposes in accordance with
resolution WHA29.35 of the Twenty-ninth World Health Assembly,
May 1976

WORLD HEALTH ORGANIZATION
GENEVA

1978

ISBN 92 4 154124 5

PRINTED IN SWITZERLAND

TABLE OF CONTENTS

To be published:

3.   RADIOLOGY AND CERTAIN OTHER APPLICATIONS OF PHYSICS
           IN MEDICINE

6 and 7.   DRUGS, MEDICAMENTS AND BIOLOGICAL AGENTS

INTRODUCTION

This Classification is intended to present in a systematic fashion the many procedures used in different branches of medicine, a task which the World Health Organization is undertaking for the first time.

The difficulties and problems encountered in preparing a Classification of Procedures in Medicine are similar to those experienced for the International Classification of Diseases, aggravated by the absence of international experience in the fields to be covered. Although certain countries have experience in these fields, especially in the classification of surgical procedures, their views and methods of approach are divergent enough to make the task of harmonizing their classifications a complicated one.

Probably these considerations motivated the cautious approach taken in the report of the International Conference for the Ninth Revision of the International Classification of Diseases, convened by the World Health Organization at WHO headquarters in Geneva from 30 September to 6 October 1975:[1]

"2. Classification of Procedures in Medicine

In response to requests from a number of Member States, the Organization had drafted a classification of therapeutic, diagnostic and prophylactic procedures in medicine, covering surgery, radiology, laboratory and other procedures. Various national classifications of this kind had been studied and advice sought from hospital associations in a number of countries. The intention was to provide a tool for use in the analysis of health services provided to patients in hospitals, clinics, outpatient departments, etc.

The Conference congratulates the Secretariat on this important development and

Recommends that the provisional procedures classifications should be published as supplements to, and not as integral parts of, the Ninth Revision of the International Classification of Diseases. They should be published in some inexpensive form and, after two or three years' experience, revised in the light of users' comments."

Subsequently the Twenty-ninth World Health Assembly, meeting in May 1976, endorsed this recommendation in resolution WHA29.35, in which it approved "the publication, for trial purposes, of supplementary classifications of Impairments and Handicaps and of Procedures in Medicine, as supplements to, but not as integral parts of, the International Classification of Diseases."

The present provisional edition of the Classification of Procedures in Medicine has been prepared by WHO in compliance with this resolution, in the hope that it will serve as a basis for further collaboration and development.

---

[1] World Health Organization. Manual of the international statistical classification of diseases, injuries and causes of death, 1975 revision, Geneva, 1977, vol. 1, p. xvii.

Preparation of the Classification

Activities for the preparation of the proposals for the International Classification of Procedures in Medicine began at about the same time as those for the Ninth Revision of the International Classification of Diseases and were carried out in parallel.

Scope and form

At a meeting of a working party convened in April 1971 in Chicago, USA, under the auspices of the American Hospital Association, the following consensus was reached on certain requisites to be fulfilled by the Classification:

(a)   it should be susceptible of expansion for those who need greater detail, but it should also offer the possibility of use in a condensed form;

(b)   it should be applicable to inpatients and outpatients;

(c)   it should include all types of procedures to be recorded for statistical, administrative, clinical or research purposes, encompassing exploratory, radiological, surgical and other procedures of a diagnostic, prophylactic or therapeutic nature.

In accordance with these recommendations, the present provisional Classification consists of nine chapters:

1.   Procedures for medical diagnosis

2.   Laboratory procedures

3.   Radiology and certain other applications of physics in medicine[1]

4.   Preventive procedures

5.   Surgical operations

6 and 7.   Drugs, medicaments and biological agents[1]

8.   Other therapeutic procedures

9.   Ancillary procedures

Structure

The International Classification of Procedures in Medicine has a structure similar to that of the International Classification of Diseases. Each volume will contain a tabular list and an alphabetical index.

The complete series of categories for the nine chapters are numbered from 1-100 to 9-823, the first digit denoting the chapter number.   The

---

[1] To be published subsequently.

Classification is significant at the three-digit level; the fourth digit provides for greater detail and precision. Optional fifth-digit subdivisions are provided for in some categories.

Sources

Chapter 1, on "Procedures for medical diagnosis", is based mainly on Physicians' current procedural terminology (American Medical Association), but other sources have been also used, such as Canada's Schedule of unit values, the Ontario Medical Association list of fees and the Nomenclature des actes professionels (France).

The classification of laboratory procedures (chapter 2) is based largely on a French project which was modified in order to take into account the ever growing number of new techniques.

The chapter on "Radiology and certain other applications of physics in medicine" (chapter 3) was originally based on a Swedish classification, a French proposal and the classification used in Switzerland by the Bureau national de la Santé et du Bien-Etre, and later modified by the WHO Radiation Medicine unit in order to take into consideration the opinion of specialists from the International Radiological Society.

Chapter 4, on "Preventive procedures", is based on reports of health centres in several countries and includes mainly methods and techniques traditionally considered as preventive and susceptible of application to individuals.

The Eighth Revision of the International Classification of Diseases (Adapted) (United States Public Health Service Publication No. 1693) served as a basis for the classification of surgical operations (chapter 5), but some items were extracted from other sources, particularly the Dutch code (Algemene Ziekenfondsen, 1968) and the Classification of the Office of Population Censuses and Surveys (England and Wales, 1974), as well as several other lists and working documents issued by hospitals and public health administrations in all regions of the world. However, the arrangement of categories is based on topography, not surgical specialty.

Two chapters are provided for the classification of drugs, medicaments and biological agents (chapters 6 and 7). They follow as closely as possible the corresponding series of categories in sections 960-979 of the Ninth Revision of ICD, which classify the toxic effects of these substances. The code numbers have been derived by omitting the ICD first digit "9" and by adding an additional digit for further detail. For example, the ICD category 960.0 Penicillins becomes 6-00 in the Drugs classification and the subdivisions 6-000 to 6-009 allow for identification of the varieties of penicillin.

Chapter 8, on "Other therapeutic procedures", as indicated by its title, includes medical therapeutic procedures not elsewhere classified. The axis chosen is the type of intervention instead of the anatomical system.

The final chapter, "Ancillary procedures" (chapter 9), contains all procedures not included in the preceding chapters. It is, therefore, a collection of marginal activities which might seem to have little relationship with the aims of most users of this classification. However, they have been included because they are, or might be, encountered as recorded procedures having a bearing on professional clinical activities.

Mode of utilization

The use of the International Classification of Procedures in Medicine should not present real problems for coders, since the steps for assigning the code numbers are similar to those followed for coding with ICD.

Evidently, the user should carefully review the arrangement of the tabular lists and the alphabetical indexes in order to become familiar with the contents and the manner of presentation and especially to become familiar with the terminology used in these classifications.

In the tabular lists the categories are numerically ordered, but some gaps will be found which are intended for greater flexibility and possible modifications if the need arises. As in ICD the fourth-digit subdivisions contain a few inclusion terms to clarify the contents of the category; exclusion notes are also used for that purpose. The reference: "Other available codes: ..." indicates to the reader the place where other related procedures have been classified.

The alphabetical indexes are organized in a way similar to the ICD Index, and are also based on lead terms which may or may not have several levels of indented modifiers. The complete terms are followed by the four-digit code. Where fourth-digit subdivisions are common for a group of three-digit categories, the fourth digit is replaced by a dash (-) and in these cases the fourth digit must be looked for in the tabular list. The optional fifth-digit subdivisions are not shown in the indexes.

For some purposes the chapters of the International Classification of Procedures in Medicine can be used separately, for example: chapter 3 by a radiotherapy department, chapter 2 by a laboratory service, chapter 4 by a preventive unit not offering treatment services, and chapters 6 and 7 by a pharmacy. Health institutions should, however, strive to use the complete set of nine chapters.

Since in the majority of circumstances a patient will be subject to more than one procedure, the principle of multiple coding appears essential, within chapters as well as between chapters. Ideally, all the procedures should be coded. This is especially advisable from the administrative standpoint (charges, accounting, etc.) and for statistical purposes. However, it is for the health institution or administration to decide how many items should be coded from each chapter and in each case.

The use of the four-digit codes will provide more precise and accurate information. Although the three-digit codes are also significant, they are less precise and offer less detail; the use of the four-digit codes is therefore preferable.

The design of the system used for gathering the data, the forms to enter the code numbers and other aspects of data processing will depend on the characteristics and needs of institutions; no attempt is therefore made here to propose such a system.

Coding with the International Classification of Procedures in Medicine is simpler than coding with ICD, since there are no special rules for coding as is the case for ICD, where we find a set of rules for single-condition coding in mortality and morbidity. Coding problems encountered with these new classifications, if any, should be dealt with in a classroom situation.

The following abbreviations are used in this volume:

NOS	not otherwise specified
NEC	not elsewhere classified

Comments and suggestions

Users of the International Classification of Procedures in Medicine are requested to forward their comments and suggestions, after an experience of two or three years, to:

Head, WHO Centre for Classification of Diseases
Office of Population Censuses and Surveys
St Catherine's House
10 Kingsway
London WC2B 6JP
United Kingdom

or

Head, WHO Center for Classification of Diseases for North
    America
National Center for Health Statistics
US Public Health Service
Department of Health, Education and Welfare
Washington, DC
United States of America

TABULAR LIST

1. PROCEDURES FOR MEDICAL DIAGNOSIS

1.   PROCEDURES FOR MEDICAL DIAGNOSIS

MEDICAL SERVICES

The term "external examination" refers to physical examination, performed by a physician by means of inspection, external palpation, percussion and auscultation where these are pertinent procedures.

The following fourth-digit subdivisions are for use with categories 1-10 to 1-18:

     0   Brief
         with short or interval history and general inspection of
           the patient

     1   Limited
         with history plus external examination referred to one
           organ or two symetric organs

     2   Intermediate
         with history plus external examination referred to one body
           system

     3   Extensive
         with history plus external examination referred to two or
           more body systems

     4   Complete
         with history plus external examination referred to the whole
           body

     9   Not otherwise specified

INITIAL MEDICAL ATTENTION

Includes: recording of:
           history
           physical examination   }   at the start of the
           intended diagnostic program   current episode
           treatment prescribed   of care

1-10   <u>Initial medical attention, outpatient</u>

1-11   <u>Initial medical attention, inpatient</u>

Excludes: newborn (1-190 to 1-192)

1-12   <u>Initial medical attention, other patient</u>

Includes: day hospital
           domiciliary
           emergency service   }
           extended care   patient
               or convalescent
           night hospital

SUBSEQUENT MEDICAL ATTENTION

Includes: recording of:
            history
            physical examinations
            other examinations   } after the start of the current
            treatment given   episode of care
            evolution
            final summary }
            diagnoses   of the current episode of care

1-13   Subsequent medical attention, outpatient

1-14   Subsequent medical attention, inpatient

1-15   Subsequent medical attention, other patient

CONSULTATION

Includes: written opinion or advice given, at the request of the
attending physician, by another physician, about
specialized evaluation or further treatment

Excludes: subsequent attentions if the consultant physician assumes
the responsibility for continuing services to the
patient (1-13 to 1-15)

1-16   Consultation, outpatient

1-17   Consultation, inpatient

1-18   Consultation, other patient

NEWBORN SERVICES

1-19   In-hospital newborn care

  1-190   Apgar scoring of newborn, without other initial medical
          evaluation

  1-191   Initial medical evaluation of newborn, without Apgar scoring

  1-192   Apgar scoring with other medical evaluation of newborn

  1-193   Recording of birthweight

  1-194   Recording of crown-heel length

  1-195   Recording of other newborn measurements

  1-198   Subsequent care of healthy newborn

  1-199   Not otherwise specified

EXAMINATION OF SPECIAL SYSTEMS

1-20   Neurological examination

  1-200   Sensory mapping and testing

  Excludes: auditory (1-23)
             visual (1-21)

  1-201   Clinical reflex testing

  1-202   Tendon reflex time recording

  1-203   Nerve conduction testing

  1-204   Determination of pain threshold

  1-205   Muscle power testing

  1-206   Examination of cerebrospinal fluid

  Diagnostic lumbar puncture or cisternal puncture

  1-207   Electroencephalography

  1-209   Other instrumental neurological examination

  Transillumination of skull

1-21   Visual testing

  1-210   Perimetry

  Color fields   Visual fields

  1-211   Visual acuity

  Reading test

  1-212   Visual acuity of infants and illiterates

  1-213   Eikonometric examination

  Prescription of aniseikonic lenses

  1-214   Dark adaptation visual acuity

  1-215   Color vision testing

  Color lanterns   Pseudoisochromatic plates

  1-216   Ocular muscle balance testing

  Binocular vision   Stereoscopic vision

1-22   <u>Other ophthalmological examination</u>

  1-220   Ophthalmoscopy

Funduscopy

  1-221   Slit lamp examination

  1-222   Photography of fundus oculi

  1-223   Photonystagmography

  1-224   Measurement of curvature of eye

Refraction with contact lenses

  1-225   Tonometry

Ophthalmodynamometry   Recording tonometry
Perilimbal suction

  1-226   Gonioscopy

  1-229   Other instrumental ophthalmological examinations

Transillumination of sclera

Excludes: fluorescent angiography of retina (1-802)

1-23   <u>Auditory and vestibular function tests</u>

  I-230   Subjective audiometry

Audiometry NOS   Bekesy 5-tone audiometry

  1-231   Impedance audiometry

Tympanogram   Stapedial reflex response

  1-232   Clinical tests of hearing

Tuning fork tests   Whispered speech

  1-233   Audiological evaluation

Barany noise machine   Equiloudness balance
Blindfold test   Masking
Delayed feedback   Weber lateralization

  1-234   Clinical vestibular function tests

Thermal tests

  1-235   Rotation tests

Barany chair

  1-239   Other auditory and vestibular function tests

Electrocochlearography

1-24   Otorhinolaryngological examinations

  1-240   Routine otoscopy

Auroscopy

  1-241   Magnifying otoscopy

  1-242   Other instrumental examination of ear

  1-243   Rhinoscopy

  1-244   Transillumination of antrum

  1-245   Other examination of nose

  1-246   Other instrumental examination of throat

  1-249   Instrumental otorhinolaryngological examination, not otherwise specified

1-25   Cardiovascular examinations

  1-250   In-depth clinical cardiovascular examination

  1-251   Heart rate recording

  1-252   Arterial pulse recording

Carotid artery tracing

  1-253   Arterial plethysmography

Blood pressure recording

  1-254   Blood flow recording

  1-255   Phonocardiography

Intracardial phonocardiology

  1-256   Ballistocardiography

  1-257   Other instrumental examination of heart

  1-259   Other instrumental examination of circulation

  Excludes: cardiac function tests (1-72)
          catheterization of heart and vessels (1-27)
          electrical response of heart (1-26)

1-26   Electrical response of heart

  1-260   Electrocardiography

ECG, EKG

1-261   Esophageal electrode

For heart monitoring

1-262   Dynamic electrocardiography

DCG
With exercise test

1-263   Vector electrocardiography

1-264   Emergency or operative methods

Epicardial recording at operation   Portable apparatus

1-265   Endocardial catheter recording

Atrioventricular bundle (AV) activity   Tripolar catheter electrode
Bundle of His (H) electrograms

1-266   Interpretation of and report on electrocardiograms

1-267   Display of electrical response

Contourograph

1-269   Other and unspecified electrical response of heart

Excludes: monitoring of fetal heart during labor (8-961)

1-27   Catheterization of heart and vessels

1-270   Jugular vein catheterization

1-271   Inferior vena cava catheterization

1-272   Central venous pressure (CVP) measurement

1-273   Intravenous catheterization of heart

Cardiac catheterization, unqualified

1-274   Transseptal cardiac catheterization

1-275   Retrograde catheterization of left heart

1-276   Myocardial oxygen consumption

1-278   Other catheterization of heart

1-279   Other diagnostic catheterization of vessels

EXAMINATION OF OTHER SPECIAL SYSTEMS

1-30   Stomatological examinations

  1-300   Dental examination

  1-301   DMF (diseased, missing, filled) charting

  1-302   Diagnostic occlusal mulds

  1-304   Buccal examination with finger

  1-309   Other examination of oral cavity

  (Other available code: sialography (see Chapter 3)

1-31   Examination of upper digestive and respiratory tract

  1-310   Pharyngeal examination with finger

  1-312   Retrieval of vomit for analysis

  1-313   Esophageal manometry

  1-319   Other instrumental examination of upper digestive tract

1-32   Gastrointestinal examination

  1-320   Digital exploration of rectum

  1-321   Electrogastrogram

  1-322   Stomal calibration

  1-329   Other instrumental examination of gastrointestinal tract

  Excludes: endoscopy with incision (1-695)
             other endoscopy (1-64)

1-33   Examination of urinary tract

  1-330   Evaluation of bladder sensation

  Detrusor   reflex testing

  1-331   Residual urinary volume

  1-332   Diagnostic catheterization of bladder

  1-333   Continuous flow cystometry

  1-334   Other cystometry

  Air cystometry
  Cystometrography

  1-335   Urethral pressure measurements

1-336   Meatal calibration

1-339   Other instrumental examination of the urinary tract

Excludes: collection of urine from single ureter (1-654)
           endoscopy (1-65)
           renal function tests (2-34)

1-34   Examination of male genital organs

1-340   In-depth clinical examination of male genital organs

1-341   Collection of semen specimen for examination

1-349   Other instrumental examination of male genital system

Excludes: examination of spermatic fluid (2-285)

1-35   Examination of female genital system

1-350   Internal clinical gynecological examination

Digital exploration through vagina   Inspection with vaginal speculum

1-351   Endocrine assessment, vaginal cytology

1-352   Endocrine assessment, endometrial cytology

1-353   Postcoital plug examination for infertility

1-354   Intrauterine pressure measurement

1-355   Placental localization

1-358   Other instrumental gynecological examination

Excludes: culdoscopy (1-696)
           insufflation of fallopian tubes (5-667)

1-359   Other instrumental obstetric examination

Excludes: amniocentesis (5-753)

1-36   Musculoskeletal examinations

1-360   In-depth clinical examination of musculoskeletal system

1-361   Measurement of limb lengths

Detection of asymmetry

1-362   Measurement of range of movement

1-363   Electromyography

1-369   Other instrumental musculoskeletal examinations

Excludes: anthropometric studies (1-950)

1-37   Examination of other systems

1-370   Skin temperature measurement

1-379   Other instrumental examinations

Excludes: electrical recording (1-960)
           medical photography (1-961)

BIOPSY

Includes: biopsy by endoscopy, punch biopsy, percutaneous
           needle biopsy and superficial smears

Excludes: biopsy by incision, open operation or excision
           of tissue (1-50 to 1-59)

1-40   Biopsy of nervous system and endocrine organs

1-400   Adrenal, percutaneous biopsy

1-401   Brain and meninges ,percutaneous biopsy

1-402   Nerve, percutaneous biopsy

1-409   Other nervous or endocrine structure, percutaneous biopsy

1-41   Biopsy of ear, eye and skin of face

1-410   External ear, biopsy

1-411   Biopsy of ear by otoscopy

1-412   Skin of eyelid or eyebrow, biopsy

1-413   Conjunctiva, biopsy

1-414   Skin of nose or face, biopsy

1-415   Biopsy of nose by rhinoscopy

1-42   Biopsy of larynx, pharynx and vascular organs

1-420   Biopsy of larynx by laryngoscopy

1-421   Oral cavity, biopsy

Tongue   Palate

Excludes: lips (1-480)

1-422   Tonsils, fauces and adenoids, biopsy

1-423   Biopsy of pharynx, gum and uvula by pharyngoscopy

1-424   Transvenous biopsy

1-425   Bone marrow biopsy

1-426   Lymphatic biopsy

Scalene node biopsy

Excludes: lymphadenectomy biopsy (5-409)

1-427   Spleen, percutaneous biopsy

1-43   Biopsy of other respiratory organs

1-430   Biopsy of trachea by endoscopy

1-431   Lung, percutaneous biopsy

1-432   Biopsy of bronchus by endoscopy

Transbronchoscopic biopsy of lung

1-433   Pleural biopsy

1-434   Biopsy of chest

1-44   Biopsy of upper alimentary tract

1-440   Biopsy of esophagus by endoscopy

1-441   Biopsy of stomach by endoscopy

1-442   Duodenal capsule biopsy

1-45   Biopsy of other alimentary organs

1-450   Biopsy of colon by endoscopy

1-451   Biopsy of sigmoid colon by endoscopy

Sigmoidoscopic biopsy

1-452   Biopsy of rectum by endoscopy

1-453   Biopsy of anus and perianal region

1-454   Liver, percutaneous biopsy

1-46   Biopsy of urinary tract and male genital organs

1-460   Kidney, percutaneous biopsy

1-461   Biopsy of ureter

1-462   Biopsy of bladder

1-463   Biopsy of prostate

1-464   Biopsy ot urethra

I-465   Biopsy of testis, epididymis and spermatic cord

1-466   Biopsy of penis

1-47   Biopsy of female genital tract

1-470   Ovary, aspiration biopsy

1-471   Endometrial biopsy

1-472   Cervical smear

(For routine screening use 4-250)

1-473   Endocervical biopsy

1-474   Ring biopsy of cervix

1-475   Other and unspecified cervical biopsy

1-476   Vaginal biopsy or smear

1-477   Biopsy of introitus

Bartholin's gland   Skene's glands
Labia

1-48   Other specified biopsy without incision

1-480   Lips, biopsy

1-481   Abdominal wall biopsy

1-482   Breast, biopsy

1-483   Skin, biopsy of other sites

Excludes: skin of nose (1-414)
            skin of ear (1-410)
            skin of eyelid or eyebrow (1-412)

1-484   Bone or joint biopsy

Drill biopsy

1-489   Other specified biopsy without incision

1-49   Biopsy of unspecified site

1-499   Biopsy, unqualified

SURGICAL BIOPSY

Includes: biopsy by incision, open operation or excision of tissue

Excludes: biopsy by endoscopy, punch biopsy, percutaneous needle biopsy
and superficial smears (1-40 to 1-49)
when incidental to excision of lesion - code the reported
excision (Chapter 5)

1-50   Skin, breast and osteomuscular system

   1-500   Skin and subcutaneous tissue

   Excludes: breast (1-501)
ear (1-530)
eyelid (1-520)
lip (1-540)
nose (1-538)
penis (1-564)
scrotum (1-569)
vulva (1-573)

   1-501   Breast

   Mammary gland

   1-502   Muscle

   Excludes: diaphragm (1-550)
eye (1-529)

   1-503   Bone

   1-504   Joint

   Arthrotomy for biopsy

1-51   Nervous system

   1-510   Intracranial tissue

   1-511   Intraspinal tissue

   1-512   Peripheral nerve

   1-519   Other

1-52   Eye

   1-520   Eyelid

   1-521   Conjunctiva

   1-522   Lacrimal gland and sac

   1-523   Cornea

   1-529   Other

1-53   **Ear, nose**

   1-530   External ear

   1-531   External auditory canal

   1-532   Ear, other

   1-537   Nose, internal

   1-538   Nose, other

1-54   **Mouth, pharynx**

   1-540   Lip

   1-541   Tongue

   1-542   Salivary glands

   1-543   Vestibule of mouth

   1-544   Palate, uvula

   1-545   Mouth, other

   1-546   Oropharynx

   1-547   Hypopharynx

   1-548   Nasopharynx

   1-549   Pharynx, other

1-55   **Other organs of the digestive system, diaphragm**

   1-550   Diaphragm

   1-551   Liver

   1-552   Extrahepatic biliary system

   1-553   Pancreas

   1-554   Stomach

   1-555   Small intestine

   1-556   Colon

   1-557   Rectum

   1-558   Anus

   1-559   Other

Intestine NOS
Peritoneum

1-56   Urinary tract and male genital organs

  1-560   Kidney

  1-561   Urethra

  1-562   Other urinary organs

  1-563   Prostate

  1-564   Penis

  1-565   Testis

  1-566   Perineum, male

  1-569   Other male genital organs

1-57   Female genital organs

  1-570   Ovary and other uterine adnexa

  1-571   Cervix

  1-572   Vagina

  1-573   Vulva

  1-574   Perineum, female

  1-579   Other

1-58   Other organs not elsewhere classified

  1-580   Pericardium

  1-581   Other mediastinal or intrathoracic organ

  1-582   Thyroid and parathyroid glands

  1-583   Other neck organs, not elsewhere classified

  1-584   Adrenal gland

  1-585   Other intra-abdominal organ, not elsewhere classified

  1-586   Superficial lymph node

  1-587   Peripheral vessel

  1-589   Other

1-59   Surgical biopsy, not otherwise specified

   1-599   Surgical biopsy

ENDOSCOPY

1-61   Laryngoscopy and pharyngoscopy

   1-610   Diagnostic laryngoscopic procedures

   1-611   Indirect laryngoscopy

   1-612   Direct laryngoscopy

   1-613   Microlaryngoscopy

   1-614   Suspension laryngoscopy

   1-615   Pharyngoscopy

1-62   Bronchoscopy and tracheoscopy

   1-620   Bronchoscopy

Excludes: biopsy (1-432)

   1-621   Tracheoscopy

Excludes: tracheoscopy via tracheostomy (1-690)

1-63   Upper alimentary tract endoscopy

   1-630   Esophagoscopy

   1-631   Esophagoscopy via stoma

   1-632   Esophagogastroscopy

   1-633   Gastroscopy

Fiberscopy of stomach

   1-634   Gastrocamera

   1-635   Gastroscopy via existing stoma

   1-636   Duodenoscopy

1-64   Lower alimentary tract endoscopy

   1-640   Intestinal endoscopy via existing stoma

   1-641   Colonoscopy

Flexible fiber endoscopy

   1-642   Sigmoidoscopy

1-643   Proctoscopy

1-644   Anoscopy

1-65   Urinary tract endoscopy

1-650   Ureteroscopy

1-651   Pyeloscopy

1-652   Cystoscopy

1-653   Panendoscopy

1-654   Collection of urine from single ureter

1-655   Urethroscopy

1-66   Endoscopy of female genital tract

1-660   Hysteroscopy

1-663   Colposcopy

Excludes: culdoscopy (1-696)

1-67   Other specified endoscopy

1-670   Cavernoscopy

Excludes: of renal pelvis (1-551)

1-679   Other specified endoscopy

1-68   Endoscopy of unspecified site

1-680   Endoscopy via orifice

1-681   Endoscopy photography

1-689   Endoscopy, unqualified

Endoscopy without incision

1-69   Endoscopy with puncture or incision

(Other available codes: biopsy 1-400 to 1-499
                         collection of parasite or micro-organism
                         1-910 to 1-919)

1-690   Bronchoscopy and tracheoscopy by means of tracheotomy

1-691   Thoracoscopy

Cardioscopy (external)   Transpleural
Mediastinoscopy

1-692   Gastroesophageal endoscopy by means of gastrotomy

1-693   Enteroscopy by abdominal route

By enterotomy   By paracentesis

1-694   Laparoscopy

Peritoneoscopy

1-695   Operative enteroscopy or other abdominal endoscopy

Choledochoscopy   Pyeloscopy
During course of operation   Ureteroscopy
Gastroscopy

1-696   Culdoscopy

1-697   Arthroscopy

1-698   Other surgical endoscopy, qualified

Endoscopy of cerebral ventricle   Spinal endoscopy

1-699   Surgical endoscopy, unqualified

Operative endoscopy

PHYSIOLOGICAL FUNCTION TESTS

1-70   Tests of immunological status

  1-700   Skin tests, not elsewhere classified

  1-701   Skin tests for susceptibility

Bacterial: brucellosis (Brucellergen)
             leprosy (lepromin, histamine lepromin)
             streptococci (Dick, Schultz-Carlton)
             tularemia   (Foshay)
Bacterial toxin diphtheria (Schick)
Virus: lymphogranuloma venereum (Frei test)

  1-702   Skin test for hypersensitivity

Delayed reaction: type III, Arthus reaction, IgE (hours)
Immediate reaction: type I, reagin, IgE (minutes)
   atopic asthma (pollen)
   rhinitis (hay fever)
Late reaction: type IV, lymphocyte mediated (days)
Metals: nickel, beryllium fungal skin reactions
Reactions for helminths (Casoni, Melcher)

  1-703   Tuberculin testing

Intradermal test, Mantoux, PPD, Monrad
Scratch test, von Pirquet

1-704   Other intradermal antigen testing

Kveim test (sarcoid), histoplasmosis

1-705   Passive transfer test
Prausnitz-Küstner reaction

1-706   Nasal challenge for allergy

1-707   Bronchial challenge for allergy

Allergic alveolitis (farmer's lung)
Bronchial edema, PMN reaction
By insufflation
Non-atopic asthma

1-708   Other specified tests

Subconjunctival   Sublingual

1-709   Allergy testing NOS

Excludes: dermal response to fungi (2-703)

1-71   Respiratory function tests

1-710   Measurement of lung volumes

Gas dilution: Spirometry:
    residual volume   tidal volume
    total lung capacity   vital capacity

1-711   Respiratory flow rates

Dynamic spirometry   Maximum breathing capacity
Forced expiratory flow rates   Peak flow rate
Forced vital capacity

1-712   Resistance to respiration

Airways conductance   Esophageal pressure
Airways resistance   Pulmonary resistance
Body plethysmography   Total flow resistance
Dynamic compliance   Total static compliance

1-713   Distribution of ventilatory airflow

Multi-breath washout   Regional ventilatory function
Nitrogen   Single breath expiration test
Radioactive gas

1-714   Distribution of circulatory bloodflow

Pulmonary vascular resistance

1-715   Gas exchange and ventilation-perfusion efficiency

Alveolar-arterial tension gradients for respiratory gases
Dead space/tidal volume ratio
Transfer factor for carbon monoxide

1-716   Ventilatory control

Response to carbon dioxide

1-719   Other respiratory function tests

Excludes: metabolic function tests (1-76)
            standardized exercise ventilation (1-724)

1-72   Cardiac function tests

1-720   Intracardiac pressures

Ventricular outflow tract pressure gradient

1-721   Cardiac output

Cardiac index

1-722   Circulation time

1-723   Detection of cardiac shunt

1-724   Exercise tolerance tests

Standardized exercise ventilation (SEV)
Step test

1-729   Not otherwise specified

1-73   Circulatory function tests

1-730   Blood flow in single artery

Renal artery flow

1-731   Blood flow in limb

1-732   Circulatory stress testing

1-733   Portal venous pressure measurement

1-734   Plethysmography of limb

1-735   Peripheral vascular resistance

Excludes: pulmonary resistance (1-714)

1-736   Thermography of skin

Temperature gradient study

1-737   Blood volume estimation

1-739   Other circulatory function tests

1-74   Urinary function tests

1-740   Water retention

Dye excretion
Salt loading test

1-741   Urinary concentration test

Vasopressin   concentration test

1-749   Other test of urinary function

Excludes: control of bladder sphincter (1-330)
            renal function tests (2-34)
            urine sampling from single ureter (1-654)

1-75   Skeletomuscular function

1-750   Bicycle dynamometer

1-751   Maximum force of muscle groups

Grip   Pull

1-759   Other skeletomuscular tests

1-76   Metabolic function tests

1-760   Basal metabolic rate (BMR)

Analysis of expired gases

1-761   Bodily oxygen consumption

At rest and during exercise

1-762   Respiratory quotient

1-769   Other metabolic function tests

Excludes: chemical metabolic function tests (2-35)

EXPLORATORY DIAGNOSTIC PROCEDURES

1-80   Diagnostic dye introduction

1-800   Subcutaneous dye introduction

1-801   Introduction of dye for angiography NEC

1-802   Orbital fluorescent angiography

1-803   Methylene blue instillation into bladder

1-809   Other diagnostic use of dye

1-82   Exploration of tissues

1-820   Magnetometer search for foreign body in brain

1-821   Other search for foreign body

Excludes: removal by operation
            search by open operation

1-83   Instrumental exploration

1-830   Probing of lacrimal passages

Canaliculus, lacrimal duct

1-831   Probing of nasolacrimal duct

1-832   Probing of bone

1-833   Probing of joint

1-84   Diagnostic puncture or aspiration

1-840   Anterior chamber of eye paracentesis

1-841   Other eye or orbit puncture

1-842   Pericardiocentesis, diagnostic

1-843   Bronchial aspiration

1-844   Puncture of pleural cavity, diagnostic

1-845   Diagnostic puncture or aspiration of liver

For cyst or hydatid

1-846   Aspiration of kidney or pelvis

1-847   Aspiration of male genital structures

Spermatocele, tunica vaginalis

1-85   Other diagnostic puncture or aspiration

1-850   Diagnostic aspiration of cyst NEC

1-851   Aspiration of ovary

1-853   Peritoneal aspiration

1-854   Diagnostic joint aspiration

1-859   Other and unspecified aspiration

1-86   Diagnostic catheterization of veins

   1-860   Selective organ sampling NEC

   1-861   Selective sampling of renal vein

   1-862   Selective adrenal sampling

   1-869   Other and unspecified diagnostic vein puncture

1-87   Diagnostic cannulation or intubation

   1-870   Diagnostic perfusion

   1-879   Other diagnostic cannulation or intubation

1-89   Other diagnostic procedures with surgical techniques

   1-890   Diagnostic surgical techniques

   1-891   Minor surgical diagnostic procedures

   1-892   Bronchospirometry

   Gas analysis from individual lobes

OTHER PROCEDURES FOR DIAGNOSIS

1-90   Procedures facilitating diagnosis

   1-901   Examination under anesthesia

   1-902   Psychotropic drug for examination

1-91   Collection of parasite or micro-organism for diagnosis

   1-910   From eye, ear, nose, mouth or throat

   1-911   From skin or skin appendages

   Perianal collection of ova   Vesicle fluid

   1-912   Sputum collection

   1-913   Stool collection

   Fecal specimen

   1-914   Blood specimen

   Paired sera

   1-915   Urinary specimen

   1-916   Other genital specimen

   Urethral   Vaginal

1-917   From wound or other source

1-92   Diagnostic psychology

1-920   Diagnostic psychology, unqualified

1-921   Initial evaluation

1-922   Diagnostic interview

1-923   Hypnosis for diagnosis

1-924   Drug sedation for diagnosis

1-925   Psychogalvanic reflex

1-929   Other diagnostic techniques

1-93   Psychological testing

1-930   Psychometric tests

1-931   Temperament testing

1-932   Personality assessment

1-933   Attitude testing

1-934   Projective tests

1-939   Other psychological tests

1-94   Psychological analysis

1-940   Psychoanalysis

1-941   Modified analysis

1-949   Other psychological analysis

1-95   Physical and nutritional assessment

1-950   Anthropometric study

Body build   Somatotypes

1-951   Dermatoglyphs

1-952   Skin fold thickness

1-953   Tests for vitamin deficiency

1-959   Other tests of nutritional state

1-96   Visual detection and recording

    1-960   Electrical recording

    1-961   Photographic recording

    Medical photography

    1-962   Transillumination, not elsewhere classified

    1-969   Other visual detection and recording

1-97   Evaluation for rehabilitation

    1-970   Medical evaluation

    1-971   Psychiatric evaluation

    1-972   Psychological testing and evaluation

    1-973   Social capabilities

    1-974   Vocational and prevocational assessment

    1-975   Fitness for physiotherapy

    1-976   Fitness for occupational therapy

    1-978   Other evaluation for rehabilitation

    1-979   Unspecified assessment for rehabilitation

1-99   Procedures related to diagnosis

    1-990   Diagnostic procedures not elsewhere classified

    1-991   Diagnostic assessment

    1-992   Clinical conference

    1-993   Writing up (for publication)

    1-999   Unspecified diagnostic procedure

---

2. LABORATORY PROCEDURES

2. LABORATORY PROCEDURES

CLINICAL CHEMISTRY OF BLOOD

2-10   Blood proteins and aminoacids

  2-100   Identification of aminoacids and metabolites

  2-101   Estimation of aminoacids

  2-102   Estimation of total protein

  2-103   Separation of protein constituents

Albumin/globulin ratio

  2-104   Estimation of albumin

  2-105   Estimation of total globulin

  2-106   Estimation of globulin fractions

Excludes: immunoglobulins (2-67)

  2-107   Estimation of other protein constituents

  2-109   Other blood protein examination

Excludes: hemoglobin (2-830)   fibrinogen (2-321)
           hemosiderin (2-839)   transferrin (2-835)

2-11   Other nitrogenous constituents of blood

  2-110   Total nonprotein nitrogen

  2-111   Ammonia in blood

  2-112   Urea in blood

  2-113   Uric acid in blood

  2-114   Creatine and creatinine in blood

  2-115   Bilirubin and related substances in blood

Bile pigments   Urobilinogen

  2-119   Other nitrogenous constituents of blood

Excludes: drugs (2-163)
           hormones (2-43)

2-12   Alkaline reserve and gaseous constituents of blood and breath

  2-120   Oxygen partial pressure of blood

Oxygen capacity   Oxygen unsaturation

2-121   Carbon dioxide partial pressure of blood

Arterial carbon dioxide

2-122   Alkaline reserve

2-123   Carbon monoxide in blood

Detection and estimation

2-124   Estimation of oxygen and carbon dioxide in exhaled breath

2-129   Other normal gaseous constituents of blood

2-13   Carbohydrate constituents of blood

2-130   Chemical estimation of glucose in blood

Plasma sugar

2-131   Enzymatic estimation of glucose in blood

2-132   Galactose in blood

2-133   Glycoprotein in blood

2-134   Mucopolysaccharides in blood

2-135   Metabolic intermediates in blood

Adenine phosphates

2-139   Other carbohydrate constituents of blood

2-14   Lipid constituents of blood

2-140   Total lipids in blood

Fasting serum lipid level

2-141   Fatty acids in blood

Free fatty acids (FFA)   Plasma neutral fats
Nonesterified fatty acids (NEFA)   triglycerides
                                          Unsaturated fatty acids

2-142   Cholesterol in blood

Free, esterified and total

2-143   Other steroids in blood

2-144   Lipoproteins in blood

Alpha-lipoprotein (high density)
Beta-lipoprotein (low density)

2-145   Phospholipids in blood

Cerebrosides   Sphingolipids

2-146   Chylomicrons in blood

Plasma turbidity

2-149   Other lipid constituents of blood

2-15   Inorganic constituents of blood

2-150   Sodium and potassium in blood

2-151   Calcium in blood

Total
Plasma ultrafiltrate

2-152   Copper in blood

Excludes: ceruloplasmin (2-106)

2-153   Lead and associated metabolites in blood

D-aminolevulinic acid

2-154   Phosphate (inorganic) in blood

2-155   Chloride in blood

2-156   Other elements in blood

Trace elements

2-159   Other inorganic estimations on blood

Excludes: carbonate (2-122)
           iodine (2-400)
           iron (2-835)

2-16   Exogenous organic substances in blood and breath

2-160   Vitamin A in blood

Carotenoids

2-161   Vitamin C in blood

Ascorbic acid saturation test

2-162   Other vitamins in blood

Excludes: cyanocobalamin (2-855)
           folic acid (2-854)

2-163   Drugs in blood

2-164　　Metallo-organic compounds in blood

Methyl mercury　　　　　　　　　　　Tetra-ethyl lead

2-165　　Ethyl alcohol in blood

2-166　　Other alcohols in blood

2-167　　Estimation of alcohol in exhaled breath

2-168　　Other exogenous organic compounds in exhaled breath

2-169　　Other exogenous organic compounds in blood

2-17　　Other organic substances in blood

2-170　　Organic acids and salts in blood

2-171　　Bile acids and salts in blood

2-172　　Products of acidosis and ketosis

2-179　　Other endogenous organic substances in blood

2-18　　Physical and other chemical blood tests

2-180　　Blood pH

2-181　　Osmolality of blood

Cryoscopy　　　　　　　　　　　　Electrical conductivity

2-182　　Density of blood

2-183　　Viscosity of blood

2-188　　Physicochemical blood tests, not elsewhere classified

2-189　　Biochemistry of blood, not otherwise specified

CLINICAL CHEMISTRY OF OTHER BODY FLUIDS

2-20　　Urinary proteins and aminoacids

2-200　　Detection of aminoacids and metabolites in urine

Excludes:　phenylketonuria (2-240)

2-201　　Estimation of aminoacids and metabolites in urine

2-202　　Clinical detection of protein in urine

2-203　　Estimation of protein in urine

Excludes:　Bence Jones protein (2-670)
　　　　　　　immunoglobulins (2-676)

2-204   Detection and estimation of albumin in urine

2-205   Detection of myoglobin and hemoglobin in urine

2-206   Estimation of plasma peptide products in urine

Bradykinin   Renin
Kallidin

2-209   Other identification of protein products in urine

2-21   Other nitrogenous constituents of urine

  2-210   Ammonia in urine

  2-211   Creatine and creatinine in urine

  2-212   Bile pigments and derivatives in urine

  2-213   Porphyrins and derivatives in urine

  2-214   Bile salts in urine

  2-215   Urea in urine

  2-216   Uric acid in urine

  2-219   Other nitrogenous constituents of urine

2-22   Carbohydrate constituents of urine

  2-220   Glucose in urine

  2-221   Galactose in urine

  2-222   Mucopolysaccharides in urine

  2-223   Reducing agents in urine

  2-224   Saccharometry of urine

  2-229   Other carbohydrate constituents of urine

2-23   Inorganic constituents of urine

  2-230   Calcium in urine

  2-231   Chloride in urine

  2-232   Potassium in urine

  2-233   Sodium in urine

  2-234   Heavy metals in urine

Arsenic   Lead
Chromium   Manganese
Copper   Nickel
Iron

2-235   Other trace elements in urine

Fluoride   Thallium
Magnesium

2-236   Other exogenous inorganic constituents of urine

2-239   Other inorganic constituents of urine

2-24   Other organic constituents of urine

2-240   Ketone bodies in urine

Acetoacetic acid   Phenylketonuria
Acetone

Excludes: formiminoglutamic acid (2-854)

(Other available code: clinical screening test for phenylketonuria
                        4-212)

2-241   Ascorbic acid in urine

2-242   Other organic acids in urine

2-243   Alcohol in urine

2-244   Drugs and their metabolized products in urine

2-248   Other exogenous organic constituents of urine

2-249   Other organic constituents of urine

2-25   Other physicochemical tests of urine

2-250   Hydrogen ion concentration of urine

Urine pH

2-251   Analysis of urinary calculus

2-252   Osmolality of urine

Depression of freezing point

2-253   Test for blood in urine

2-254   Microscopic examination of urinary sediment

Birefringent bodies

Excludes: cast and cells (2-914)

2-255   Routine clinical urinalysis

2-258   Other physicochemical properties of urine

Chemical tests for bacteriuria   Volume
Density

2-259   Biochemistry of urine, not otherwise specified

2-26   <u>Examination of intestinal tract contents</u>

2-260   Aminoacids in feces

2-261   Other fecal nitrogen excretion

2-262   Lipids in feces

2-263   Detection of occult blood in feces

2-264   Enzymes in feces

2-269   Other constituents of feces

Excludes: intestinal digestive function (2-31)

2-27   <u>Cerebrospinal fluid examination</u>

2-270   Blood in cerebrospinal fluid

2-271   Electrolytes in cerebrospinal fluid

2-272   Glucose in cerebrospinal fluid

2-273   Urea in cerebrospinal fluid

2-274   Protein in cerebrospinal fluid

2-275   Tests for abnormal protein in cerebrospinal fluid

Colloidal gold curve   Turbidity
Electrophoresis

2-276   Aminoacids in cerebrospinal fluid

2-278   Other constituents of cerebrospinal fluid

Enzymes

2-279   Cerebrospinal fluid examination, not otherwise specified

2-28   <u>Examination of other body fluids</u>

2-280   Lymph examination

2-281   Gastric contents examination

Excludes: forensic (2-943)
             gastric function (2-30)

2-282   Pleural fluid examination

2-283   Peritoneal fluid examination

2-284   Sweat examination and function

Chloride sodium

2-285   Spermatic fluid examination

Excludes: microscopic examination (2-915)

2-286   Amniotic fluid examination

Excludes: alpha-fetoprotein (2-632)

2-288   Examination of other body fluids

2-289   Biochemistry, other and unspecified

CHEMICAL FUNCTION TESTS

2-30   <u>Gastric function</u>

2-300   Fasting gastric aspirate

Basal acid output

2-301   Insulin response

2-302   Response to other stimulation of gastric secretion

Augmented histamine test

2-303   Tubeless gastric analysis

2-304   Gastric ferments

Pepsin   Trypsin
Rennin

2-305   Stomach transit time

2-309   Other tests of gastric function

2-31   <u>Intestinal digestive function</u>

2-310   Analysis of duodenal fluid aspirate

2-311   Lactose absorption from bowel

Blood glucose response to milk ingestion
Lactose tolerance with ethanol administration

2-312   D-xylose absorption from bowel

2-313   Fat absorption from bowel

2-314   Secretin production by bowel

2-315   Disaccharidase activity of bowel

Lactase   Sucrase
Maltase

2-319   Other intestinal digestive function tests

2-32   Hepatic function tests

2-320   Biliary obstruction tests

Excludes: bilirubin in blood (2-115)
            urinary excretion (2-113 to 2-115)

2-321   Protein dysfunction

Blood fibrinogen   Turbidity tests
Precipitation tests

Excludes: albumin/globulin ratio (2-103)

2-322   Deaminization and hepatic detoxication tests

Aminoacid tolerance   Santonin excretion
Hippuric acid excretion

2-323   Carbohydrate metabolism disorder

Galactose tolerance   Levulose tolerance

Excludes: blood sugar (2-130)

2-324   Biliary dye excretion tests

Azorubin-S   Rose bengal
Bromsulphthalein (BSP)

2-325   Analysis of biliary calculus

2-326   Liver profile

Drug metabolizing capacity   Suite of function tests
Plasma half-life of drug

2-329   Other tests of biliary function

Excludes: enzymes (2-450 to 2-489)

2-33   Pancreatic function tests

2-330   Glucose metabolism

Glucose tolerance   Insulin tolerance

2-331   Plasma insulin

2-332   Plasma glucagon

2-333   Secretin response

2-334   Serum gastrin

2-335   Cholecystokinin-pancreatozymin in serum

2-336   Pancreatic aspirate

Enzyme activity

2-339   Other tests of pancreatic function

2-34   <u>Renal function</u>

2-340   Aminoacid clearance pattern

2-341   Clearance of endogenous substance

Creatinine clearance   Urea clearance
P-amino hippuric acid clearance   Urea/creatinine excretion ratio
Phosphate clearance

2-342   Clearance of exogenous substances

Insulin clearance   Phenol red excretion
Mannitol clearance   Phenolsulfonphthalein test (PSP)

2-343   Glomerular filtration rate (GFR)

2-344   Tubular reabsorption tests

2-345   Other chemical tests of function

2-346   Microscopic examination of urine

Casts, red blood cells   Sediment count (Addis)

2-349   Other tests of renal function

2-35   <u>Chemical metabolic function tests</u>

2-350   Nitrogen balance

2-351   Electrolyte balance

Potassium balance   Sodium balance

2-352   Body water balance and composition

Body cell mass   Chemical dissection of body
Body densitometry   Total body water

2-353   Fat balance

Fat loading test

2-354   Adrenal function tests

Ascorbic acid depletion method   Water loading test

Excludes: corticotrophin stimulation (2-420)

2-359   Other metabolic function tests

Excludes: basal metabolic rate (1-760)

2-36   Bone metabolism tests

  2-360   Calcium balance

  2-361   Phosphate balance

  2-362   Calcium phosphate balance

  2-364   Parathyroid hormone (PTH)

  2-365   Vitamin D

  2-369   Other bone metabolism tests

ENDOCRINE FUNCTION TESTS AND ENZYMES

2-40   Thyroid function

  2-400   Protein-bound iodine in serum

  2-401   Thyroxine-binding globulin

  2-402   Total serum thyroxine (T-4)

Competitive protein binding   Saturation analysis

  2-403   Iodine uptake and conversion

Circulating tri-iodothyronine   Tri-iodothyronine (T-3) uptake

  2-404   Free thyroxine index

Effective thyroxine ratio (ETR)   Normalized thyroxine ratio (NTR)
Non-protein-bound thyroxine   Serum free thyroxine (T-4)

  2-405   Thyroid urinary excretion

  2-406   Plasma thyrotrophin

Dynamic response to hypothalamic   Immunoassay of TSH
   releasing factor (TRH)   Thyroid stimulating hormone (TSH)

  2-407   Other chemical tests of thyroid function

Long-acting thyroid stimulator (LATS)   Thyroid clearance

  2-409   Other tests of thyroid function

Excludes: basal metabolic rate (1-760)
         tendon reflex time (1-202)

2-41   Pituitary function tests

  2-410   Response to metyrapone

  2-411   Response to antidiuretic hormone

2-412   Serum follicle stimulating hormone (FSH)

2-413   Serum human growth hormone (HGH)

2-414   Adrenocorticotrophin assay

2-415   Luteinizing hormone response

2-416   Thyrotrophic release factor assay (TRF)

2-417   Other examination of pituitary hormones

Cigarette test for diabetes insipidus

2-419   Pituitary function test, not otherwise specified

2-42   <u>Hypothalamic-pituitary-adrenocortical axis function</u>

2-420   Adrenocorticotrophin stimulation response

2-421   Growth hormone response to hypoglycemia

2-422   Plasma glucocorticoids

2-423   Aldosterone activity

2-424   Response to gonadotrophins

2-425   Steroid suppression test

2-429   Other tests of hypothalamic-pituitary-adrenocortical axis
        function

2-43   <u>Blood hormones and steroids</u>

2-430   Adrenal cortex hormones in blood

2-431   Adrenal medulla hormones in blood

Adrenalin (epinephrine)   Noradrenalin, levarterenol

Excludes: plasma renin (2-344)

2-432   Estrogens in blood

2-433   Pregnancy hormones in blood

Chorionic somatomammotropin   Pregnancy lactogen
Plasma chorionic gonadotropin   Progesterone

2-439   Other blood steroids and hormones

Caval sampling

2-44   <u>Urinary hormones and steroids</u>

2-440   Pituitary hormones in urine

2-441   Adrenal cortex hormones in urine

2-442   Other adrenal hormones in urine

Aldosterone   Urinary catecholamines

2-443   Estrogens in urine

2-444   Pregnancy hormones in urine

Chorionic gonadotropin (HCG)   Pregnanediol
Gonadotropin inhibiting factor   Pregnanetriol
   in urine   Progesterone

2-449   Other urinary hormones and steroids

2-45   Oxidoreductase enzymes

2-450   Serum lactate dehydrogenase

Isoenzymes (LDHS)

2-451   Homogentisate oxygenase

2-452   Tyrosinase (o-diphenol oxidase)

2-453   Glucose-6-phosphate dehydrogenase

2-454   Phenylalanine-4-hydroxylase

I labile   II stable

2-458   Other oxidoreductases

2-459   Oxidoreductase , not otherwise specified

2-46   Transferase enzymes

2-460   Aspartate transaminase (Asp-AT)

Serum glutamic oxaloacetic (SGOT)

2-461   Alanine transaminase (Ala-AT)

Serum glutamic pyruvic (SGPT)

2-462   Creatine kinase

Creatine phosphokinase (CPK)

2-463   Glycogenolytic enzymes

Type I: glycogen synthetase
            glycose-6-phosphatase
Type III: dextrin transglucosylase
                (Forbes, glycogen storage)
Type IV: glucan branching glycosyl
                transferase
            brancher enzyme (Andersen's)
Type V: glycogen phosphorylase
                (McArdle's)

2-468   Other hepatic transferases

2-469   Transferase, not otherwise specified

Hepatic enzyme

2-47   <u>Hydrolase enzymes</u>

2-470   Amylase

(Somogyi units)

2-471   Lipase

Lipoprotein lipase   Triglyceride lipase

2-472   Alkaline phosphatase (ALPS)

(King-Armstrong units)

2-473   Acid phosphatase

Formol stable (FSAP)   Tartrate resistant
Tartrate labile (TLAP)   Total (TAP)

2-474   Cholinesterase

2-478   Other hydrolases

Excludes: urinary betaglycosidase

2-479   Hydrolase, not otherwise specified

2-48   <u>Other enzymes</u>

2-480   Fructose diphosphate aldolase

2-481   Argininosuccinate lysase

2-482   Other lysases

2-483   Isomerases

Methylcrotonyl GA carboxylase

2-484   Other synthetase

Cyclic AMP   Lysozyme

2-489   Other and unspecified enzymes

Enzyme profile

Excludes: bacterial (2-513)
            cerebrospinal fluid (2-278)
            fecal (2-264)
            gastric secretion (2-304)
            intestinal (2-315)
            leucocytic (2-887)
            tissular (2-904)

2-49   Chemical analytical methods

Note: to be used a)   as additional code, if desired, to identify the
                        method used
                  b)   as single code when no other information is available

2-490   Colorimetric analysis

Infrared   Ultraviolet
Photometric   Visual

2-491   Flame photometry

Emission spectrometry

2-492   Chromatography

Gas/liquid (GLC-EC)   Thin layer (TLC)
Paper

2-493   Microscopic examination for chemical identification

Birefringence   Crystal form

2-494   Other optical methods

Fluorometry   Rotation of polarized light
Nephelometry

2-495   Continuous flow analysis

Autoanalyzer

2-496   Electrophoresis

2-499   Other chemical analysis

MICROBIOLOGY

2-50 Detection and isolation of micro-organisms

2-500 Unstained microscopic examination

Bacterial count   Motility
Hanging drop   Slide examination

2-501 Dark-ground (dark-field) examination

For Treponema and Leptospira

2-502 Other optical examination

Phase contrast   Polarized light

2-503 Gram stained smear

2-504 Detection of acid-fast bacilli

Carbol fuchsin   Ziehl-Neelsen stain
Concentration methods (sputum)

2-505 Culture of Mycobacterium tuberculosis

Enrichment media

2-506 Culture of aerobic bacteria

Broth culture   Plate culture
Culture unspecified   Selective culture media

2-507 Culture of anaerobic bacteria

Absorption of oxygen   Inert gas or vacuum
Added milk or meat   Sealed media

2-508 Dye tests

Methylene blue (reductase test)

2-509 Other detection and isolation of micro-organisms

2-51 Identification of micro-organisms

2-510 Specific culture media

2-511 Carbohydrate fermentation tests

Acid and gas production

2-512 Aminoacid utilization

Liquefaction of gelatin

2-513 Other chemical results of enzyme activity

2-514   Physical changes to bacteria

Clumping factor   Coagulase

2-515   Hemolysin production

2-516   Animal inoculation for identification

2-517   Electron microscopy

2-519   Other methods of identification of micro-organisms

Excludes: serological methods (2-60 to 2-62)

2-52   Typing and virulence testing

2-520   Nature of growth on culture

Rough/smooth variants

2-521   Somatic and flagellar agglutinins

2-522   Typing by precipitins

2-523   Fluorescent antibody identification of types

2-524   Typing by cellular response

Bacteriophage   Phagocytosis

2-525   Identification by toxin production

Gravis/mitis strains of diphtheria   Yersinia

2-526   Other animal virulence tests

2-527   Separation of antigenic components

2-529   Other typing and virulence testing

2-53   Susceptibility of bacteria to antibiotics

2-530   Qualitative exploration

Agar diffusion technique   Antibiotic spectrum

2-531   Quantitative determination

Bactericidal   Minimal inhibiting concentration
Bacteriostatic

2-532   Susceptibility to combinations of antibiotics

2-533   Transferable resistance factor

R + fecal strains

2-539   Other tests of antibiotic susceptibility

2-54   <u>Detection and isolation of viruses</u>

  2-540   Demonstration by light microscopy

Cytopathic effect   Syncytial formation
Inclusion bodies

  2-541   Demonstration by electron microscopy

Negative staining

  2-542   Isolation by organ culture

Human embryo lung

  2-543   Isolation by tissue cell culture

Human diploid: Lung fibroblast
   embryo   Monkey kidney
   neoplastic

  2-544   Isolation by animal passage

  2-545   Culture on chick embryo chorioallantoic membrane (CAM)

  2-549   Other detection and isolation of viruses

2-55   <u>Identification of viruses</u>

  2-550   Hemagglutination

  2-551   Neuraminidase surface antigens

  2-552   Immunodiffusion against hyperimmune sera

  2-553   Counter immunoelectrophoresis

  2-554   Complement fixation test

  2-555   Phage typing

  2-556   Extraction of viral antigen

  2-558   Other serological identification of virus

  2-559   Other identification of virus

2-56   <u>Other diagnosis and culture of infectious organisms</u>

  2-560   Postmortem diagnosis of infectious organism in brain

  2-561   Postmortem diagnosis of infectious organism in respiratory tract

  2-562   Postmortem diagnosis of infectious organism in other organs

  2-563   Xenodiagnosis

2-564   Production of vaccine

Autogenous vaccine

2-57   Microbiological assay

2-570   Assay of vitamin B12

Euglena gracilis   Lactobacillus leichmannii

2-571   Assay of folic acid

Lactobacillus casei   Streptococcus faecalis

2-572   Other microbiological assay of vitamins

2-573   Animal test for chemical substances

Histamine

2-579   Other microbiological assay

SEROLOGY AND IMMUNOLOGY

2-60   Serological diagnosis of treponemal diseases

2-600   Complement fixation test on blood

Protein antigen (Reiter) (RPCF)   Wassermann reaction

2-601   Flocculation and precipitin tests on blood

VDRL (qualitative) slide test

2-602   Quantitative tests on blood

Kahn   Quantitative VDRL

2-603   Complement fixation tests on cerebrospinal fluid

2-604   Treponema immobilization

2-605   Fluorescent Treponema antibody absorption (FTA-ABS)

Treponema hemagglutination (TPHA)

2-609   Other serological tests for syphilis

2-61   Direct serological reactions with micro-organisms

2-610   Assay of Salmonella agglutinins

Ohne Haut (O), Haut (H) and
      Virulent (Vi)

2-611   Detection of incomplete antibodies

2-612   Other bacterial agglutination

Microscopic slide test (MST)   Microscopic agglutination test
                                                      (MAT)

2-613   Agglutination against other micro-organisms

Rickettsial (Proteus OX)(Weil-Felix)

2-614   Agar gel diffusion precipitation technique (Ouchterlony)

2-615   Direct immunofluorescent reactions

2-619   Other direct serological reactions with micro-organisms

Colostrum antibodies

2-62   Other serological reactions to micro-organisms

2-620   Neutralization of virus

2-621   Hemagglutination inhibition (HI, HAI)

2-622   Indirect hemagglutination (passive)

2-623   Enzyme inhibition

Neuraminidase inhibition antibody

2-624   Other neutralizing activity of serum

2-625   Serum antibodies against streptococci

Antifibrolysin   Antistreptolysin
Antistreptokinase

2-626   Complement fixation of viral antigen (CFT)

2-627   Other antiviral antibodies

Absorption of complement   Warm immune antibodies
Precipitation of antigen-antibody
    complex

2-628   Other fluorescent antibody reactions

Immunofluorescent methods

2-629   Other serological tests of infective state

Dye test (toxoplasmosis)

2-63   Identification of other antigenic determinants

2-630   Antibodies to plant and animal antigens

Pollen   Pigeon antigen

2-631   Sensitized tanned red cell agglutination

Serum milk protein antibody   Thyroglobulin antibody

2-632   Fetal proteins and antigens

Alpha-fetoprotein in amniotic fluid

2-639   Other identification of antigenic determinants

Excludes: skin tests (1-700 to 1-704)

2-64   Incompatibility reactions

2-640   Lymphocytotoxicity

HL-A compatibility/antileucocytic   Leucocytotoxic antisera
    serum (ALS)

2-641   Other serotyping of leucocytes

Leucocytic migration

2-642   Lymphocyte transfer test

2-643   Serum haptoglobins

2-644   Antibodies to normal tissue varieties

2-645   Urinary rejection products

2-646   Tissue evidence of rejection

Fluorescent antibody staining   Transplantation test

2-648   Other evidence of rejection or incompatibility

Antireticulin antibodies   Hemolysin and hemagglutinin

2-649   Other incompatibility reactions

2-65   Indications of altered reactivity

2-650   Cold agglutinins

2-651   Heterophile antibodies

2-652   Hematological reactions

Eosinophilia   Mast cell degranulation

2-653   Detection of blocking antibody

Irregular agglutinins

2-654   Identification of blocking antibody

Wight's serodiagnostic test

2-655   Serum (hemolytic) complement level

2-659   Other tests of altered reactivity

Antitrypsin activity of serum

2-66   <u>Other tissue reactivity</u>

2-660   Autoimmune antibodies

2-661   Tumor antibodies

2-662   Assay of carcinoembryonic antigen (CEA)

2-663   Latex fixation test

Agglutination of sensitized particles

2-664   Sheep cell

Agglutination test   Rose-Waaler rheumatic factor

2-665   Antinuclear factors (ANF) (ANA)

Anti-DNA antibody   Mitochondrial antibody (AMA)
Leucocyte nucleoprotein   Smooth muscle antibody (SMA)

2-666   Immunological pregnancy test

2-667   Serum anti-alpha-fetoprotein (AFP)

2-669   Other serological response to non-infectious disease

Liver-kidney microsomal antibody (LKM)

2-67   <u>Detection and estimation of immunoglobulins in blood and urine</u>

2-670   Identification of Bence Jones protein in urine

L (light) chains

2-671   Identification of heavy chain (H) protein in urine

2-672   Identification of immunoglobulins by agar gel diffusion (AGD)

2-673   Counter electroimmunophoresis (CEP)

2-674   Indirect hemagglutination inhibition (HAI)

Blocking of antibody-coated Rhesus-   Determination of allotypes
    positive red blood cells   InV, Gm

2-676   Complement fixation (CF) of immunoglobulins

2-678   Other methods of immunoglobulin estimation

2-679   Other tests for immunoglobulins

2-68   Other immunology of body fluids

  2-680   Detection and assay of meningococcal antibody

  2-681   Other immunofluorescent methods

  2-682   Bacteriostatic power of serum

  2-689   Other antigenic reactions of other body fluids

MYCOLOGY AND PARASITOLOGY

2-70   Mycological examinations

  2-700   Microscopic examination for fungus

  Stained   Unstained

  2-701   Culture of fungus

  Sabouraud's medium

  2-702   Identification of fungus

  Fermentation reactions   Production of auxines (growth
                                        factors)

  2-703   Sensitivity reactions to fungi

  2-704   Detection of fungus by ultraviolet light

  Wood's light

  2-705   Animal inoculation of fungus

  2-706   Postmortem isolation of fungus

  2-709   Other mycological examination

2-71   Examination for intestinal parasites

  2-710   Microscopic examination of feces

  2-711   Microscopic examination after ova concentration

  2-712   Microscopic examination of feces stained for ova

  2-713   Microscopic examination of feces, other staining

  2-714   Macroscopic examination of feces

  2-715   Identification of helminths and ova

  2-716   Examination of rectal wall scraping

2-717   Culture of parasite ova or larvae

Hookworm   Schistosome

2-719   Other examination for intestinal parasites

2-72   Examination of circulating body fluids for parasites

2-721   Examination of blood film for parasites

Thin film   Thick (hemolysed film)

2-722   Blood centrifugation technique for parasites

2-723   Culture of blood parasites

2-724   Examination of lymph gland fluid for parasites

2-725   Examination of cerebrospinal fluid for parasites

2-726   Examination of other body fluid for parasites

2-727   Identification of blood parasites

2-73   Other examination for parasites

2-730   Examination of ocular tissues for parasites

2-731   Examination of sputum for parasites

2-732   Examination of skin and subcutaneous tissue for parasites

2-733   Examination of urine for parasites

2-734   Examination of vaginal secretion for parasites

2-735   Organ puncture for parasites

2-736   Postmortem examination for parasites

2-737   Identification of other parasites

2-739   Other examination for parasites

Blood incubation infectivity test (BIIT)

2-74   Culture of parasites

2-740   Culture of protozoa in vitro

2-741   Culture of protozoa by animal passage

2-742   Culture of helminths in vitro

2-743   Culture of helminths by animal passage

2-744   Cultivation of arthropods

2-745   Xenodiagnosis of parasites

2-749   Other culture of parasites

Insects   Ticks
Mites

2-75   Serology of parasites

2-750   Detection of parasite antigen

Toxocara ova   Toxoplasma

2-751   Separation of parasite antigen

2-752   Latex agglutination of parasites

Trypanosoma cruzi

2-753   Immunofluorescent serology of parasites

2-754   Indirect hemagglutination of parasites

2-755   Labelled antibody of parasites

Ferritin (electron microscopy) for
    Leishmania

2-759   Other serology of parasites

HEMATOLOGY

2-80   Cytology of blood

2-800   Blood cell precursors

Bone marrow examination   Spleen pulp smear
Lymph node smear

2-801   Blood count

In counting chamber of stained   Total:
    smear   white and red
Ratio

2-802   Platelet count

2-803   Examination for abnormal morphology

2-804   Staining for reticulocytes

Vital staining

2-805   Other staining for abnormal morphology

2-806   Size of red blood cells

Halometry

2-807   Automated blood count

2-809   Other blood cytology

2-81   <u>Other examination of red blood cells</u>

2-810   Erythrocyte sedimentation rate

2-811   Hematocrit (HCT)

Packed cell volume

2-812   Red cell fragility

2-813   Red cell volume

2-814   Splenic blood pool

2-819   Other examination of red blood cells

Excludes: blood volume estimation (1-737)

2-82   <u>Blood groups and other hemolytic factors</u>

2-820   Cross matching

Pre-transfusion compatibility test

2-821   Major blood groups

ABH, Rhesus

2-822   Subgroups and other minor groups

       A_1 A_2 D_u C c E Kell Duffy (FY) MNS

2-823   Test for antibodies

Pooled anti-D

2-824   Coombs test

Indirect antiglobulin test (IAGT)

2-825   Hemagglutinins

2-826   Enzyme test for blood groups

Salivary enzymes

2-829   Other investigation of hemolysis

2-83   <u>Hemoglobin and iron analyses</u>

2-830   Estimation of total hemoglobin

2-831   Corpuscular hemoglobin

2-832   Chemical differentiation of hemoglobin components

Carboxyhemoglobin   Oxyhemoglobin
Cyanhemoglobin   Sulfhemoglobin
Methemoglobin

2-833   Iron-binding capacity

2-834   Hematin detection

Porphyrins

2-835   Estimation of iron

Transferrin

2-836   Detection of blood in body fluids

2-839   Other analyses of iron and compounds

2-84   Varieties of hemoglobin

   2-840   Sickling

   2-841   Electrophoretic separation of hemoglobin

   2-842   Familial studies of hemoglobin inheritance

   2-843   Detection of red blood cells containing Hb-F

   Kleihauer test

   2-849   Other investigations on varieties of hemoglobin

2-85   Erythrokinetics

   2-850   Iron absorption

   2-851   Red cell survival time

   Cohort labelling   Rate of destruction

   2-852   Site of red cell destruction

   2-853   Plasma iron transport rate

   2-854   Folic acid metabolism

   2-855   Cyanocobalamin metabolism (Vitamin B12)

   2-856   Thrombokinetic studies

   2-859   Other studies on production and destruction of red blood cells

2-86   Hemostasis and coagulation defects

  2-860   Rapid screening tests

Bleeding time (BT)   Clot retraction (CR)
Capillary resistance test (CRT)   Coagulation (CT)

  2-861   Control of anticoagulant therapy

Heparın assay   Thrombin clotting time (TCT)

  2-862   Prothrombin tests

One-stage prothrombin test (PT)
Partial prothromboplastin time (PTT)
Prothrombin time (with Russell's viper venom) (PTV)
Prothrombin and proconvertin (Owren) (P&P)

  2-863   Quantitative tests

Accelerator globulin ACG (Factor V),proaccelerin
Platelet defects
Platelet life span
Prothrombin consumption test
Specific coagulation defects

  2-864   Graphical record

Coagulogram   Thromboelastogram

  2-865   Tests of fibrinolytic activity

Fibrinogen-fibrin related antigen (FR)
Products of fibrinogen degeneration (FDP)
Thromboplast in generation test (TGT)

Excludes: fibrinogen titre (FGT) (2-321)

  2-866   Other tests for blood components

Platelet aggregation time (PAT)

  2-869   Other tests of hemostasis and coagulation of blood

2-87   Lymphocytes

  2-870   Thymus- dependent lymphocytes

EAC cells   E-binding lymphocytes

  2-871   Reactive B-lymphocytes

Membrane-associated immunoglobulins   Membrane-staining techniques

  2-872   Lupus erythematosus (L.E.) cells

2-873   Lymphocyte transformation test

Stimulation of mitosis by culture with
        phytohemagglutinin (PHA)

2-874   Lymphocyte rosette inhibition test

2-875   Antibody-dependent toxicity

2-876   Hamazaki-Wesenberg bodies in lymph nodes

2-879   Other examinations of lymphocytes

2-88   Other leukocytes

2-880   Total leukocyte count

2-881   Differential leukocyte count

2-882   Staining for eosinophils

2-883   Indirect staining of leukocytes

2-884   Classification of polymorphonuclear cells by lobulation

2-885   Nitro blue tetrazolium test (NBT)

2-886   Migration inhibition

Macrophage electrophoretic mobility (MEM)
Opsonic index

2-887   Enzyme activity of leukocytes

2-889   Other examination of leukocytes and blood

GENERAL PATHOLOGY

2-90   Histology

2-900   Unfixed section, unstained

2-901   Optical microscopy by special techniques

Polarizing microscopy   Reflexion microscopy

2-902   Stained sections

Hematoxylin and eosin   Reticulum stain

2-903   Histochemistry

2-904   Enzyme cytology of tissue

Pentose shunt in epithelial smear (G-6 PD)
Tartrate-resistant acid phosphatase

2-905   Immunofluorescence in sections

2-906   Electron microscopy of tissues and cells

Computer image analysis

2-907   Examination of biopsy material from digestive tract

Jejunal biopsy   Rectal mucosal bipsy

2-909   Other biopsy examination

2-91   <u>Cytology</u>

2-910   Examination of cerebrospinal fluid cells

2-911   Examination of smears from respiratory tract

Bronchial   Nasal

2-912   Examination of stomach washings

2-913   Examination of intestinal washings for cells

Colonic   Feces

2-914   Examination of urinary cells

2-915   Examination of spermatic fluid

Spermiogram
Volume, count, motility, differential count

Excludes: forensic examination (2-942)

2-916   Examination of vaginal or cervical smear

Papanicolaou stain

2-917   Cytological examination of other body fluids

Amniotic fluid   Peritoneal fluid
Ascitic fluid   Pleural fluid

2-919   Other cytological examination

2-92   <u>Examination of cell nuclear structure and chromosomes</u>

2- 920   Nucleus/cytoplasm ratio

2-922   Sex chromatin

Barr drumstick

2-923   Karyotyping of chromosomes

Chromosome aberrations

2-924   Banding and fluorescent staining of chromosomes

2-925   Cell culture and stimulation of mitosis

Quinacrine mustard staining

2-926   Computer assisted chromosome analysis

2-93   Culture and examination of tissues

2-930   Culture of tissue for diagnosis

2-931   Hormone assay of tissue susceptibility

2-932   Extraction of transfer factor

2-933   Fibroblast culture

Cystic fibrosis factor activity (CFFA)

2-934   Malignant tissue culture for chemosensitivity

2-939   Other examination of tissue

2-94   Forensic examinations and chemical analysis

2-940   Heavy metals in dermal appendages

2-941   Identification of blood stains

2-942   Examination of seminal stains

2-943   Chemical analysis of gastric contents

2-944   Other forensic chemical analysis of tissues

2-946   Microscopic examination

2-949   Other forensic examination

Lead in paint work

2-95   Gross pathology

2-950   Naked eye examination of organ or tissue

Dissection of specimen   Whole organ section (lung)

2-951   Macroscopic examination of gastric contents

2-952   Chemical analysis of tissue

2-953   Immunofluorescence of tissue

2-954   Digestion of tissue for examination of parasites

2-959   Other pathological examination

2-97   <u>Postmortem procedures</u>

  2-970   Postmortem examination, general

  2-971   Postmortem examination, brain

  2-972   Postmortem examination, chest

  2-973   Other limited postmortem examination

  2-979   Other postmortem procedures

———

4. PREVENTIVE PROCEDURES

4. PREVENTIVE PROCEDURES

CERTAIN HEALTH EXAMINATIONS

4-10   <u>Prenuptial examination</u>

   4-100   Prenuptial   health examination, male

   4-101   Prenuptial   health examination, female

4-11   <u>Geriatric health care</u>

   4-110   Health examination, old person

   4-119   Other geriatric care

4-12   <u>Health examination related to employment</u>

   4-120   Health examination before employment

   4-122   Periodical occupational health examination

   4-125   Health examination for retirement

   4-129   Occupational health examination, not otherwise specified

4-13   <u>Other adult health examination</u>

   4-130   Adult health examination under own initiative

   4-131   Recall health examination

   4-139   Adult health examination, not otherwise specified

4-14   <u>Psychiatric assessment for legal purposes</u>

   4-140   Determination of legal responsibility

   4-149   Other psychiatric assessment

4-15   <u>Physical examination for legal purposes</u>

   4-150   Medical examination of rape victim

   4-156   Medical examination of victim of other aggression

   4-159   Medical examination for legal purpose, not otherwise specified

4-16   <u>Other health examination for administrative purposes</u>

   4-160   For induction in armed forces or police

   4-161   For driving licence

   4-162   For licence as food handler or vendor

4-163　　For licence in other personal services

Beauticians　　　　　　　　　　　　　　Domestics

4-169　　Medical examination for administrative purpose, not otherwise
　　　　　　　specified

4-17　Other commissioned health examination

4-170　　For health insurance proposal

4-171　　For health insurance compensation

4-179　　Other commissioned health examination

4-19　Other health examination

4-190　　Other specified health examination

4-199　　Health examination, not otherwise specified

SCREENING EXAMINATION

4-20　Prenatal screening investigation

4-200　　Cardio-ergodynamography of fetal heart

4-201　　Pregnancy stress tests

4-202　　Examination of fetoplacental products

Placental lactogen
Urinary estrogens

Excludes:　amniocentesis (5-753)
　　　　　　　ultrasonic cephalography (see Chapter 3)

4-209　　Other prenatal screening

4-21　Neonatal screening for abnormality

4-210　　Determination of immaturity

4-211　　Screening for congenital hip disease

4-212　　Screening for phenylketonuria

4-213　　Screening for hemoglobinopathies

Sickling, Hb-S　　　　　　　　　　　　Thalassemia

4-214　　Screening for galactosemia

4-215　　Screening for other biochemical disorders

4-22   Other infancy screening examination

   4-220   Screening for cot death liability

   4-221   Screening for battered baby suspect

   4-229   Other infancy screening examination

4-23   Childhood screening examination

   4-230   Screening for deafness

   4-231   Screening for other physical disabilities

   4-232   Psychological screening

   4-233   Screening for infectious conditions

Pediculosis   Plantar warts

   4-239   Other childhood screening examination

4-24   Adult screening examination

   4-240   Screening by chest radiography

Excludes: mass miniature radiography (see Chapter 3)

   4-249   Other adult screening

4-25   Cancer screening examination

   4-250   Prophylactic smear for cytology

   4-251   Routine cervical smear

   4-259   Screening for cancer

4-26   Biochemical screening

   4-260   Screening for biochemical changes

4-27   Other screening examination

   4-270   Multiphasic screening

   4-279   Screening examination

PREVENTION AND CONTROL OF INFECTIOUS DISEASES

4-30   Isolation on account of infection

   4-300   Isolation of patient with infectious disease

   4-301   Isolation of contact of infected patient

   4-302   Isolation of carrier of infection

4-303   Isolation of immunosuppressed patient

4-309   Isolation, unqualified

4-31   <u>Surveillance and investigation for infection</u>

4-310   Surveillance of contact

4-311   Surveillance of carrier

4-312   Search for new cases

4-313   Tracing and investigation of contact

4-314   Investigation of carrier

4-319   Surveillance for infectious disease, not otherwise specified

4-32   <u>Immunization against bacterial disease</u>

4-320   Cholera immunization

4-322   Immunization against Salmonella group

TAB (C)

4-323   Plague immunization

4-324   Meningococcal immunization

4-329   Unspecified bacterial immunization

4-33   <u>Immunization against other bacterial disease</u>

4-330   Tuberculosis immunization

BCG vaccination

4-331   Brucellosis immunization

4-332   Tularemia immunization

4-333   Diphtheria immunization

4-334   Whooping cough immunization

Bordetella pertussis vaccination

4-335   Tetanus immunization

4-336   DPT immunization

4-339   Other bacterial immunization

4-34   <u>Immunization against viral disease</u>

4-340   Smallpox vaccination

4-341   Yellow fever immunization

4-342   Rabies immunization

4-343   Influenza immunization

4-344   Typhus immunization

4-35   Immunization against other viral and unspecified disease

4-350   Measles immunization

4-351   Rubella immunization

4-352   Mumps immunization

4-353   Poliomyelitis immunization

4-358   Other viral immunization

4-359   Other immunization

4-36   Drug protection against protozoal and helminth infection

4-360   Antimalarial drug prophylaxis

4-361   Antiamebic drug prophylaxis

4-362   Antischistosomal drug prophylaxis

4-363   Antifilarial drug prophylaxis

4-369   Anthelminthic drug prophylaxis

4-37   Drug protection against other infections

4-370   Antibiotic prophylaxis against rheumatic fever

4-371   Other antibiotic prophylaxis

4-373   Chemoprophylaxis against tuberculosis

Administration of medicaments after tuberculin conversion without sign
    of disease

4-374   Drug prophylaxis for meningococcal carrier

4-379   Drug prophylaxis against infection

4-38   Other prophylaxis against infection

4-389   Prophylaxis against infection, not otherwise specified

PROPHYLAXIS AND CONTROL OF OTHER GENERAL DISEASES

4-40   Alteration of immunological status

4-400   Administration of gammaglobulin

4-402   Enhancement of immunity by other means

4-409   Other alteration of immunological status

Excludes: immunosuppression for transplant (9-220)

4-43   Removal of potential source of infection

4-430   Prophylactic dental extraction

4-439   Other removal of potential source of infection

Excludes: appendectomy (5-470):
           optional (5-982)
           tonsillectomy (5-281)

4-44   Alteration of hematological status

4-440   Prophylactic administration of anti-D (Rhesus) globulin

4-441   Prophylactic administration of anticoagulants

4-449   Other prophylactic alteration of hematological status

4-45   Hormonal prophylaxis and control

4-450   Steroid prophylaxis

4-452   Psychiatric control by endocrine prophylaxis

4-459   Other endocrine prophylaxis

4-46   Dietary prophylaxis

4-460   Low carbohydrate diet, prophylactic

4-461   Low calory diet, prophylactic

4-462   Low salt or salt-free diet, prophylactic

4-463   Low protein diet, prophylactic

4-464   Unsaturated fat diet, prophylactic

4-469   Other dietary prophylaxis

4-47   Prophylaxis by inorganic salts or vitamins

4-470   Goitre prophylaxis with iodine

Excludes: iodized salt (4-471)

4-471   Use of iodized salt

4-472   Vitamin D supplements

4-473   Other vitamin supplements

4-479   Inorganic salt supplements

4-48   Other specified prophylaxis

  4-480   Specified prophylaxis, not elsewhere classified

4-49   Unspecified prophylaxis

  4-499   Unspecified prophylaxis

CONTROL OF LOCAL CONDITIONS

4-50   Surveillance and notification of disease

  4-500   Notification of ophthalmia

  4-501   Surveillance of local disease

  4-509   Notification of local disease

4-52   Surgical dental prophylaxis

  4-520   Dental debridement

  Plaque removal

  4-521   Dental scaling and polishing

  4-529   Prophylactic dental surgery

4-53   Other dental prophylaxis

  4-530   Anti-tooth-decay serum

  4-531   Fluoride dentifrice

  4-532   Topical fluoride application

  Excludes: water fluoridation (4-533)

  4-533   Use of fluoridated water

  4-539   Other dental prophylaxis

4-55   Home control of vectors

  4-550   Control of flies

  4-551   Control of mosquitos

  4-552   Control of bedbugs

  4-553   Control of other arthropods

  4-554   Control of rodents

  4-555   Control of other mammals

  4-559   Not otherwise specified

MATERNAL AND CHILD HEALTH CARE

4-60   Initial ambulatory medical attention, current pregnancy

   4-601   Prenatal, first trimester

   4-602   Prenatal, second trimester

   4-603   Prenatal, third trimester

4-61   Initial medical ambulatory attention after delivery

   4-610   Postnatal, case having had prenatal care

   4-612   Postnatal, case not having had prenatal care

4-62   Subsequent medical attention, current pregnancy

   4-620   Prenatal

   4-622   Postnatal

4-63   Public health nurse care

Includes: services provided by:
                graduate or registered nurse (with public health training)
                midwife with university degree or equivalent

   4-630   Registration for initiation of care

   Prenatal

   4-631   Registration for initiation of care

   Postnatal

   4-632   At health center, prenatal care

   4-633   At health center, postnatal care

   4-635   At home, prenatal visit

   4-636   At home, postnatal visit

4-65   Contraceptive procedures

   4-650   Contraceptive instruction

   4-651   Prescription of oral contraceptive

   4-652   Prescription of intrauterine device

   4-653   Insertion of intrauterine device

   4-658   Other contraceptive procedures

Excludes: male surgical sterilization (5-981)
                surgical operation for female sterilization (5-980)

4-659 Contraceptive procedure, not otherwise specified

4-66   <u>Eugenic procedures</u>

 4-660 Genetic counselling

 4-662 Prevention of specific congenital abnormalities

 4-669 Other eugenic procedure

4-67   <u>Child medical guidance</u>

 4-670 Child medical guidance

4-69   <u>Participation in other health activities</u>

 4-690 Individual general mothercraft instruction

 4-691 General mothercraft instruction to group

 4-692 Nutrition information and demonstration

 4-695 Other health education activities

 4-697 Exercising in preparation for delivery

 4-698 Other health activities related to maternal or child care

4-70   <u>Premature care at home</u>

 4-700 Incubator

 4-702 Other

4-71   <u>Well baby health care</u>

 4-710 Initial medical attention

 4-712 Subsequent medical attention

 4-715 First nurse-parent(s) conference at health center

 4-716 Subsequent nurse-parent(s) conferences at health center

 4-717 First nurse home visit related to baby

 4-718 Subsequent nurse home visits related to baby

4-72   <u>Preschool child health care</u>

 4-720 Initial medical attention

 4-721 Subsequent medical attention

 4-725 First nurse-parent(s) conference at health center

 4-726 Subsequent nurse-parent(s) conferences at health center

 4-727 First nurse home visit related to child

 4-728 Subsequent nurse home visits related to child

4-73   <u>School child health care</u>

  4-730   Entrance medical examination, primary school student

  4-731   Other medical examination, primary school student

  4-732   Entrance medical examination, other school student

  4-733   Other medical examination, other school student

  4-736   Interview nurse-parent(s) at health center or school

  4-737   Interview nurse-child at health center or school

  4-738   Nurse home visit related to student

Note: preferably, categories 4-78 and 4-79 should be used only when the health unit provides no care by professional personnel of the types considered or implied under 4-60 to 4-63 and 4-70 to 4-73.

4-78   <u>Health care by other personnel</u>

Includes: services provided at the health unit

  4-780   First prenatal attention, current pregnancy

  4-781   Subsequent prenatal attention, current pregnancy

  4-782   First postnatal attention

  4-783   Subsequent postnatal attention

  4-784   Well baby, first attention

  4-785   Well baby, subsequent attention

  4-786   Preschool child, first attention

  4-787   Preschool child, subsequent attention

  4-788   School child, first attention

Includes: services provided at the school premises

  4-789   School child, subsequent attention

4-79   <u>Home health care by other personnel</u>

  4-790   Home visit related to pregnancy or puerperium

  4-791   Home visit related to care of baby

  4-792   Home visit related to care of preschool child

  4-793   Home visit related to care of school child

5.   SURGICAL PROCEDURES

5 - SURGICAL PROCEDURES

Excludes: biopsies (1-4 and 1-5), performed as independent procedures

OPERATIONS ON THE NERVOUS SYSTEM

5-01   Incision and excision of skull, brain and meninges

5-010   Cranial puncture

Aspiration (drainage)   Ventriculopuncture

(Other available code: cisternal puncture 1-206)

5-011   Craniotomy

Burr holes   Removal of unwanted material
Craniectomy   Reopening of craniotomy
Decompression, cranial   Trephination

Excludes: decompression of fracture (5-020)
           removal of plate (5-020)
           strip craniectomy (5-020)

5-012   Incision of brain and meninges

Electrocoagulation   Lobotomy
Leucotomy   Tractotomy

Excludes: division of cortical adhesions (5-029)

5-013   Operations on thalamus and globus pallidus

Incision   Ansa
Excision   Cingulus
Destruction   Globus pallidus
                                         Thalamus

5-014   Other excision or destruction of brain and meninges

Decortication   Marsupialization
Lobectomy   Resection

5-015   Excision of lesion of skull

5-02   Other operations on skull, brain and meninges

5-020   Cranioplasty

Elevation of bone fragments   Removal of bone or plate
Linear craniectomy   Repair with graft or plate
Opening cranial suture

5-021   Repair of cerebral meninges

Graft of dura   Repair of encephalocele
Ligation, meningeal artery   or meningocele
Ligation, venous sinus

5-022   Ventriculostomy

Anastomosis, ventricle to cisterna magna
Ventriculocisternal drainage

5-023   Extracranial ventricular shunt

Anastomosis, ventriculo-atrial
              ventriculo-pleural
              ventriculo-caval

5-024   Revision of ventricular shunt

Removal or replacement of valve or catheter

Excludes: irrigation of shunt (8-151)

5-029   Other operations on skull, brain and meninges

Freeing of intracranial adhesions

Excludes: hypophysectomy (5-075)
           operations on pineal gland (5-074)

5-03   Operations on spinal cord and spinal canal structures

5-030   Exploration of spinal canal

Laminectomy   Reopening of laminectomy site
Laminotomy

5-031   Division of intraspinal nerve root

5-032   Chordotomy

Electrocoagulation   Stereotaxis
Percutaneous division of cord   Tractotomy

5-033   Excision or destruction of spinal cord and meninges

5-034   Plastic operations on spinal cord and meninges

Elevation of bone fragments   Removal of granulation tissue
Repair of spina bifida   Suture of meninges

5-035   Freeing adhesions of spinal cord and nerve roots

5-036   Spinal drainage

Drainage by puncture
Drainage by shunt of spinal theca

(Other available code: diagnostic spinal puncture 1-206)

5-037   Injection of destructive agent into spinal canal

(Other available code: injection of other drugs 8-570)

5-039   Other operations on spinal cord and canal structures

Insertion of neuropacemaker

Excludes: excision of intervertebral disc (5-803)
           other operations on vertebral column (5-78, 5-80 and 5-810)

5-04   Operations on cranial and peripheral nerves

5-040   Division and excision of nerve

Crushing   Ramisection

Excludes: glossopharyngeal nerve (5-299)
           opticociliary neurectomy (5-133)
           spinal nerve roots (5-031)
           superior laryngeal nerve (5-319)
           sympathetic ganglia (5-051)

5-041   Other destruction of nerve

5-042   Suture of nerve

Reanastomosis of divided nerve

5-043   Freeing of adhesions and decompression of nerve

Release of nerve in carpal tunnel

5-044   Nerve graft

5-045   Transposition of nerve

5-046   Other neuroplasty

Cross anastomosis, nerve   Repair of old injury
New attachment of nerve

5-047   Injection into nerve

(Other available code: anesthesia for operation 8-571)

5-049   Other operations on cranial and peripheral nerves

5-05   Operations on sympathetic nerves or ganglia

Includes: parasympathetic nervous system

Excludes: sympathetic nerves to:
adrenals (5-073)   uterus (5-694)
eye (5-133)   vascular bundles (5-399)
tympanum (5-209)

5-050   Division of sympathetic nerve or ganglion

Crushing   Splanchnicotomy

5-051   Sympathectomy

Excision of nerve or ganglion
Presacral neurectomy

Excludes: periarterial stripping (5-397)
tympanosympathectomy (5-209)

5-052   Injection into sympathetic nerve or ganglion

5-053   Other operations on sympathetic nerves or ganglia

Gangliorrhapy   Suture of nerve

5-059   Other operations on the nervous system

OPERATIONS ON ENDOCRINE SYSTEM

5-06   Operations on thyroid and parathyroid glands

5-060   Incision of thyroid field

Drainage
Exploration   Thyroglossal tract
Reopening wound   Thyroid gland

5-061   Unilateral thyroid lobectomy

Hemithyroidectomy

5-062   Other partial thyroidectomy

Excision of adenoma
Isthmectomy   Thyroidectomy, unqualified

5-063   Complete thyroidectomy

5-064   Substernal thyroidectomy

Partial   Total

5-065   Excision of lingual thyroid

5-066   Excision of thyroglossal tract

5-067   Partial parathyroidectomy

Excision of adenoma
Excision of ectopic parathyroid

5-068   Complete parathyroidectomy

5-069   Other operations on thyroid and parathyroid glands

Division of thyroid isthmus
Ligation of thyroid arteries

5-07   <u>Operations on other endocrine glands</u>

5-070   Exploration of adrenal glands

5-071   Partial adrenalectomy

Excision of lesion   Unilateral excision of adrenal

5-072   Bilateral adrenalectomy

Removal of remaining gland

Includes: associated oophorectomy

5-073   Other operations on adrenal glands

Division of nerves to adrenal glands
Ligation of adrenal artery

5-074   Operations on pineal gland

5-075   Hypophysectomy

Ablation of pituitary   Section of hypophyseal stalk
Cryohypophysectomy

(Other available code: interstitial irradiation - see Chapter 3)

5-076   Other operations on hypophysis

Drainage of Rathke's pouch

5-077   Thymectomy

5-078   Transplantation of thymus

5-079   Other operations on endocrine glands

Excludes: aortic and carotid bodies (5-398)
           ovaries (5-650 to 5-659)
           pancreas (5-520 to 5-529)
           testis (5-620 to 5-629)

OPERATIONS ON THE EYES

5-08   Operations on lacrimal apparatus

  5-080   Incision of lacrimal gland

  Removal of foreign body

  5-081   Excision of lacrimal gland or lesion

  Dacryoadenectomy

  5-082   Other operations on lacrimal gland

  5-083   Removal of lesion of lacrimal passages

  Removal of calculus

  5-084   Incision of lacrimal sac and passages

  Drainage   Splitting of lacrimal papillae

  5-085   Excision of lacrimal sac or lesion

  Dacryocystectomy   Destruction of sac

  5-086   Repair of canaliculus and punctum

  Correction of everted punctum   Repair of punctum
  Plastic operation   Suture of canaliculus

  5-087   Dacryocystorhinostomy

  D.C.R.   Intubation
  Fistulization into nose   Nasolacrimal anastomosis

  5-088   Conjunctivorhinostomy

  Canthocystostomy   Conjunctivodacryocystorhinostomy
                                              Dacryocystostomy

  5-089   Other operations on lacrimal apparatus

  (Other available code: catheterization of lacrimal duct 8-141)

5-09   Operations on eyelids

  5-090   Incision of eyelid

  Blepharotomy   Drainage of hordeolum
  Drainage of chalazion

  5-091   Excision or destruction of eyelid

  Excision of cilia base   Tarsectomy
  Excision of Meibomian gland

  5-092   Operations on canthus and tarsus

  Epicanthus repair   Palpebral fissure repair

5-093   Correction of entropion or ectropion

5-094   Correction of blepharoptosis

5-095   Blepharorrhaphy

Suture of eyelid   Tarsorrhaphy

Excludes: canthorrhaphy (5-092)

5-096   Other repair of eyelids

Repositioning of cilia base
Transplantation of hair follicles

5-099   Other operations on eyelids

(Other available codes: epilation of eyelid 8-181
                        removal of foreign body 8-102)

5-10   Operations on ocular muscles

5-100   Myotomy and tenotomy of ocular muscles

5-101   Excision of ocular muscle or tendon
             with recession or advancement of same muscle

5-102   Advancement or recession of ocular muscle

5-103   Transposition of ocular muscle

Excludes: transposition for correction of ptosis (5-094)

5-104   Other shortening of ocular muscle

5-105   Freeing of adhesions of ocular muscle

5-109   Other operations on ocular muscle

5-11   Operations on conjunctiva

5-110   Removal of foreign body from conjunctiva by incision

Excludes: magnet extraction (5-120)
          other (8-101)

5-111   Other incision of conjunctiva

Expression of follicles   Peritomy

5-112   Excision of lesion of conjunctiva

Curettage of follicles   Peritectomy

5-113   Conjunctivoplasty

Conjunctival flap   Mucosal graft

5-114   Freeing of adhesions of conjunctiva and eyelid

5-115   Suture of conjunctiva

5-119   Other operations on conjunctiva

5-12   Operations on cornea

5-120   Magnetic removal of foreign body from cornea

5-121   Incision of cornea

Keratotomy   Saemisch section

5-122   Excision of pterygium

Includes: with graft or transposition

5-123   Excision or destruction of lesion of cornea

Fistulectomy   Keratectomy

5-124   Suture of cornea

5-125   Corneal transplant

Lamellar keratoplasty   Penetrating keratoplasty

5-126   Other repair of cornea

Collar stud prosthesis   Refractive keratoplasty
Insertion of keratoprosthesis

5-129   Other operations on cornea

Tattooing of cornea

5-13   Operations on iris, ciliary body and anterior chamber

5-130   Removal of foreign body from anterior eye by incision

Foreign body penetrating cornea

5-131   Magnetic removal of foreign body from anterior eye

Anterior chamber, ciliary body, iris

5-132   Relief of intraocular tension

Filtering procedure   Sclerectomy
Iridencleisis   Sclerotomy

Excludes: exploratory sclerotomy (5-139)

5-133   Facilitation of intraocular circulation

Diminution of ciliary body: (irido-)cyclectomy
Improved internal drainage:
  ciliarotomy   goniopuncture
  cyclotomy   trabeculotomy
Reduction of formation of aqueous:
  cycloanemization   Opticociliary injection
  cyclodiathermy   Opticociliary neurectomy

(Other available code: injection into eye or orbit 8-572)

5-134   Destruction of lesion of iris, ciliary body or sclera

Excision of prolapsed iris or ciliary body

(Other available code: laser beam destruction - see Chapter 3)

5-135   Other iridectomy or iridotomy

Iridosclerostomy   Optical iridectomy
Iridosclerotomy   Sphincterotomy of iris
Iridocystectomy (peripheral)   Transfixion of iris

5-136   Iridoplasty

Freeing of adhesions in anterior segment of eye
Repair of uveal hernia

5-137   Scleroplasty

Repair of sclera   With graft
Suture of sclera

5-139   Other operations on iris, ciliary body and anterior chamber

Exploratory sclerotomy

(Other available codes: aspiration of anterior chamber 8-152
                        injection into anterior chamber 8-572)

5-14   Operations on lens

5-140   Magnetic removal of foreign body from lens

5-141   Removal of foreign body from lens by incision

5-142   Linear extraction of lens

Curette evacuation

5-143   Discission of lens and capsulotomy

Needling of capsule

5-144   Intracapsular extraction of lens

Cryoextraction   Forceps extraction
Erysiphake extraction   Suction extraction

5-145   Extracapsular extraction of lens

Includes: combined, or with iridectomy

5-146   Other cataract extraction

Phakoemulsification

5-147   Insertion of prosthetic lens

5-148   Removal of implanted lens

5-149   Other operations on lens

Capsulectomy

5-15   <u>Operations on retina, choroid and vitreous</u>

5-150   Removal of foreign body from posterior eye by incision

Removal of encircling tube

5-151   Magnetic removal of foreign body from posterior eye

5-152   Scleral buckling with implant

Buckling with vitreous implant

5-153   Other scleral buckling

Constriction of globe   Scleral resection

5-154   Other operations for repair of retina

5-155   Destruction of lesion of retina or choroid

5-156   Other operations on retina or choroid

(Other available codes: laser beam destruction - see chapter 3
                          laser beam production of adhesions-see chapter 3
                          other photocoagulation 8-622)

5-157   Operations on vitreous

Replacement of vitreous

5-16   <u>Operations on orbit and eyeball</u>

5-160   Orbitotomy

Decompression   Drainage

5-161   Removal of foreign body from eye or orbit NEC

Excludes: removal of nonpenetrating foreign body (8-102)

5-162   Evisceration of eyeball

Removal of ocular contents
With implant into scleral shell

5-163   Removal of eyeball

Includes: implant into Tenon's capsule

5-164   Excision or destruction of orbital contents

5-165   Insertion of orbital implant

Reinsertion of extruded implant

5-166   Removal of orbital implant

5-167   Repair of orbit

Permanent lid closure

5-169   Other operations on orbit and eye

(Other available code: therapeutic injection into eye or orbit 8-572)

OPERATIONS ON THE EAR

5-18   Operations on external ear

5-180   Incision of external ear

Drainage of furuncle

(Other available code: puncture of furuncle 8-150)

5-181   Excision or destruction of lesion of external ear

Curettage   Excision of preauricular fistula

5-182   Other excision of external ear

Amputation of ear   Radical excision of ear

5-183   Suture of external ear

5-184   Surgical correction of prominent ear

Cartilage graft   Otoplasty

5-185   Reconstruction of external auditory canal

Correction of meatal atresia   Skin graft lining

5-186   Other repair of external ear

Reconstruction of auricle of ear

5-189   Other operations on external ear

(Other available codes: removal of cerumen 8-171
                         removal of foreign body in meatus 8-103)

5-19   Reconstructive operations on middle ear

   5-190   Stapes mobilization

Crurotomy of stapes
Division of otosclerotic material
Remobilization

   5-191   Stapedectomy

With fenestration of footplate
With graft of vein or fat
With wire prosthesis

   5-192   Revision of stapedectomy

   5-193   Other operations on ossicular chain

   5-194   Myringoplasty

Construction of tympanum   Type I tympanoplasty
Repair of eardrum

   5-195   Other tympanoplasty

Type II, graft against incus or malleus
Type III, myringostapediopexy
Type IV, leaving mobile foot plate
Type V, graft covering semicircular canal

   5-196   Revision of tympanoplasty

   5-199   Other repair of middle ear

Closure of mastoid fistula

5-20   Other operations on middle and inner ear

   5-200   Myringotomy

Insertion of tympanotomy tube   Paracentesis tympani

   5-201   Removal of tympanostomy tube

Removal of grommet

   5-202   Incision of mastoid and middle ear

Atticotomy   Exploration, transtympanic
Drainage of mastoid antrum   Hypotympanotomy

   5-203   Mastoidectomy

Attico-antrotomy   Mastoid antrotomy

(Other available codes: skin grafting 5-893
                          tympanoplasty 5-194, 5-195)

5-204   Other excision of middle ear

Excision of cholesteatoma   Removal of outer attic wall
Excision of petrous apex cells

5-205   Fenestration of inner ear

With partial ossiculectomy
With skin or vein graft

5-206   Revision of fenestration

5-207   Incision and destruction of inner ear

Drainage   Labyrinthotomy
Endolymphatic shunt   Sacculotomy
Excision, glomus jugulare tumor   Vestibulotomy

5-209   Other operations on middle and inner ear

Revision of mastoidectomy   Tympanosympathectomy

(Other available codes: insufflation of Eustachian tube 8-173
                         tympanic injection 8-573
                         ultrasonic destruction - see chapter 3)

OPERATIONS ON NOSE, MOUTH AND PHARYNX

5-21   Operations on nose

5-210 Control of epistaxis

By cautery, cryosurgery, suture

Excludes: ligation of artery (5-387)

(Other available code: nasal packing 8-501)

5-211   Incision of nose

Drainage   Septotomy
Removal of foreign body   Turbinotomy

Excludes: removal of foreign body by rhinoscopy (8-104)

5-212   Excision or destruction of lesion of nose

Polypectomy   Snaring

Excludes: cauterization (5-911)
           electrocoagulation (5-920)
           freezing (5-944)
           ionization (5-931)
           ostectomy of facial bone (5-772)

5-213   Resection of nose

(Other available code: rhinoplasty 5-217)

5-214   Submucous resection of nasal septum

5-215   Turbinectomy

Electrocoagulation

(Other available code: infraction of turbinate 8-210)

5-216   Open reduction of fracture of nasal bone

Excludes: closed reduction of fracture (8-210)

(Other available code: correction of displacement, nasal 8-201)

5-217   Repair and plastic operations on nose

Closure, septal perforation   Reconstruction
Graft or implant   Suture

Excludes: suture or graft of skin of nose (5-890 to 5-897)

(Other available code: manipulation of displaced septum 8-201)

5-219   Other operations on nose

Separation of adhesions

5-22   Operations on nasal sinuses

5-220   Puncture of nasal sinus

With irrigation

5-221   Intranasal antrotomy

Antrum window operation

5-222   External maxillary antrotomy

Canine fossa approach

Includes: associated antrum window operation

5-223   Frontal sinusotomy and sinusectomy

Decompression   Excision of lesion
Drainage of mucocele

5-224   Other nasal sinusotomy

Combined sinuses   Sphenoidotomy
Ethmoidotomy

5-225   Other nasal sinusectomy

Ethmoidectomy
Sphenoidectomy   With removal of turbinates

5-226   Repair of nasal sinus

Plastic operation on sinus   Repair of oro-antral fistula

Excludes: elevation of fractured bone:
           frontal sinus (5-767)
           maxillary sinus (5-763)

5-229   Other operations on nasal sinuses

Excludes: excision of neoplasm of antrum (5-771)

5-23   Removal and restoration of teeth

5-230   Forceps extraction of tooth

5-231   Surgical removal of tooth

Excision of buried root   With odontotomy or dental flap
Removal of impacted tooth

5-232   Restoration of tooth by filling

With drilling of cavity

(Other available code: temporary dressing 9-300)

5-233   Restoration of tooth by inlay

Gold inlay

5-234   Other dental restoration

Crown: ceramic, gold   Fixed bridge

5-235   Reimplantation of tooth

5-236   Prosthetic dental implant

Endosseous implant

5-237   Apicectomy and root canal therapy

Canal filling   Pulpectomy
Nerve extirpation

5-24   Other operations on gums and alveolus

5-240   Incision of gum or alveolar bone

Drainage of dental abscess   Drainage of pulp canal

5-241   Gingivoplasty

With graft of bone or soft tissue

5-242   Other operations on gum

Curettage of periodontium   Suture of gingiva
Excision of epulis or granuloma of gum

5-243   Excision of dental lesion of jaw

Dental cyst   Odontome

5-244   Alveoloplasty

Alveolectomy   Vestibuloplasty
Reconstruction of alveolar ridge

5-245   Exposure of tooth

5-246   Application of orthodontic appliance

Arch bars   Orthodontic wiring
Obturator   Periodontal splint

(Other available codes: insertion of orthodontic appliance 8-350
                         wiring of teeth 8-334)

5-247   Other orthodontic operation

Equilibration   Repair of dental arch

5-249   Other dental operation

(Other available codes: dental prophylaxis 4-520 to 4-529
                         removable denture or appliance 9-301 to 9-303)

5-25   Operation on tongue

5-250   Excision or destruction of lesion of tongue

Excision of benign neoplasm   Frenumectomy

Excludes: frenotomy of tongue (5-258)

5-251   Partial glossectomy

Glossectomy, unqualified   Wedge resection of tongue

5-252   Complete glossectomy

(Other available code: regional lymph node excision 5-402)

5-253   Radical glossectomy

Commando removal of tongue and jaw

(Other available code: radical cervical lymphadenectomy 5-403)

5-254   Repair of tongue and glossoplasty

Fascial sling   Fusion to lip
Freeing of adhesions   Graft, skin or mucosa

5-258   Frenotomy, lingual

5-259   Other operations on tongue

Incision and drainage

(Other available code: radiotherapy, volume implant - see chapter 3)

5-26   Operations on salivary glands and ducts

5-260   Incision of salivary gland or duct

Drainage of abscess   Sialoadenotomy
Enlargement of duct orifice   Sialolithotomy

5-261   Excision of lesion of salivary gland

Excision of benign neoplasm
Marsupialization of sublingual cyst

5-262   Other excision of salivary gland

Lobectomy of parotid gland

5-263   Repair of salivary gland or duct

Closure of fistula   Sialodochoplasty
Revision of scar of duct   Transplantation of duct opening

5-269   Other operations on salivary glands and ducts

(Other available codes: dilation of duct 8-223
                          removal of calculus 8-110)

5-27   Other operations on mouth and face

5-270   Drainage of face or floor of mouth

Drainage of facial abscess   Drainage of Ludwig's angina

Excludes: drainage of thyroglossal tract (5-060)

5-271   Incision of palate

Drainage of abscess   Fenestration of palate

5-272   Excision of palate

5-273   Excision of other parts of mouth

Excludes: excision of tongue (5-251 to 5-253)

5-274   Plastic repair of mouth

Closure of fistula   Stomatoplasty
Correction of buccal deformity   With graft of skin or mucosa

Excludes: closure of oro-antral fistula (5-226)
            correction of microstoma or macrostoma (5-898)
            repair of cleft lip (5-898)

5-275   Palatoplasty

Repair of cleft palate   Suture
Reconstruction of palate   With bone or skin graft

5-276   Operations on uvula

5-279   Other operations on mouth and face

Labial frenotomy with suture

(Other available code: removal of foreign body
                            from mouth or palate 8-110)

5-28   Operations on tonsils and adenoids

5-280   Oral drainage of pharyngeal abscess

Parapharyngeal   Retropharyngeal
Peritonsillar   Tonsillar

5-281   Tonsillectomy (without adenoidectomy)

5-282   Tonsillectomy with adenoidectomy

5-283   Excision of tonsil tag

5-284   Excision of lingual tonsil

5-285   Adenoidectomy (without tonsillectomy)

Excision of adenoid tag

5-289   Other operations on tonsils or adenoids

Excision of lesion

(Other available code: control of hemorrhage after tonsillectomy 8-894)

5-29   Operations on pharynx

5-290   Pharyngotomy

Aspiration of diverticulum   Removal of foreign body

Excludes: drainage of retropharyngeal abscess (5-280)

(Other available code: removal of foreign body
                            without incision 8-110)

5-291   Excision of branchial cleft vestiges

Excludes: excision of thyroglossal tract (5-066)

5-292   Excision or destruction of lesion of pharynx

Diverticulectomy   Pharyngectomy
Excision or closure of fistula (except branchial)

Excludes: laryngopharyngectomy (5-304)

5-293   Plastic operation on pharynx

Correction of atresia   Reconstruction

5-294   Other repair of pharynx

Division of adhesions or web   Invagination of diverticulum

(Other available code: dilation 8-224)

OPERATIONS ON RESPIRATORY SYSTEM

5-30   Excision of larynx

5-300   Excision or destruction of lesion of larynx

Excision of lesion of epiglottis   Stripping of vocal cords

Excludes: endoscopic application of caustic (5-981)

5-301   Hemilaryngectomy

5-302   Other partial laryngectomy

Arytenoidectomy   Laryngectomy, unqualified
Cricothyroidectomy   Submucous excision of cord
Epiglottidectomy

5-303   Complete laryngectomy

5-304   Radical laryngectomy

Includes: radical neck dissection

5-31   Other operations on larynx and trachea

5-310   Injection into larynx

Injection of vocal cord

5-311   Temporary tracheostomy

Emergency cricothyroidotomy   Tracheostomy, unqualified

5-312   Permanent tracheostomy

5-313   Other incision of larynx or trachea

Drainage   Laryngotomy
Exploration   Thyrotomy

5-314   Local excision or destruction of trachea

Bronchoscopic electrocoagulation   Resection with reanastomosis

5-315   Repair of larynx

Closure of fistula   Insertion of plate or keel
Cordopexy   Transposition of cords

5-316   Repair and plastic operations on trachea

Closure of tracheostomy   Tracheoplasty
Construction of artificial larynx   Tracheorrhaphy
Reconstruction of trachea

Excludes: closure of tracheo-esophageal fistula (5-427)

5-319   Other operations on larynx and trachea

Dilation   Removal of plate
Division of adhesions or web

(Other available codes: injection into trachea 8-574
                         removal of tracheostomy tube 8-109
                         replacement of tracheostomy tube 8-700)

5-32   Excision of lung and bronchus

5-320   Excision or destruction of lesion of bronchus

Bronchoscopic destruction   Local excision

5-321   Other excision of bronchus

En bloc resection   Sleeve resection

5-322   Excision or destruction of lesion of lung

Excision of tumor   Removal of cyst

5-323   Segmental excision of lung

Apicectomy   Partial lobectomy
Lingulectomy   Wedge resection

5-324   Lobectomy of lung

Partial pneumonectomy

5-325   Complete pneumonectomy

Extended pneumonectomy   Radical (mediastinal) dissection
Pneumonectomy, unqualified

5-329   Other excision of lung and bronchus

Excludes: pulmonary decortication (5-344)

5-33   Other operations on lung and bronchus

5-330   Incision of bronchus

Exploration   Removal of foreign body
                                              by incision

Excludes: removal of foreign body by bronchoscopy (8-107)

5-331   Incision of lung

Drainage   Removal of foreign body

5-332   Surgical collapse of lung

Destruction of phrenic nerve   Thoracoplasty
Plombage

Excludes: therapeutic pneumothorax (8-731)

5-333   Freeing of adhesions of lung and chest wall

Pneumonolysis   Thoracolysis

5-334   Repair and plastic operation on lung and bronchus

Anastomosis to trachea   Reconstruction
Closure of fistula   Suture

5-335   Lung transplant

5-339   Other operations on lung and bronchus

Dilation of bronchus   Ligation of bronchus
Excludes: ligation of vascular pedicle (5-387)

(Other available code: aspiration of lung 8-156)

5-34   <u>Operations on chest wall, pleura, mediastinum and diaphragm</u>

5-340   Incision of chest wall and pleura

Exploration   Rib resection for drainage
Hemostasia   Thoracotomy

5-341   Incision of mediastinum

Drainage   Removal of foreign body
Exploration

5-342   Excision or destruction of mediastinal lesion

5-343   Excision or destruction of chest wall lesion

Costectomy for thoracic disease   Resection of chest wall

Excludes: costectomy for disease of rib (5-783)
           excision of skin lesion of chest wall (5-884, 5-885)

5-344   Pleurectomy

Excision of pleural lesion   Pulmonary decortication

5-345   Scarification of pleura

Obliteration of pleural cavity   Poudrage

5-346   Repair of chest wall

Correction of pectus excavatum

5-347   Operations on diaphragm

Drainage   Resection
Excision of lesion   Suture

Excludes: repair of diaphragmatic hernia (5-537 and 5-538)

5-349   Other operations on thorax

Excludes: lysis of adhesions (5-333)
           thoracocentesis (5-962)

OPERATIONS ON THE CARDIOVASCULAR SYSTEM

5-35   Operations on valves and septum of heart

5-350   Closed heart valvotomy

Commissurotomy, transventricular   Digital opening of valve

5-351   Open heart valvotomy

Division of chordae tendinae   Open commissurotomy
Division of papillary muscle   Removal of leaflets or cusps
Infundibulectomy   Sculpturing of valve

5-352   Replacement of heart valve

Graft or prosthesis   Partial or total

5-353   Heart valvuloplasty (without replacement)

Annuloplasty   Mobilization or hinging
Bicuspidization   Repair of cusp

5-354   Other repair of defects of heart valves

Reattachment of papillary muscle
Repair of sinus of Valsalva aneurysm

5-355   Production of septal defect in heart

Enlargement of foramen

5-356   Other repair of valve or septum with prosthesis

Outflow prothesis   Tube prosthesis for
Plastic patch implant   pulmonary artery

5-357   Other repair of valve or septum (without prosthesis)

Auricular ligation   Repair of endocardial defect
Closure of septal fenestration   Repair with tissue graft
Interatrial baffle (pericardial)

5-359   Other operations on valves and septum of heart

5-36   Operations on vessels of heart

5-360   Removal of coronary artery obstruction

Coronary endarterectomy

Includes: venous graft or patch repair

5-361   Bypass anastomosis for heart revascularization

Aortocoronary anastomosis   Internal mammary to coronary
Direct revascularization   anastomosis

5-362   Heart revascularization by arterial implant

Implantation of aortic branches
Implantation of internal mammary artery into heart muscle
Indirect vascularization

5-363   Other heart revascularization

Abrasion of epicardium   Introduction of irritants
Cardio-omentopexy   Poudrage

5-369   Other operations on vessels of heart

Ligation of coronary arteriovenous fistula

5-37   Other operations on heart and pericardium

5-370   Pericardiocentesis

(Other available codes: cardioscopy 1-691
                          diagnostic pericardial aspiration 1-842
                          drainage aspiration of pericardial cavity 8-153
                          pericardial injection 8-575)

5-371   Pericardiotomy

Division of adhesions   Pericardial window operation
Evacuation of hematoma   Removal of foreign body

5-372   Pericardiectomy

Decortication   Excision of cyst
Excision of adhesions or scar

5-373   Excision of lesion of heart

Atrial appendectomy   Excision of aneurysm
Excision of akinetic area   Myocardiectomy of infarct

5-374   Other repair of heart and pericardium

Ligation   Suture
Repair of ruptured aneurysm

5-375   Heart transplant

5-376   Implant of heart assist system

Artificial heart   Intra-aortic balloon pump

Includes: removal, replacement or repair of system

5-377   Implant of cardiac pacemaker

Implant of epicardial electrodes
Implant of pulse generator (battery)
By thoracotomy or mediastinotomy

(Other available codes: cardiac pacing 8-650 to 8-658
                         electrical conversion of cardiac rhythm
                           8-640 to 8-649
                         intravenous endocardial electrode 8-840)

3-378   Removal or replacement of implanted cardiac pacemaker

Excludes: replacement of battery (5-973)

5-379   Other operations on heart or pericardium

Open chest cardiac massage

Excludes: replacement or removal of transvenous electrodes (8-882)

5-38   Incision, excision and occlusion of vessels

Optional anatomical subdivision, fifth digit:

    1   intracranial   5   abdominal arteries
    2   other head and neck   6   abdominal veins
    3   upper limb vessels   7   lower limb arteries
    4   thoracic vessels   8   lower limb veins

Excludes: heart vessels (5-360 to 5-369)

5-380   Incision of vessel

Embolectomy   Exploration

Excludes: catheterization of vessel (8-830 to 8-839)
           puncture of vessel (8-840 to 8-849)

5-381   Endarterectomy

Thromboendarterectomy

Includes: removal of thrombus
            temporary bypass during operation
            vein patch closure

5-382   Resection of vessel with reanastomosis

Correction of coarctation of aorta
Excision of aneurysm with reanastomosis

5-383   Resection of vessel with replacement

Graft or synthetic bypass
Graft or synthetic implant

5-384   Ligation and stripping of varicose veins

5-385   Other excision of vessels

Aneurysmectomy   Excision of vein for graft
Excision of lesion of vessel

Excludes: aneurysmectomy of heart (5-373)

5-386   Plication of vena cava

Antiembolic filter   Ligation

5-387   Other surgical occlusion of vessels

Banding or ligation   Suture of aneurysmal
Division   sacculation

Excludes: adrenal artery (5-073)
           coronary artery (5-369)
           gastric or duodenal vessel (ulcer) (5-443)
           meningeal vessels (5-021)
           thyroid artery (5-069)

5-39   Other operations on vessels

5-390   Systemic to pulmonary arterial shunt

Anastomosis:
  aorta-pulmonary artery
  left to right shunt
  pulmonary-innominate artery
  subclavian-pulmonary artery

5-391   Intra-abdominal venous anastomosis

Anastomosis:
  mesenteric-caval
  portacaval
  portal decompression
  splenorenal
Portal venous shunt

5-392   Other shunt or vascular bypass

Arterial bypass graft (venous) (saphenous)
Arteriovenous anastomosis
Prosthetic bypass graft

Excludes: extracorporeal cardiopulmonary bypass
               (during operation) (5-396)

5-393   Suture of vessel

Excludes: suture of aneurysm (5-395)
               see also exclusions to 5-387

5-394   Revision of vascular procedure

Control of hemorrhage   Replacement of vascular graft
Removal of clots or infected tissue

3-395   Other repair of vessel

Aneurysmorrhaphy   Prosthetic patch to artery
Patch graft to artery   Re-entry operation, aorta

5-396   Extracorporeal cardiopulmonary bypass

Artificial heart and lung

(Other available code: hemodialysis (8-853)

5-397   Periarterial sympathectomy

Decortication or denervation of artery

5-398   Operation on carotid and other vascular bodies

Chemodectomy   Insertion of pacemaker

Excludes: glomus jugulare operation (5-207)

5-399   Other operations on vessels

Freeing of adherent tissue in vascular bundle

OPERATIONS ON THE HEMIC AND LYMPHATIC SYSTEMS

5-40   Operations on lymphatic system

5-400   Incision of lymphatic structures

Drainage   Lymphadenotomy
Incision of cystic hygroma   Lymphangiotomy

5-401   Simple excision of lymphatic structure

Excision of cystic hygroma   Excision of lymph node

5-402   Regional lymph node excision

5-403   Radical excision of cervical lymph nodes

Resection down to muscle and deep fascia

5-404   Other radical excision of lymph nodes

5-405   Operations on thoracic duct

Closure of fistula   Ligation of thoracic duct

(Other available code: withdrawal of body fluid 8-829)

5-409   Other operations on lymphatic structures

Excision of lymphedema   Transplantation of lymphatics
Lymph node graft

(Other available code: injection into lymphatic vessel 8-577)

5-41   Operations on spleen and bone marrow

5-410   Bone marrow transplant

(Other available code: removal of bone marrow 8-154)

5-411   Puncture of spleen

(Other available code: contrast radiography - see Chapter 3)

5-412   Splenotomy

Drainage of abscess   Exploration

5-413   Splenectomy

Excision of lesion   Total splenectomy
Partial splenectomy

5-418   Other operations on bone marrow

5-419   Other operations on spleen

Excision of accessory spleen   Transplant of spleen
Fixation, suture or repair

Excludes: freeing of adhesions of spleen (5-544)

OPERATIONS ON THE DIGESTIVE SYSTEM

5-42   Operations on esophagus

5-420   Esophagotomy

Drainage   Removal of foreign body by incision
Exploration by incision   Rupture of esophageal web

Excludes: cardiomyotomy (5-426)
           removal of foreign body by esophagoscopy (8-111)

5-421   Esophagostomy

External fistulization   Exteriorization of pouch

5-422   Local excision or destruction of lesion of esophagus

5-423   Excision of esophagus   With end-to-end anastomosis

Esophagectomy
Esophagogastrectomy

5-424   Anastomosis of esophagus (intrathoracic)

Anastomosis with stomach or bowel
Interposition of jejunum or colon

5-425   Antesternal anastomosis of esophagus

Presternal graft or prosthesis
Production of subcutaneous tunnel with anastomosis

5-426   Esophagomyotomy

Cardiomyotomy   Esophagogastromyotomy
Division of cardiac sphincter

5-427   Other repair of esophagus

Cardioplasty
Closure of fistula or stoma
Production of subcutaneous tunnel without anastomosis

Excludes: repair of diaphragmatic hernia (5-537 and 5-538)

5-428   Manipulation within esophagus

Dilation   Removal of foreign body
Intubation   Tamponade

5-429   Other operations on esophagus

Injection of esophageal varices
Ligation of blood vessels

5-43   Incision and excision of stomach

5-430   Gastrotomy

Exploration   Removal of foreign body

5-431   Temporary gastrostomy

Fine calibre tube gastrostomy

5-432   Permanent gastrostomy

Tubulovalvular fistula

5-433   Pyloromyotomy

5-434   Excision or destruction of lesion of stomach

Excision of diverticulum   Wedge resection of lesion
Excision of ulcer

5-435   Partial gastrectomy with anastomosis to esophagus

Cardiectomy   Proximal (subtotal)gastrectomy

5-436   Partial gastrectomy with anastomosis to duodenum

Antrectomy   Pylorectomy

5-437   Partial gastrectomy with anastomosis to jejunum

Gastroduodenectomy (partial)

5-438   Other partial gastrectomy

Fundusectomy   With gastrogastrostomy
Gastrectomy, unqualified   With jejunal interposition

5-439   Total gastrectomy

Complete gastroduodenectomy   With esophagoduodenostomy
Radical gastrectomy   With esophagojejunostomy

5-44   Other operations on stomach

  5-440   Vagotomy

Selective vagotomy   Transection of vagus

  5-441   Pyloroplasty

  5-442   Gastroenterostomy (without gastrectomy)

Bypass gastrojejunostomy

  5-443   Suture of gastric or duodenal ulcer site

Closure of perforated ulcer   Ligation of bleeding vessel

  5-444   Revision of gastric anastomosis

Conversion of anastomosis   Pantaloon operation
Jejunal interposition

  5-445   Other repair of stomach

Closure of gastrostomy   Other suture of stomach
Gastroplasty   Repair of gastrocolic fistula
Invagination of diverticulum

Excludes: suture of ulcer (5-443)

5-449   Other operations on stomach

Reduction of gastric volvulus

Excludes: cryosurgery of stomach (5-434)

(Other available code: gastric cooling 8-613)

5-45   Incision, excision and anastomosis of intestine

5-450   Enterotomy

Drainage   Removal of foreign body
Exploration

Excludes: duodenocholedochotomy (5-513 and 5-514)
          exteriorized intestine (5-460)
          proctotomy (5-480)

5-451   Excision or destruction of lesion of small intestine

Excision of diverticulum   Redundant mucosa, ileostomy
Polyps   Ulcer (duodenal)

5-452   Excision or destruction of lesion of large intestine

Excision of diverticulum   Polyps
Intestine, unqualified   Redundant mucosa, colostomy

Excludes: segmental excision of intestine with lesion (5-455)

5-453   Isolation of intestinal segment

Resection for interposition   Reversal of segment

5-454   Other excision of small intestine

Duodenectomy   Jejunectomy
Enterectomy   With end-to-end anastomosis
Ileectomy   With excision of lesion

Excludes: enterocolectomy (5-455)
          gastroduodenectomy (5-436 and 5-439)
          pancreatoduodenectomy (5-524 to 5-526)

5-455   Excision of large intestine, partial

Excision with end-to-end anastomosis

Excludes: proctosigmoidectomy (5-483 to 5- 485)

5-456   Total colectomy

Excision of cecum, colon and sigmoid colon

5-457   Anastomosis, small to small intestine

Bypass shunt of: duodenum, ileum or jejunum

5-458   Anastomosis, small to large intestine

Colon exclusion   Intestinal bypass

5-459   Anastomosis, large to large intestine

Bypass shunt of: cecum, colon or sigmoid, colon and rectum

5-46   <u>Other operations on intestine</u>

5-460   Exteriorization of intestine

Loop colostomy   Resection and formation of stoma

5-461   Colostomy

Cecostomy   Sigmoidostomy

5-462   Ileostomy

Formation or transplantation of stoma site

5-463   Other enterostomy

Duodenostomy   Jejunostomy

5-464   Repair of intestinal stoma

Release of scar tissue   Revision, reconstruction

Excludes: excision of redundant mucosa (5-451)

5-465   Closure of intestinal stoma

5-466   Fixation of intestine

To abdominal wall   To liver

5-467   Other repair of intestine

Closure of fistula or perforated ulcer

Excludes: closure of perforated duodenal ulcer (5-443)
           closure of vesical fistula (5-578)

5-468   Intra-abdominal manipulation of intestine

Malrotation   Torsion
Reduction of intussusception   Volvulus

5-469   Other operations on intestine

Revision of anastomosis   Sigmoid myotomy

(Other available codes: dilation of stoma 8-225
                         intubation of small intestine 8-124)

5-47   Operations on appendix

  5-470   Appendectomy

  Includes: appendectomy with drainage

  5-471   Drainage of appendix abscess

  5-479   Other operations on appendix

  Appendicostomy   Closure of fistula

5-48   Operations on rectum

  5-480   Proctotomy

  Decompression   Proctovalvotomy
  Exploration   Removal of foreign body
                                               by incision

  5-481   Proctostomy

  5-482   Local excision or destruction of rectum

  Cauterization   Excision of rectal mucosa

  5-483   Pull-through excision of rectum

  5-484   Abdominoperineal excision of rectum

  Combined synchronous excision

  5-485   Other excision of rectum

  Protosigmoidectomy   With end-to-end anastomosis
  Sphincter saving operation

  5-486   Repair of rectum

  Closure of fistula, internal   Suture
  Closure of proctostomy   With graft or wiring
  Fixation

  Excludes: repair of rectovaginal fistula (5-706)

  5-487   Incision or excision of perirectal tissue

  Drainage of pelvirectal tissue   Incision of rectovaginal septum
  Excision of external fistula

  5-489   Other operations on rectum and perirectal tissue

  Freeing of adhesions

  (Other available codes: dilation of rectum 8-225
                           irrigation 8-127
                           manual reduction of prolapse 8-242
                           removal of foreign body by endoscopy 8-113
                           removal of impacted feces 8-127)

5-49   Operations on anus

5-490   Incision or excision of perianal tissue

Drainage of abscess   Undercutting for denervation

5-491   Incision or excision of anal fistula

5-492   Other local excision or destruction of anus

Cryptectomy   Papillectomy
Fissurectomy   Removal of anal tags

5-493   Hemorrhoidectomy

Cauterization   Ligation
Crushing

Excludes: injection (5-973)

(Other available code: ringing 8-341)

5-494   Division of anal sphincter

5-495   Other excision of anus

5-496   Repair of anus

Cerclage   Sphincteroplasty
Closure of fistula   Suture
Repair of imperforate anus   Wiring

5-499   Other operations on anus

Evacuation of thrombosed hemorrhoids

(Other available codes: control of postoperative hemorrhage 8-896
                         dilation of anus 8-225
                         irrigation 8-127
                         manual reduction of hemorrhoids 8-243

5-50   Operations on liver

5-500   Hepatotomy

Drainage   Removal of foreign body
Exploration   With packing

5-501   Local excision or destruction of liver

Marsupialization   Partial hepatectomy

5-502   Lobectomy of liver

5-503   Total hepatectomy

5-504   Liver transplant

5-505   Repair of liver

Hemostatic suture   Hepatopexy

5-509   Other operations on liver

(Other available code: percutaneous aspiration of abscess 8-158)

5-51   Operations on gallbladder and biliary tract

5-510   Cholecystotomy

Drainage   Removal of foreign body or
Exploration   calculus from gallbladder

5-511   Cholecystectomy

Includes: drainage and lithotomy

5-512   Anastomosis of gallbladder or bile duct

Includes: anastomosis to:
                intestine
                pancreas
                stomach

5-513   Incision of bile ducts, for relief of obstruction

For calculus, stricture or tumor

5-514   Other incision of bile ducts

For drainage, endoscopy, exploration, radiography

5-515   Local excision or destruction of bile ducts

Excision of ampulla (of Vater), with reimplantation of ducts
Resection, with end-to-end anastomosis of duct

5-516   Repair of bile ducts

Closure of artificial opening   Suture

5-517   Removal of prosthetic appliance from bile duct

5-518   Operation on sphincter of Oddi

5-519   Other operations on biliary tract

Repair of gallbladder   Repair of gallbladder fistula

Excludes: freeing of adhesions (5-544)

5-52   Operations on pancreas

5-520   Pancreatotomy

Drainage (external)   Removal of calculus
Exploration

5-521   Local excision or destruction of pancreas

5-522   Marsupialization of pancreatic cyst

5-523   Internal drainage of pancreatic cyst

5-524   Partial pancreatectomy

Fistulectomy

Includes: associated duodenectomy

5-525   Total pancreatectomy

Includes: associated duodenectomy

5-526   Radical pancreaticoduodenectomy

With anastomosis to stomach or jejunum

5-527   Anastomosis of pancreatic duct

Anastomosis to stomach, jejunum or ileum
Implant of tube

Excludes: anastomosis with bile duct (5-512)

5-528   Transplant of pancreas

5-529   Other operations on pancreas

Dilation of duct (of Wirsung)   Repair of duct
Removal of tube   Suture

Excludes: freeing of adhesions (5-544)

5-53   Repair of hernia

5-530   Repair of inguinofemoral hernia

5-531   Repair of inguinofemoral hernia with graft or prosthesis

5-532   Bilateral repair of inguinofemoral hernia

5-533   Bilateral repair of inguinofemoral hernia with graft or
          prosthesis

Fascial graft   Synthetic mesh fabric

5-534   Repair of umbilical hernia

Omphalocele   Paraumbilical hernia

5-535   Repair of other hernia of anterior abdominal wall

5-536   Repair of other hernia of anterior abdominal wall with graft
          or prosthesis

Epigastric hernia   Incisional hernia
Gastroschisis   Ventral hernia

5-537   Repair of diaphragmatic hernia

Abdominal approach
Para-esophageal hernia   Parahiatal hernia

5-538   Repair of diaphragmatic hernia, thoracic approach

Parasternal hernia   With thoraco-abdominal approach

5-539   Other hernia repair

Excludes: freeing of intestinal adhesions (5-544)
            relief of strangulated hernia with exteriorization of
              bowel (5-460)
            repair of enterocele in female (5-707)

5-54   Other operations in abdominal region

Includes: inguinal region   Male pelvic cavity

Excludes: female pelvic cavity (5-65, 5-66)
            retroperitoneal tissue (5-590)
            superficial tissues (5-880 to 5-908)

5-540   Incision of abdominal parietes

Extraperitoneal drainage   Removal of foreign body
Extraperitoneal exploration

5-541   Laparotomy

Celiotomy   Reopening of recent laparotomy
Drainage, peritoneal   site

Excludes: culdocentesis (5-700)
            drainage of appendix abscess (5-471)
            reopening wound for hemorrhage (8-896)

5-542   Excision or destruction of abdominal wall and umbilicus

Excludes: size reduction (5-901)
            skin of abdominal wall (5-883 to 5-885)

5-543   Excision or destruction of peritoneum

Mesentery   Omentum

5-544   Division of peritoneal adhesions

Adhesions surrounding intraperitoneal organs

Excludes: fallopian tube and ovary (5-647)
            kidney, ureter and retroperitoneal (5-590)

5-545   Suture of abdominal wall and peritoneum

Closure of burst abdomen   Secondary suture
Delayed closure

5-546   Other repair of abdominal wall and peritoneum

Detorsion of omentum
Fixation of intestine
Grafting of omentum

Plication of intestine
Suture or mesentery and
    ligaments

5-549   Other operations in abdominal region

Removal of foreign body in peritoneal cavity
Repair of multiple injuries to abdominal organs

Excludes: paracentesis abdominis (5-963)

(Other available code: aspiration of abdominal cavity 8-157)

OPERATIONS ON THE URINARY TRACT

5-55   Operations on kidney

5-550   Nephrotomy and nephrostomy

Drainage
Exploration

Removal of calculus or foreign
    body

5-551   Pyelotomy and pyelostomy

Drainage
Exploration

Removal of calculus in renal
    pelvis

Excludes: removal of calculus via ureter (5-560)

5-552   Local excision or destruction of kidney

5-553   Partial nephrectomy

Calycectomy
Heminephrectomy

Wedge resection

5-554   Total nephrectomy

Nephro-ureterectomy

5-555   Transplant of kidney

5-556   Nephropexy

Fixation of movable kidney

5-557   Other repair of kidney

Anastomosis: kidney and pelvis to ureter or kidney
Correction of pelviureteral junction
Nephroplasty and pyeloplasty
Reduction of torsion
Suture

5-559   Other operations on kidney

Decapsulation
Implantation of artificial kidney

Excludes: freeing of perirenal adhesions (5-590)

(Other available codes: aspiration of renal cyst or pelvis 8-160
                         radiographic puncture- see chapter 3)

5-56   Operations on ureter

5-560   Transurethral clearance of ureter and renal pelvis

Removal of: Removal of:
   blood clot   foreign body
   calculus

5-561   Ureteral meatotomy

Modification of ureterovesical junction

5-562   Ureterotomy

Exploration   Removal of calculus
Implantation of electronic   Ureteral splinting
   stimulator

5-563   Ureterectomy

Excision of lesion
Resection with end-to-end anastomosis

5-564   Cutaneous uretero-ileostomy

Ileal bladder   Ileal conduit

5-565   Other external urinary diversion

Implantation of ureter into skin

5-566   Urinary diversion to intestine

Implantation of ureter into: ileum, colon, rectum

Includes: associated colostomy

5-567   Other anastomosis or bypass of ureter

Nephrocystanastomosis
Pyeloureterovesical anastomosis
Reimplantation of ureter into bladder
Revision of anastomosis

5-568   Repair of ureter

Closure of fistula   Graft
Freeing of internal adhesions   Suture

5-569   Other operations on ureter

Ligation

Excludes: denervation (5-051)
            ureteral catheterization and dilation (5-598)

5-57   Operations on urinary bladder

5-570   Transurethral clearance from bladder

Aspiration of blood clot   Crushing and removal of calculus

(Other available codes: bladder washout 8-133
                          other aspiration 8-161
                          removal of foreign body 8-114)

5-571   Cystotomy

Drainage (suction)   Removal of calculus, clot or
Exploration   foreign body
Implantation of electronic   Suprapubic catheterization
    stimulator

5-572   Cystostomy

(Other available code: removal or replacement of tube 8-136)

5-573   Transurethral excision or destruction of bladder

Bladder neck   Papilloma
Diathermy fulguration   Punch operation
Electroresection   Ulcer

Excludes: instillation of cytotoxic drug (5-965)

(Other available code: radioactive implant - see chapter 3)

5-574   Other excision or destruction of bladder

Diverticulectomy
Excision of urachal cyst
Open operation for resection or fulguration of tumor

5-575   Partial cystectomy

Dome of bladder   Wedge resection
Trigonectomy

5-576   Complete cystectomy

Cystoprostatectomy   Radical cystectomy
Pelvic clearance, in male   With removal of urethra

5-577   Reconstruction of urinary bladder

Augmentation of bladder   Ileocystoplasty
Colocystoplasty   Replacement of bladder

5-578   Other repair of urinary bladder

Closure of fistula   Sphincteroplasty
Cystocolic anastomosis   Suture
Cystoplasty

Excludes: closure of vesicorectal fistula (5-486)
            closure of vesicovaginal fistula (5-706)
            operation for stress incontinence (5-592 to 5-597)
            repair of cystocele (5-704)

5-579   Other operations on urinary bladder

Freeing of internal adhesions

Excludes: freeing of external adhesions (5-544)

(Other available codes: aspiration by puncture 8-161
                          distension 8-226
                          removal of foreign body, endoscopic 8-114
                          replacement of cystostomy tube 8-136)

5-58   Operations on urethra

5-580   External urethrotomy

Exploration   Urethrostomy
Removal of calculus by incision

5-581   Urethral meatotomy

5-582   Excision or destruction of urethra

Excision of: Excision of:
  congenital valve   fistula
  diverticulum   stricture

5-583   Repair of urethra

Closure of urethrostomy   Reconstruction
End-to-end anastomosis   Suture

Excludes: closure of urethrorectal fistula (5-486)
            closure of urethrovaginal fistula (5-706)
            repair of epispadias or hypospadias (5-643)
            repair of obstetric laceration (5-756)
            repair of urethrocele (5-704)

5-584   Freeing of stricture of urethra

Internal urethrotomy

5-585   Dilation of urethra

Calibration of urethra

5-589   Other operations on urethra

Drainage of bulbourethral gland
Incision and excision of periurethral tissue

5-59   Other operations on urinary tract

5-590   Dissection of retroperitoneal tissue

Drainage
Exploration
Freeing of adhesions

Perirenal tissue
Periureteral tissue

5-591   Incision of perivesical tissue

Drainage
Exploration

Perineal tissue
Retropubic tissue

5-592   Plication of urethrovesical junction

Kelly-Stoeckel plication or stitch

5-593   Levator muscle operation

Ingleman-Sundberg operation

Pubococcygeoplasty or sling

5-594   Suprapubic sling operation

Fascia lata sling

5-595   Retropubic urethral suspension

Marshall-Marchetti-Kranz operation
Suture of paraurethral tissue to symphysis pubis

5-596   Periurethral suspension and compression

Pereyra operation
Suspension of urethrovesical junction

5-597   Other repair of urinary incontinence

Urethrovesicopexy

Excludes: operation with colporrhaphy (5-704)

5-598   Ureteral catheterization

Dilation, ureteral meatus

Excludes: removal of calculus from kidney (5-560)

(Other available codes: retrograde pyelography - see chapter 3
                        sampling of single kidney 1-554)

5-599   Other operations on urinary system

Excludes: replacement or removal of external urinary drain (5-982)

OPERATIONS ON MALE GENITAL ORGANS

Excludes: surgical operations to produce male sterilization (5-981)

5-60   Operations on prostate and seminal vesicles

   5-600   Incision of prostate

   Drainage   Removal of calculus by incision

   5-601   Transurethral prostatectomy

   Cutting loop   Punch resection

   5-602   Suprapubic prostatectomy

   Transvesical

   5-603   Retropubic prostatectomy

   Transcapsular retropubic resection

   5-604   Radical prostatectomy

   By any approach   Prostatovesiculectomy

   Excludes: cystoprostatectomy (5-576)

   5-605   Other prostatectomy

   Perineal (transcapsular)   Transcapsular prostatectomy
   Prostatectomy, unqualified

   5-606   Operations on seminal vesicles

   Spermatocystectomy

   Excludes: prostatovesiculectomy (5-604)

   5-607   Incision or excision of periprostatic tissue

   Drainage

   5-608   Other operations on prostate

   Control of hemorrhage by endoscopy

5-61   Operations on scrotum and tunica vaginalis

   5-610   Incision of scrotum and tunica vaginalis

   Drainage

   5-611   Excision of hydrocele (of tunica vaginalis)

   Repair of hydrocele

5-612   Excision or destruction of scrotal lesion

Fistulectomy of scrotum   Resection of scrotum
Reduction of elephantiasis

5-613   Repair of scrotum and tunica vaginalis

Eversion or inversion   Suture
Reconstruction

5-619   Other operations on scrotum and tunica vaginalis

Removal of foreign body

5-62   Operations on testis

5-620   Incision of testis

Drainage   Removal of foreign body

5-621   Excision or destruction of testis lesion

5-622   Unilateral orchiectomy

5-623   Bilateral orchiectomy

Castration   Removal of remaining testis
Removal of ovotestis

5-624   Orchiopexy

Exploration for abdominal testis
Mobilization and replacement in scrotum

5-625   Repair of testis

Excludes: reduction of torsion (5-634)

5-626   Insertion of testicular prosthesis

5-629   Other operations on testis

(Other available codes: aspiration of hydrocele 8-163
                         injection of hydrocele 8-582)

5-63   Operations on spermatic cord, epididymis and vas deferens

5-630   Excision of varicocele and hydrocele of spermatic cord

Ligation of spermatic veins   Varicocelectomy
Repair of hydrocele of cord

5-631   Excision of cyst of epididymis

Spermatocelectomy

5-632   Excision of other lesion of spermatic cord and epididymis

5-633   Other epididymectomy

Excludes: that with orchiectomy (5-622 and 5-623)

5-634   Repair of spermatic cord and epididymis

Detorsion of spermatic cord   Transplantation of cord
Suture of spermatic cord

Excludes: that with orchiopexy (5-624)

5-635   Vasotomy

Drainage and exploration   Removal of foreign body

5-636   Vasectomy

For excision of lesion

5-637   Repair of vas deferens and epididymis

Anastomosis or reconstruction   Removal of ligature or valve
Epididymovasostomy   Suture

5-639   Other operations on spermatic cord, epididymis and vas deferens

(Other available code: aspiration of spermatocele 8-163)

5-64   Operations on penis

5-640   Circumcision

5-641   Local excision or destruction of penis

5-642   Amputation of penis

5-643   Repair and plastic operation on penis

Balanoplasty   Release of chordee
Reconstruction   Repair of epispadias, hypospadias
                                     Suture

5-644   Operations for sex transformation, not elsewhere classified

Operations with indeterminate sex

5-649   Other operations on male genital organs

Division of adhesions   Irrigation, corpus cavernosum
Drainage

OPERATIONS ON FEMALE GENITAL ORGANS

Excludes: surgical operations to produce female sterilization (5-980)

5-65   Operations on ovary

   5-650   Oophorotomy

   Drainage (abscess) (cyst)   Salpingo-oophorotomy
   Rupture of cyst

   5-651   Local excision or destruction of ovary

   Ovarian cystectomy   Wedge resection
   Partial oophorectomy

   5-652   Unilateral oophorectomy

   Oophorectomy, unqualified

   5-653   Unilateral salpingo-oophorectomy

   5-654   Bilateral oophorectomy

   Castration, female   Removal of remaining ovary

   5-655   Bilateral salpingo-oophorectomy

   Removal of remaining ovary and tube

   5-656   Repair of ovary

   Autotransplant of ovary   Salpingo-oophoroplasty
   Oophoropexy   Suture
   Oophoroplasty

   Excludes: homotransplant of ovary (5-659)
               salpingo-oophorostomy (5-666)

   5-657   Freeing of adhesions of ovary and fallopian tube

   5-659   Other operations on ovary

   Ovarian homograft

   (Other available code: aspiration of ovary 8-164)

5-66   Operations on fallopian tube

Excludes: tube with ovary, see 5-65

   5-660   Salpingotomy

   Drainage

   5-661   Total salpingectomy (unilateral)

5-662   Total bilateral salpingectomy

Removal of remaining tube

Excludes: bilateral salpingo-oophorectomy (5-655)

5-663   Bilateral endoscopic destruction or occlusion of fallopian tubes

By culdoscopy   Crushing
By laparoscopy   That of remaining tube
Cauterization

5-664   Other bilateral destruction or occlusion of fallopian tubes

Partial removal   That of remaining tube
Resection or transection

5-665   Other salpingectomy

Cornual resection   Excision of lesion
Destruction of lesion   Fimbriectomy

5-666   Repair of fallopian tube

Anastomosis   Salpingo-oophorostomy
Implantation into uterus   With graft or prosthesis
Reconstruction

Excludes: salpingo-oophoroplasty (5-656)
           salpingo-oophororrhaphy (5-656)

5-667   Insufflation of fallopian tubes

With air, gas, saline or dye

(Other available codes: hysterosalpingography - see chapter 3)

5-669   Other operations on fallopian tubes

Unilateral ligation and division (not of remaining tube)

5-67   Operations on cervix

5-670   Dilation of cervical canal

Excludes: dilation and curettage (5-690)
           termination of pregnancy (5-752)

5-671   Conization of cervix

Cold (knife) excision of cervix

5-672   Other excision or destruction of lesion of cervix

Cryoconization   Excision of polyp
Electroconization

5-673   Amputation of cervix

Cervicectomy   Hysterotrachelectomy
Excision of cervical stump   With colporrhaphy

5-674   Repair of internal cervical os

Encirclement suture   Wedge excision with suture
Supporting suture in pregnancy

5-675   Other repair of cervix

Late repair of obstetric laceration
Repair of nonobstetric laceration

Excludes: repair of lacerations during the immediate
              postpartum period (5-755)

5-679   Other operations on cervix

(Other available code: radioactive implant - see chapter 3)

5-68   Other incision and excision of uterus

5-680   Hysterotomy

(Hystero) trachelotomy

Excludes: embryectomy (5-744)
            myomectomy (5-681)

5-681   Excision or destruction of lesion of uterus

Division of endometrial synechiae
Endometrectomy
Myomectomy

(Other available code: radioactive implant - see chapter 3)

5-682   Subtotal abdominal hysterectomy

Fundectomy   Supravaginal
Supracervical

Excludes: hysterotrachelectomy (5-673)

5-683   Total abdominal hysterectomy

Extended hysterectomy   Panhysterectomy
Hysterectomy, unqualified

5-684   Vaginal hysterectomy

Colpohysterectomy

5-685   Radical abdominal hysterectomy

Includes: hysterocolpectomy
            modified radical hysterectomy
            removal of upper vagina and cellular tissues

5-686   Radical vaginal hysterectomy

5-687   Pelvic evisceration

En masse excision of ovaries, tubes, uterus, vagina
      bladder and urethra

(Other available codes: radical lymph node dissection 5-404
                           regional lymph node dissection 5-402
                           removal of tubes or ovaries 5-652 to 5-662
                           repair of cystocele and rectocele 5-704
                           repair to pelvic floor 5-693)

5-69   Other operations on uterus and supports

5-690   Dilation and curettage (of uterus)

Removal of: Removal of:
  mole   retained products of conception
  missed abortion   following delivery or
                                               abortion

Excludes: termination of pregnancy (5-752)

5-691   Vaginal removal of intrauterine foreign body

Removal of intrauterine contraceptive device

5-692   Excision or destruction of uterine supports

Broad ligament   Hematoma
Canal of Nuck   Hydrocele
Cyst (parovarian)   Round ligament

5-693   Repair of uterine supports

Fixation   Broad ligament
Plication   Cardinal ligaments
Reattachment   Endopelvic fascia
Shortening   Uterosacral ligament
Ventrosuspension

5-694   Paracervical uterine denervation

Division of uterosacral ligament

5-695   Repair of uterus

Hystero(trachelo)rrhaphy
Repair of nonobstetric laceration

5-699   Other operations on uterus, cervix and supporting structures

Removal of encircling suture of cervix

Excludes: obstetric dilation or incision of cervix (5-739)
            obstetric insertion of bag or pack (5-758)

(Other available codes:　insertion of intrauterine contraceptive
appliance 4-653
menstrual regulation 8-165
paracervical nerve block 8-891)

5-70　Operations on vagina

5-700　Culdocentesis

Aspiration of cul-de-sac

Excludes:　culdoscopy (5-916)

5-701　Incision of vagina

Colpotomy	Exploration
Culdotomy	Hymenotomy
Drainage, pelvic abscess	Vaginoperineotomy

5-702　Local excision or destruction of vagina

Colpectomy, partial
Excision of:　　　　　　　　　　　Excision of:
  cyst　　　　　　　　　　　　　　　polyp
  hymen　　　　　　　　　　　　　　septum

Excludes:　fistulectomy (5-706)

5-703　Obliteration and total excision of vagina

Colpectomy, total　　　　　　　Colpocleisis

5-704　Repair of cystocele and rectocele

Repair of:　　　　　　　　　　　Repair of:
  pouch of Douglas　　　　　　　　vaginal wall (anterior,
  urethrocele　　　　　　　　　　　　posterior)

5-705　Vaginal reconstruction

Colpopoiesis　　　　　　　　　　With graft (skin, colon)

5-706　Other repair of vagina

Colpoperineorrhaphy　　　　　　Freeing of adhesions
Excision and closure of fistula　Hymenorrhaphy
Fixation　　　　　　　　　　　　Suture

Excludes:　repair of vagina during the immediate postpartum period
　　　　　(5-756)

5-707　Obliteration of vaginal vault

Repair of enterocele
Suture to obliterate cul-de-sac

5-709　Other operations on vagina

Removal of foreign body by incision

(Other available codes: dilation of vagina 8-228
                         packing to control hemorrhage, nonobstetric
                         8-503)

5-71   Operations on vulva and perineum

Includes: Bartholin's gland   labia (minora, majora)
           clitoris   Skene's gland

Excludes: hymen (5-701 to 5-709)

   5-710   Incision of vulva and perineum

Drainage   Exploration
Enlargement of introitus   Removal of foreign body by
                                           incision

   5-711   Operations on Bartholin's gland

Drainage   Marsupialization

Excludes: perineal cauterization (5-912)

   5-712   Other local excision or destruction of vulva and perineum

Division of Skene's gland   Excision of redundant mucosa

Excludes: perineal cauterization (5-912)

   5-713   Operations on clitoris

Amputation of clitoris

   5-714   Radical vulvectomy

   5-715   Other vulvectomy

Bilateral (simple)   Partial (unilateral)

   5-716   Repair of vulva and perineum

Closure of perineal fistula   Perineorrhaphy
Perineoplasty

Excludes: repair of vulva and perineum during the immediate
              postpartum period (5-756)

   5-719   Other operations on female genital organs

(Other available code: dilation of introitus 8-228)

OBSTETRIC OPERATIONS

5-72   Breech and instrumental delivery

   5-720   Low forceps delivery (without episiotomy)

5-721   Low forceps delivery with episiotomy

5-722   Mid forceps delivery

5-723   High forceps delivery

5-724   Forceps rotation of fetal head

5-725   Breech extraction

Version with breech extraction

5-726   Forceps application to aftercoming head

5-727   Breech delivery

5-728   Vacuum traction on fetal scalp

5-729   Other and unspecified instrumental delivery

5-73   Other operations inducing or assisting delivery

5-730   Artificial rupture of membranes

5-731   Other surgical induction of labor

Insertion, hydrostatic bag or bougie

5-732   Internal version and extraction

Cephalic version   Combined version

5-733   Failed forceps

Trial forceps

5-734   Operations on fetus to facilitate delivery

Cleidotomy   Drainage of hydrocephalus

5-738   Episiotomy

With repair

5-739   Other operations assisting delivery

Dilation or incision of cervix   Symphysiotomy
Pubiotomy

Excludes: removal of encircling suture (5-699)

(Other available codes: external version 8-251
                          medical induction of labor 9-250
                          other manipulations 8-250 to 8-259
                          oxytocic drugs 7-500 to 7-509
                          replacement of cord 8-254)

5-74   <u>Cesarean section and removal of fetus</u>

  5-740   Classical cesarean section

  Upper uterine segment, transperitoneal

  5-741   Cervical cesarean section

  Lower uterine segment, transperitoneal

  5-742   Extraperitoneal cesarean section

  Supravesical, without opening peritoneal cavity

  5-743   Removal of intraperitoneal embryo

  Abdominal (ectopic) pregnancy
  Ovarian pregnancy
  Ruptured tubal pregnancy

  5-744   Other removal of embryo

  By hysterotomy   Hysterectomy during pregnancy
  Embryectomy
  Excludes: removal of uterine mole (5-690)
             termination of pregnancy (5-750 to 5-752)

  (Other available code: menstrual extraction 8-165)

  5-748   Other cesarean section

  5-749   Cesarean section, not otherwise specified

5-75   <u>Other obstetric operations</u>

  5-750   Amniotic injection for termination of pregnancy

  Injection of:
    prostaglandin
    saline

  Excludes: for induction of labor (9-250)

  5-751   Vacuum aspiration for termination of pregnancy

  5-752   Other termination of pregnancy

  Excludes: by hysterotomy (5-744)

  5-753   Amniocentesis

  Excludes: amnioscopy (5-925)

  5-754   Intrauterine transfusion

  Exchange transfusion in utero
  Intraperitoneal blood transfusion exchange

5-755   Other intrauterine operations on fetus

Biopsy specimen and blood sampling
Correction of fetal defects
Scalp electrodes

5-756   Removal of retained placenta

Manual removal of placenta and membranes

5-757   Repair of obstetric laceration of uterus

Repair of ruptured uterus   Suture of torn cervix

5-758   Repair of other obstetric lacerations

Episiorrhaphy   Secondary repair of laceration
Perineorrhaphy

Excludes: late repair, not in immediate postpartum period (5-706 and
              5-716)
            repair of routine episiotomy (9-263)

5-759   Other obstetric operations

Evacuation of hematoma of vulva
Exploration of uterine cavity, postpartum
Surgical correction of inverted uterus:
  incision of cervix
  transsection of cervix
Tamponade of uterus, obstetric

Excludes: episiotomy (5-738)

(Other available codes: expression of placenta 8-510
                          external version 8-251
                          manipulations of fetus or uterus 8-250 to 8-259
                          manual replacement of inverted uterus 8-256
                          manual replacement of retroverted gravid uterus
                            8-252)

OPERATIONS ON THE MUSCULOSKELETAL SYSTEM

5-76   Reduction of facial fractures

   5-760   Closed reduction of zygomatic fracture

   5-761   Open reduction of zygomatic fracture

   5-762   Closed reduction of maxillary and mandibular fracture

   5-763   Open reduction of maxillary and mandibular fracture

   5-764   Open reduction of alveolar fracture

5-765   Open reduction of orbital fracture

With graft or implant

5-766   Other closed reduction of facial fracture

(Other available codes: jaw traction 8-473
                          nasal bone 8-200
                          wiring of teeth 8-334)

5-767   Other open reduction of facial fracture

Excludes: nasal bone (5-216)

(Other available code: dental wiring 8-334)

5-77   Other operations on facial bones and joints

5-770   Incision of facial bone

Drainage   Removal of foreign body
Exploration   Removal of sequestrum

5-771   Excision or destruction of facial bone lesion

Excludes: excision of odontogenic lesion (5-243)

5-772   Partial ostectomy of facial bone, except mandible

With bone graft or prosthesis

5-773   Excision and reconstruction of mandible

With bone graft or prosthesis

5-774   Temporomandibular arthroplasty

Condylectomy (intracapsular)   Removal of joint structures
Meniscectomy

5-775   Other facial bone repair and osteoplasty

Condylotomy   Ramisection of jaw
Genioplasty

5-779   Other operations on facial bones and joints

Excludes: accessory nasal sinuses (5-220 to 5-229)
            nasal bones (5-211 to 5-219)

(Other available codes: injection of therapeutic substances 8-584
                          and 8-585
                          manipulation of temporomandibular joint 8-211)

5-78   Operations on other bones

5-780   Incision of bone

Drainage   Removal of foreign body
Drilling, exploration   Removal of sequestrum

5-781   Division of bone

Condylotomy   Osteotomy
Displacement   With muscle transfer

Excludes: clavicotomy of fetus (5-734)
           pubiotomy to assist delivery (5-739)

5-782   Ostectomy for hallux valgus

Bunionectomy   Excision of metatarsal head or
Excision of bunionette (5th toe)   phalanx
                                         Exostectomy of hallux

5-783   Excision of bone lesion

With bone graft or bone chips

Excludes: removal of bone fragments of compound fracture (5-795)

5-784   Partial ostectomy

Excision of bone for (homo)graft
Wedge resection
With bone graft or metallic fixation

5-785   Total ostectomy

Excludes: excision of sesamoid bone (5-833)

5-786   Bone graft

Autogenous graft   Homograft
Heterogenous transplant   With metallic fixation

5-787   Internal fixation of bone (without fracture reduction)

Insertion or reinsertion of fixation appliance

Excludes: spine (5-810)

5-788   Removal of internal fixation appliance

Excludes: removal of traction pin or wire (8-460)

5-789   Other operations on bone

Fusion of bone   Reconstruction
Lengthening of bone   Shortening of bone

For details, refer to index and to the following sections:
  amputation (5-840 to 5-849)   nasal sinus (5-220 to 5-229)
  bone marrow (5-410)   rib (5-340 to 5-343)
  face (5-760 to 5-779)   skull (5-010 to 5-029)
  fracture (5-790 to 5-794)   sesamoid bone (5-833)
  jaw (5-762 to 5-764,   spine (5-030, 5-810)
      5-770 to 5-779)   thumb (5-826)
  joint, bone ends (5-800 to 5-812)
  nasal bone (5-212 to 5-219)

5-79   Reduction of fracture and dislocation

Excludes: facial bones (5-760 to 5-767)
            nasal bones (5-217)
            skull (5-020)

(Other available codes: closed reduction of dislocation 8-206
                          closed reduction of fracture 8-200 to 8-205
                          skeletal and other traction 8-400 to 8-430,
                             8-470 to 8-479)

  5-790   Closed reduction of fracture with internal fixation

  (Other available code: nailing of bone 8-362)

  5-791   Open reduction of fracture (without internal fixation)

  5-792   Open reduction of fracture with internal fixation

  Band, plate, screw, wire

  5-793   Closed reduction of separated epiphysis

  (Other available code: closed nailing of epiphysis 8-362)

  5-794   Open reduction of separated epiphysis

  5-795   Toilet of open fracture site

  Removal of bone fragments

  5-796   Open reduction of dislocation of joint

  5-797   Operations for multiple fractures and injuries, not elsewhere
          classified

Fracture of bones in two or more limbs
Fracture of limb bone with fracture of skull, thorax or pelvis
Fracture of thorax or pelvis with internal injuries

5-80   Incision and excision of joint structures

Excludes: temporomandibular joint (5-774)

(Other available codes: injection for radiography - see chapter 3
                          injection of therapeutic substance into joint
                             or ligament 8-584
                          therapeutic aspiration 8-166)

5-800   Arthrotomy

Drainage   Removal of loose or
Exploration   foreign body

5-801   Division of joint capsule, ligament or cartilage

Chondrotomy   Freeing of external adhesions
Desmotomy

Excludes: carpal tunnel nerve decompression (5-043)
           pubiotomy (symphysiotomy) in delivery (5-739)

5-802   Excision or destruction of lesion of joint

Curettage or cartilage

Excludes: ganglion (5-822)

5-803   Excision of intervertebral disc

With laminectomy or bone graft

5-804   Excision of semilunar cartilage of knee

Meniscectomy

Excludes: excision or removal of cruciate ligament or
           loose body (5-800, 5-802)

5-805   Synovectomy of joint

Villusectomy

5-809   Other excision of joint structure

Arthrectomy   Excision of capsule or ligament
Condylectomy

5-81   Repair and plastic operations on joint structures

Includes: repair and reconstruction of:
           capsule, cartilage, joint cavity, synovial membrane
           graft for bone, cartilage, tendon
           internal or external fixation or prosthetic appliance

5-810   Spinal fusion

Arthrodesis of spine   Spondylosyndesis

Excludes: sacroiliac joints (5-812)

5-811   Arthrodesis of foot and ankle

Correction of hammer toe deformity
Fusion of bone of foot
Subtalar or triple arthrodesis

5-812   Arthrodesis of other joints

Excision of bone ends and compression
Production of ankylosis

5-813   Arthroplasty of foot and toe

Capsuloplasty   Reconstruction
Chondroplasty

5-814   Arthroplasty of knee

Capsuloplasty   Reconstruction
Chondroplasty

5-815   Total hip replacement

Replacement of head of femur and acetabulum by prosthesis

5-816   Other arthroplasty of hip

Acetabuloplasty   Replacement of head of femur
Reconstruction

5-817   Arthroplasty of hand and finger

Capsuloplasty   Reconstruction
Chondroplasty

5-818   Arthroplasty of shoulder

Capsulorrhaphy   Reconstruction
Chondroplasty

5-819   Other repair of joint structure

Arthroplasty of other joints   Suture of ligament
Repair of capsule, not involving
    joint cavity

Excludes: temporomandibular joint (5-774)

5-82   Operations on muscle, tendon and fascia of hand

5-820   Incision of muscle, tendon fascia and bursa of hand

Drainage   Incision of tendon sheath
Exploration   Irrigation of tendon sheath
Incision of palmar whitlow   Removal of rice bodies,
                                             foreign bodies

(Other available code: aspiration of bursa 8-167)

5-821   Division of muscle, tendon and fascia of hand

Release of tendon or muscle   Transection of tendon or muscle
Retinaculotomy (phalangeal)

5-822   Excision of lesion of muscle, tendon and fascia of hand

Excision of:
  ganglion, lesion of tendon sheath, myositis ossificans

5-823   Other excision of muscle, tendon and fascia of hand

Bursectomy   Excision of tendon for graft
Excision of Dupuytren's contracture

5-824   Suture of muscle, tendon and fascia of hand

Myosuture   Repair of tendon

5-825   Transplantation of muscle and tendon of hand

Advancement of tendon   Recession of tendon
Reattachment of tendon

5-826   Reconstruction of thumb

Cocked hat procedure
Digital transfer to act as thumb
Pollicization. with neurovascular bundle
Toe to thumb transfer
With bone graft, skin graft or island graft

5-827   Plastic operation on hand with graft or implant

Opponens plasty   With graft of fascia,
Tendon pulley reconstruction   muscle or tendon

5-828   Other plastic operations on hand

Fixation of tendon   Pollicization of finger
Lengthening of tendon   Shortening of tendon
Plication of fascia

5-829   Other operations on muscle, tendon and fascia of hand

Freeing of adhesions

Excludes: decompression of carpal tunnel (5-043)

(Other available codes: stretching of fascia, muscle
                        or tendon 8-215 and 8-216)

5-83   Operations on other muscles, tendons, fascia and bursae

Excludes: diaphragm (5-347)
            eyelid (5-090 to 5-099)
            muscles of eye (5-100 to 5-109)
            muscles of hand (5-820 to 5-829)

5-830   Incision of muscle, tendon, fascia and bursa

Drainage
Exploration
Incision of tendon sheath
Removal of:
  calcareous deposit in bursa
  foreign body
  rice bodies in tendon sheath

5-831   Division of muscle, tendon and fascia

Tenotomy   Transection

5-832   Excision of lesion of muscle, tendon, fascia and bursa

Removal of: Removal of:
  Baker's cyst   myositis ossificans
  heterotopic bone   synovial cyst
  hydatid cyst

5-833   Other excision of muscle, tendon and fascia

Excision of: Excision of:
  aponeurosis   tendon sheath
  sesamoid bone

Excludes: excision of patella (5-785)

5-834   Excision of bursa

5-835   Suture of muscle, tendon and fascia

Myosuture   Rotator cuff repair
Repair of diastasis recti

Excludes: secondary suture of abdominal wall (5-545)

5-836   Reconstruction of muscle and tendon

Advancement   Recession
Reattachment   Transposition

5-837   Other plastic operations on muscle, tendon and fascia

Fixation (suture for)   Plication
Grafting   Shortening
Lengthening

5-839   Other operations on muscle, tendon, fascia and bursa

Freeing of adhesions

(Other available codes: aspiration of bursa 8-167
                          injection into bursa or tendon 8-585
                          stretching of fascia 8-216
                          stretching of muscle or tendon 8-215)

5-84   Amputation and disarticulation of limbs

Includes: revision of current amputation for trauma

Excludes: revision of amputation stump (5-850)

   5-840   Amputation and disarticulation of fingers

   5-841   Amputation and disarticulation of thumb

   5-842   Amputation of forearm and hand

   Disarticulation at wrist   Metacarpal amputation

   5-843   Disarticulation at elbow and amputation through humerus

   5-844   Disarticulation at shoulder and interthoracoscapular amputation

   5-845   Amputation and disarticulation of toes

   5-846   Amputation and disarticulation of foot

   Between tarsus and metatarsus
   Midtarsal amputation or disarticulation
   With heel flap

   5-847   Amputation of lower leg or ankle

   Below knee amputation
   Site of election
   Supramalleolar amputation
   With patellar tendon weight bearing

   5-848   Amputation of thigh and disarticulation at knee

   Above-knee (supracondylar) amputation
   Patellar tendon weight bearing

   5-849   Abdominopelvic amputation and disarticulation at hip

   Hemicorporectomy
   Hemipelvectomy
   Hindquarter amputation

5-85   Other operations on musculoskeletal system

   5-850   Revision of amputation stump

   Secondary closure
   Trimming of stump

   Excludes: further amputation for current injury (5-840 to 5-849)

   5-851   Reattachment of fingers and thumb

   5-852   Other reattachment of upper limb

   5-853   Reattachment of toes and foot

   Excludes: toe to thumb transfer (5-826)

5-854   Other reattachment of lower limb

5-855   Implantation of prosthetic limb appliance

Bioelectric prothesis
Cineplastic prosthesis
Replacement of prosthesis

5-859   Other operations on musculoskeletal and multiple system

Amputation, unqualified
Separation of conjoined twins

(Other available codes: injection 8-584 to 8-589
                          manipulation 8-210 to 8-219)

OPERATIONS ON THE BREAST

5-86   Excision of the breast

5-860   Local excision of lesion of breast

Excision of lesion of duct   Partial mastectomy
Excision of mammary lesion

Excludes: excision of nipple (5-872)

5-861   Complete mastectomy

Simple mastectomy
Total excision, limited to breast

5-862   Extended simple mastectomy

Modified radical mastectomy
With regional lymphadenectomy

5-863   Radical mastectomy

With excision of regional lymph nodes and pectoral muscles

5-864   Extended radical mastectomy

Excision of breast and regional lymph nodes and also:
    clavicular and supraclavicular lymph nodes
    intrathoracic lymph nodes
    other extensions of growth beyond pectoral muscles

5-865   Subcutaneous mastectomy with implantation of prosthesis

Removal of breast tissue with preservation of nipple and skin

5-869   Other excision of breast

Excision for gynecomastia
Excision of supernumerary breast
Mastectomy, unqualified
Subcutaneous mastectomy (without implant)

5-87   Other operations on breast

5-870   Aspiration of breast

(Other available code: diagnostic aspiration 1-859)

5-871   Mastotomy

Drainage   Removal of foreign body
Exploration

5-872   Breast nipple operation

Excision of nipple   Transposition of nipple
Graft or plastic operation

5-873   Augmentation mammoplasty

Graft
Implant: prosthesis, silicone

5-874   Reduction mammoplasty

Excludes: mastectomy for gynecomastia (5-869)

5-875   Other repair and plastic operation on breast

Mastopexy   Suture
Skin graft

5-879   Other operations on breast

OPERATIONS ON SKIN AND SUBCUTANEOUS TISSUE

Excludes: skin of: anus (5-490 to 5-499)
                     breast (5-860 to 5-869)
                     ear (5-180 to 5-189)
                     eyelid (5-090 to 5-099)
                     female perineum (5-710 to 5-719)
                     nose (5-210 to 5-219)
                     penis (5-640 to 5-649)
                     scrotum (5-610 to 5-619)
                     vulva (5-710 to 5-719)

5-88   Incision and excision of skin and subcutaneous tissue

5-880   Tattooing or insertion into skin and subcutaneous tissue

Injection of filling material
Pigmentation of skin

5-881   Incision of pilonidal sinus

Drainage, sacrococcygeal cyst
Exploration of sinus

5-882   Other incision of skin and subcutaneous tissue

Drainage   Removal of foreign body
Exploration   Undercutting of hair follicle

Excludes: drainage of face or floor of mouth (5-270)

5-883   Surgical toilet of wound or infected tissue

Removal of slough

Excludes: site of open fracture (5-795)

5-884   Local excision or destruction of skin and subcutaneous tissue

Excision of fistula   Excision of lesion with Z-plasty

Excludes: adipectomy (5-901)
           cauterization (5-913)
           cryosurgery (5-949)
           electrolysis (5-930 to 5-933)

(Other available codes: dermabrasion 8-182
                         laser beam - see chapter 3)

5-885   Radical excision of skin lesion

Excludes: excision of elephantiasis of scrotum (5-612)

5-887   Excision of pilonidal sinus

Exteriorization, marsupialization

5-888   Excision of skin for graft

5-89   Repair and reconstruction of skin and subcutaneous tissue

5-890   Suture of skin and subcutaneous tissue

Repair of open wound (without skin graft)
Resuture of wound
Skin plasty for repair of wound

5-891   Relaxation of scar or contracture of skin

5-892   Free skin graft to hand

Excision of: full thickness, partial thickness, or
              split thickness graft

5-893   Other free skin grafts

Excludes: construction of artificial vagina (5-705)

5-894   Cutting and preparation of flap or pedicle graft

Advancement of flap or tube

5-895   Attachment to hand of flap or pedicle graft

Cross finger flap   Pocket flap
Double pedicled flap

Excludes: pollicization (5-826 and 5-828)

5-896   Attachment to other sites of flap or pedicle graft

Transfer of pedicle

5-897   Revision of flap or pedicle graft

Defatting

5-898   Plastic operations on lip and external mouth

Cheilostomatoplasty   With flap, pedicle or free skin
Reconstruction for cleft lip   graft

Excludes: cleft palate operation (5-275)
           cutting and preparation of flap or pedicle graft (5-894)

5-899   Other repair and reconstruction of skin and subcutaneous tissue

Correction of syndactyly

Excludes: genoplasty with bone graft (5-775)

5-90   Other operations on skin and subcutaneous tissue

5-900   Facial rhytidectomy

Face   Fascial sling for facial weakness

5-901   Size reduction plastic operation

Adipectomy
Panniculectomy
Reduction of adipose tissue of:
  abdominal wall
  arms
  buttocks
  thigh

Excludes: breast (5-874)

5-902   Hair transplant

Graft of hair-bearing skin

5-903   Removal of superficial skin layers

Keratotomy

(Other available codes: removal of tattoo marks 8-184
                         dermabrasion 8-182
                         whirling brush 8-183)

5-904   Chemosurgery of skin

Caustic application with surgical removal
Chemical exfoliation

5-908   Other operations on skin and subcutaneous tissue

Excludes: electrolysis (5-933)

(Other available code: aspiration 8-150)

5-909   Other operations

Operation on calculus, cyst or tumor of ill defined location
Removal of foreign body, unqualified

DISRUPTION OF TISSUE

5-91   <u>Cauterization</u>

  5-910   Corneal cauterization

  5-911   Nasal cauterization

Excludes: for epistaxis control (5-210)

  5-912   Perineal cauterization

  Bartholin's gland   Perianal
  Condyloma acuminata   Vulva

  5-913   Skin cauterization

  5-914   Electrocautery

5-92   <u>Surgical diathermy</u>

Excludes: for eye conditions

  5-920   Nasal electrocoagulation

Excludes: for turbinectomy (5-215)

  5-921   Cystoscopic electrocoagulation

  5-922   Electrocoagulation of skin

  Warts   Nevi

  5-929   Other coagulation

Excludes: endoscopic electrocoagulation of tracheal lesion (5-314)

5-93   <u>Other electrical destruction</u>

Includes: electrolysis   iontophoresis
           ionization

5-930   Electrolysis of eyelash

5-931   Nasal ionization

5-932   Fulguration of lesion

5-933   Ionization or electrolysis, unqualified

5-94   Cryosurgery

5-949   Cryosurgery, not elsewhere classified

Excludes: for eye conditions

5-95   Caustics and other chemicals

5-950   Topical application of caustic

5-951   Endoscopic application of caustic

5-952   Injection of caustic into tissue

Excludes: prostatic injection of caustic (8-581)

5-953   Endoscopic injection of caustic

5-954   Chemopeel

5-955   Boiling water injection

5-96   Cytotoxic drug therapy

5-960   Subarachnoid injection of cytotoxic drug

5-961   Arterial injection into head of cytotoxic drug

5-962   Other arterial injection of cytotoxic drug

5-963   Pleural instillation of cytotoxic drug

5-964   Peritoneal instillation of cytotoxic drug

5-965   Bladder instillation of cytotoxic drug

5-966   Superficial application of cytotoxic drug

5-969   Other cytotoxic drug therapy

By injection
By mouth

5-97   Sclerosing injection

5-970   Intravenous sclerosing injection

5-971   Sclerosis of veins of leg

Production of thrombosis
Varicose vein injection

5-972   Compression sclerosis

5-973   Sclerosing injection of hemorrhoids

5-974   Sclerosing injection of peritoneum

5-975   Sclerosing of vulval veins

5-976   Sclerosing of hemangioma

5-979   Other sclerosing injection

Excludes: sclerosing injection of spleen (5-411)

OPTIONAL SURGERY

5-98   Optional surgery

5-980   Surgical operations to produce female sterilization

5-981   Surgical operations to produce male sterilization

5-982   Other surgical operations for preventive purposes

5-988   Other optional surgical procedures

ILL-DEFINED OPERATIONS

5-99   Ill-defined operations

5-990   Endoscopic destruction of lesion, not otherwise specified

5-991   Destruction of lesion, not otherwise specified

5-994   Operation abandoned before onset

5-995   Operation not completed (abandoned during progress of operation)

5-999   Surgical procedure not otherwise specified

8.   OTHER THERAPEUTIC PROCEDURES

8.   OTHER THERAPEUTIC PROCEDURES

REMOVAL OF UNWANTED MATERIAL

8-10   <u>Removal of object</u>

Includes: removal of foreign body, calculus and parasite
            by endoscopy

  8-100   Removal of object from orifice or by endoscopy

  8-101   Removal of object from conjunctiva or cornea

  Excludes: foreign body penetrating cornea

  8-102   Removal of object from eyelid or orbit

  8-103   Removal of object by auroscopy and from meatus

  8-104   Removal of object by rhinoscopy

  8-105   Removal of body by laryngoscopy

  8-106   Removal of object by tracheoscopy

  8-107. Removal of object by bronchoscopy

  8-108   Removal of object by thoracoscopy

  8-109   Other removal from respiratory tract

  Removal of tracheostomy tube

8-11   <u>Other removal of object</u>

  8-110   Removal of object from mouth and nasopharynx

  From tonsil, adenoid or salivary duct

  8-111   Removal of object by pharyngoscopy and esophagoscopy

  8-112   Removal of object by gastroscopy

  8-113   Removal of object by endoscopy of lower bowel

  8-114   Removal of object by cystoscopy

  8-115   Removal of object from vagina

  8-116   Removal of object from specified dermal site

  8-117   Removal of parasite from tissue

  Extraction of Dracunculus medinensis or helminth larva

  8-118   Removal of object from anus

8-119   Other removal of foreign body

Excludes: foreign body penetrating tissue - see site in Chapter 5
           uterine foreign body (5-691)

8-12   Evacuation of contents of alimentary tract

8-120   Gastric intubation

8-121   Gastric decompression

8-122   Gastric drainage

Use of stomach pump

Excludes: test meal

8-123   Gastric irrigation

Lavage

8-124   Intestinal intubation

8-125   Intestinal decompression

8-126   Intestinal drainage

8-127   Removal of impacted fecal contents

Removal of impacted feces
Removal of meconium
Simple enema

8-13   Evacuation of contents of urinary bladder

8-130   Catheterization of bladder

Urethral catheterization

8-131   Drainage of bladder

8-132   Irrigation of bladder

8-133   Manipulation with urethral catheter

Removal of blood clot or calculus by suction

8-134   Insertion of indwelling catheter

8-135   Replacement of urethral catheter

Replacement of indwelling catheter

Excludes: aspiration of bladder by puncture (8-161)

8-136   Replacement of cystostomy tube

8-14   Other irrigation, catheterization or cannulation

   8-140   Catheterization, unqualified

   8-141   Lacrimal duct catheterization

   8-142   Catheterization of nasal sinus

   8-143   Catheterization of bronchus

   8-144   Peritoneal cannulation

   8-145   Intrauterine catheterization

   8-149   Percutaneous catheterization, unqualified

8-15   Therapeutic aspiration, puncture and evacuation

Includes: removal of fluid without incision

   8-150   Aspiration of hygroma, cyst or abscess

   Excludes: aspiration from sites specified in the index

   8-151   Aspiration from brain ventricular shunt or spine

Aspiration of spinal cyst
Irrigation of ventricular shunt

   Excludes: aspiration or drainage of brain (5-010)

   8-152   Aspiration of eye

Anterior chamber

   8-153   Aspiration of pericardial sac

   8-154   Aspiration of bone marrow

   8-155   Aspiration of pleural cavity

   8-156   Aspiration of lung

   8-157   Aspiration of peritoneal cavity

Lavage
Tapping of ascites

   8-158   Aspiration of liver

   8-159   Other alimentary aspiration

Aspiration of digestive organ

8-16   <u>Other therapeutic aspiration, puncture and evacuation</u>

  8-160   Aspiration of kidney

  Aspiration of:
    renal cyst
    renal pelvis

  8-161   Aspiration of bladder

  Excludes: aspiration of blood clot or calculus (8-133)

  8-162   Aspiration of prostate

  Aspiration of prostatic abscess

  8-163   Aspiration of male genital organs

  Spermatocele   Hydrocele
  Tunica vaginalis

  8-164   Aspiration of ovary

  8-165   Aspiration of uterus

  Menstrual extraction

  Excludes: vacuum aspiration to terminate pregnancy (5-751)

  8-166   Aspiration of joint

  8-167   Aspiration of other musculoskeletal structures

  Aspiration of bursa

  8-169   Other aspiration of fluid

  Excludes: breast (5-870)

8-17   <u>Evacuation by syringing or irrigation, insufflation</u>

  8-170   Syringing of lacrimal sac or duct

  8-171   Syringing of aural canal

  Removal of cerumen

  8-172   Syringing of middle ear

  Suction clearance of middle ear

  8-173   Insufflation of Eustachian tube

  8-174   Irrigation of nasal sinus

  Antral lavage

  8-175   Lavage of bronchus or trachea

8-179   Other syringing or irrigation

Continuous suction drainage

Excludes: irrigation of bowel (8-127)

8-18   Removal of dermal appendages

8-180   Epilation, unqualified

8-181   Epilation of eyelash

8-182   Dermabrasion

8-183   Whirling brush on skin

8-184   Removal of tattoo marks

8-185   Other removal of skin blemishes

8-186   Removal of nail

Avulsion of nail

8-187   Ligation of dermal protuberance

Supernumerary digit   Wart

8-19   Wound cleaning and dressing

8-190   Wound cleaning, unqualified

8-191   Toilet of wound, unqualified

Removal of: contaminated and necrotic tissue⎫
             debris, foreign matter   ⎬ without incision
                                             ⎭

8-192   Dressing of wound

8-193   Dressing of ulcer

Elastic bandaging

8-194   Dressing of burn

CORRECTION OF MISPLACEMENT

8-20   Correction of fracture or dislocation

8-200   Closed reduction of fracture of nasal bone

8-201   Correction of displacement of nasal bone or septum

8-202   Closed reduction of fracture of upper arm

Elbow   Shoulder
Humerus

8-203   Closed reduction of fracture of forearm and hand

Finger or thumb   Radius and ulna
Metacarpus   Wrist

8-204   Closed reduction of fracture of upper leg

Femur   Knee
Hip

8-205   Closed reduction of fracture of lower leg and foot

Ankle   Tibia and fibula
Metatarsus   Toe or hallux

8-208   Closed reduction of other fracture

8-209   Closed reduction of dislocation of joint

8-21   Forcible correction of adhesions or deformity

8-210   Infraction of turbinate or nasal bone

8-211   Manipulation of temporomandibular joint

8-212   Forced extension of limb

Hyperextension of joint

8-213   Refracture of bone

Osteoclasis

8-214   Rupture of joint adhesions

8-215   Stretching of muscle or tendon

8-216   Stretching of fascia

8-217   Manipulation under anesthesia

8-219   Other forcible correction of deformity

8-22   Gradual correction of abnormality

8-220   Endoscopic dilation, unqualified

8-221   Dilation of frontonasal duct

8-222   Dilation of lacrimonasal duct

8-223   Dilation of salivary duct

8-224   Dilation of pharynx

8-225   Dilation of bowel or artificial anus

Anal sphincter   Ileostomy opening
Colostomy opening   Pecten band
Hemorrhoids

8-226 Distension of urinary bladder

8-227 Stretching of foreskin

8-228 Dilation of introitus and vagina

8-229 Other dilation

Excludes: dilation of: cervix uteri (5-670), esophagus (5-428)
           ureter (5-598), urethra (5-585)

8-23 Correction by appliance

8-230 Wedging of plaster

8-231 Orthopedic compensation for deformity

8-24 Replacement of displaced organ

8-240 Reimplantation of tooth

8-241 Manual reduction of hernia

8-242 Reduction of prolapsed rectum

8-243 Reduction of hemorrhoids

8-249 Other replacement of displaced organ

8-25 Manipulation of fetus or pregnant uterus

8-250 Antenatal manipulation, unqualified

8-251 External version

Bipolar version   Correction of breech presentation

8-252 Correction of retroverted gravid uterus

8-253 Reposition of fetus

Conversion of face-to-pubis presentation
Manual flexion of head or rotation of head

8-254 Reposition of cord

8-255 Manually assisted vaginal delivery

8-256 Manual replacement of inverted puerperal uterus

8-259 Other obstetric manipulation

8-29 Other manipulations

8-290 Chiropraxy

8-291 Osteopathy

8-292 Osteopathic manipulation

8-299   Manipulation, unqualified

IMMOBILIZATION AND SUPPORT

8-30   Bandaging and sling support

   8-300   Bandaging

   8-301   Application of sling

   8-302   Pelvic sling

   8-303   Immobilization by bandaging or sling

   8-309   Other specified support of limb

8-31   Immobilization by cast

Includes: plaster of Paris

   8-310   Application of cast

   8-311   Application of plaster jacket

   8-312   Application of moulded neck support

   Minerva cast

   8-313   Replacement of cast or jacket

   8-319   Cast or plaster immobilization

8-32   Immobilization by splinting

   8-320   Splinting of hand

   8-321   Splinting of finger

   8-322   Splinting of dislocated hip

   8-323   Splinting for knee

   Tray splint

   8-324   Splinting for fracture

   8-329   Other splinting for immobilization

8-33   Other rigid support

   8-330   External fixation of fractured bone

   8-331   Other external fixation of bone

   8-332   Other immobilization of bone

   8-333   Immobilization of wound

8-334   Wiring of teeth

8-335   Other splinting of teeth

8-34   Compression

8-340   Compression union of fracture

8-341   Ringing of hemorrhoids

8-35   Other restraint by appliance

8-350   Orthodontic arch bands

8-351   Pneumatic splinting

8-359   Other restraint by appliance

8-36   Internal support

8-360   Urethral splinting

8-361   Uterovaginal pessary

8-362   Nailing of bone

Arthrodesis   Separated epiphysis
Fracture of femur

8-369   Internal prosthesis

8-37   Bodily support

8-370   Bodily support

8-371   Spinal frame

8-372   Corset support

Trunk corset

8-373   Special bed

Cardiac bed

8-374   Water bed

8-375   High air loss bed

8-38   Removal of fixation and support

8-380   Removal of cast, mold or support

8-381   Removal of splint

8-382   Removal of support or brace

8-389   Removal of other fixation

SKELETAL AND OTHER TRACTION

8-40   Traction by bone fixation

  8-400   Infixed bone pin

  8-401   Kirschener wire

  Böhler stirrup   Through tibial condyle

  8-402   Balanced skeletal traction

  90-90 traction

  8-403   Intermittent skeletal traction

8-41   Spinal traction

  8-410   Spinal extension

  8-411   Halo traction of skull

  Caliper tongs

  8-412   Other cervical traction

  8-413   Lumbar traction

8-42   Skin and soft tissue traction of limbs

  8-420   Skin traction

  Adhesive tape traction

  8-421   Boot traction

  8-422   Thomas' splint traction

  8-423   Gallows traction

  8-424   Plaster cast traction

8-43   Balanced suspension

  8-430   Balanced suspension

  Buck's suspension

8-45   Soft tissue traction on neck

  8-450   Cervical collar for head traction

8-46   Removal of traction device or support

  8-460   Removal of infixed bone pin

8-47   Other traction

  8-470   Extension, unqualified

8-471   Bone traction

8-472   Traction for closed fracture

8-473   Traction for fracture of jaw

8-474   Traction for dislocation

8-475   Hinged traction

8-476   Abduction traction

8-477   Intermittent traction

8-479   Traction, other and unqualified

8-48   Orthopedic procedures

8-480   Application of orthopedic appliance

8-481   Removal of orthopedic appliance

8-489   Orthopedic procedure

OTHER MECHANICAL PROCEDURES

8-50   Control of hemorrhage by packing

Excludes: packing for puerperal uterine hemorrhage (5-759)
            postoperative dental hemorrhage (8-894)

8-500   Control of hemorrhage by packing

8-501   Control of nasal hemorrhage

Excludes: postoperative hemorrhage (8-894)
          surgical control (5-210 and 5-387)

8-502   Control of rectal hemorrhage

8-503   Control of non-obstetric uterine hemorrhage

8-504   Control of vaginal hemorrhage

8-51   Expression of placenta

8-510   Credé expression

Excludes: manual removal of placenta (5-756)

8-52   Cardiac massage

8-520   Closed cardiac massage

8-53   Other external manipulation or compression

8-530   External manipulation

8-531   Other immobilization of fractured bone

Antral pack

8-532   Manipulation of salivary calculus

8-533   Endoscopic manipulation

8-534   Abdominal manipulation

8-535   Prostatic massage

8-536   Skeletal massage

Pneumatic compression

8-539   Massage, unqualified

8-54   Vibration and acupuncture

8-540   Acupuncture

8-541   Acupuncture for anesthesia

Whirling acupuncture

8-542   Rhythmic percussion

To neuroma of amputation stump

8-543   Vibration of cervix

8-544   Venous flow stimulator

Electronic gaiter
Intermittent compression of calf

8-55   Hydrotherapy and aerotherapy

8-550   Hydrotherapy

8-551   Assisted exercise in pool

8-552   Free exercises in pool

8-553   Whirlpool therapy

8-554   Therapeutic insufflation

Excludes: Eustachian insufflation (8-173)
            fallopian insufflation (5-667)

8-56   Internal or external prosthesis

8-560   Palatal obturator

8-561   Dental obturator

8-562   Fitting of prosthesis

8-563   Application of prosthesis

8-564   Fitting of artificial limb

8-565   Application of limb prosthesis

8-566   Repair, revision or readjustment of prosthesis

8-57   Injection for local action

8-570   Injection into spinal canal

Spinal anesthesia

Excludes: injection of destructive agent (5-037)

8-571   Injection into nerve

8-572   Other injection into eye or orbit

Subconjunctival injection

Excludes: opticociliary injection (5-133)

8-573   Injection into tympanum

8-574   Injection into trachea

8-575   Injection into pericardial sac

8-576   Injection into heart

8-577   Injection into lymphatics

Lymphatics of breast

Excludes: diagnostic injection into lymphatics (1-801)

8-578   Injection into bone marrow

8-58   Further injection for local action

8-580   Injection into kidney

8-581   Injection into prostate

8-582   Injection into hydrocele

8-583   Injection into breast

8-584   Injection into joint or ligament

8-585   Injection into muscle, tendon or bursa

Injection of trigger point

8-586   Injection into skin and subcutaneous tissue

8-587   Injection into other specified tissue

Excludes: vessels (8-849), spleen (5-411)

8-589   Injection, for local action, unqualified

OTHER THERAPY BY PHYSICAL AGENTS

8-60   <u>Heating</u>

8-600   Local heating

Infra-red irradiation

8-601   General warming of body

Whole body hyperthermia

8-602   Hot packs

8-603   Baths

Contrast bath   Paraffin bath

8-604   Medical diathermy

Short wave therapy

8-605   Radiant heat

Infra-red physiotherapy

8-606   Moxibustion

Acupuncture with smouldering moxa

8-61   <u>Cooling</u>

8-610   Hypothermia, unqualified

8-611   General cooling

Whole body hypothermia

8-612   Local cooling

Excludes: cryosurgery (5-949)

8-613   Gastric cooling

8-614   Hypothermia with hypotension

8-62   <u>Radiation and phototherapy</u>

8-620   Phototherapy

8-621   Ultraviolet light therapy

General bodily effect   Sun tan

8-622   Photocoagulation therapy of retina

Arc light coagulation of retina

8-623   Destruction of lesion by ultraviolet light

8-624   Other light coagulation

Excludes: laser beam coagulation - see Chapter 3

8-63   <u>Electrical stimulation of nervous system</u>

8-630   Electroconvulsive therapy

Electronarcosis   E.C.T.

8-631   Faradism

8-64   <u>Electrical conversion of cardiac rhythm</u>

8-640   External electrode stimulation

External cardioversion

8-641   Internal electrode stimulation

Intravenous electrode   Transvenous electrode

8-642   Conversion to sinus rhythm

8-643   Operative cardiac stimulation

8-644   Carotid sinus stimulation

8-649   Other conversion of cardiac rhythm

8-65   <u>Cardiac pacing</u>

8-650   Cardiac pacing, unqualified

8-651   Emergency pacemaker

Transvenous catheter electrode

8-652   Permanent pacemaker

8-653   Asynchronous pacemaker

Fixed-rate ventricular stimulator

8-654   Triggered pacemaker

Atrial synchronous pacing   Non-competitive pacing
Demand pacing

8-655   Atrial overdrive pacing

8-656   Controlled atrial fibrillation

8-657   Other atrial stimulation

8-658   Evaluation of pacemaker function

Excludes: insertion (8-880)   } of intravenous
            removal or replacement (8-882)   }   electrode
            replacement of implanted battery
               or pulse generator (8-881)

8-66   Other electrical stimulation

8-660   Cardiac arrest during cardiovascular bypass

8-661   Spinal neuropacemaker

8-662   Urinary bladder stimulator

8-663   Skeletal muscle stimulator

Soleus stimulator

8-668   Other specified stimulation

8-669   Electrical stimulation, unqualified

8-69   Other and unspecified physical agents

8-690   Other physical agent

8-699   Physical agent, not otherwise specified

RESPIRATORY PROCEDURES

8-70   Endotracheal intubation

8-700   Insertion of endotracheal tube

8-701   Emergency laryngeal intubation

Transglottal intubation

Excludes: transcricoid intubation (5-311)

8-702   Endotracheal anesthesia

8-709   Tracheal intubation, unqualified

8-71   Mechanical assistance to respiration

8-710   Mechanical ventilation

8-711   Endotracheal respiratory assistance

8-712   Intermittent positive pressure respiration

8-72   Other methods of resuscitation

  8-720   Manual resuscitation

  8-721   Mouth-to-mouth resuscitation
Kiss of life

  8-722   Artificial respiration

  8-723   Other respiratory assistance
External counter pulsation (ECP)

  8-724   Operative resuscitation

  8-729   Resuscitation, unqualified

8-73   Production of collapse of lung

  8-730   Collapse therapy, nonsurgical
Excludes: surgical collapse (5-332)

  8-731   Therapeutic pneumothorax

  8-732   Controlled atelectasis

  8-733   Pneumoperitoneum

  8-739   Collapse therapy

8-74   Prevention of collapse of lung

  8-740   Pleural drainage
Underwater seal

  8-741   Plugging of flail chest

  8-742   Relief of tension pneumothorax

  8-749   Prevention of collapse of lung

8-75   Respiratory medication

  8-750   Mist therapy

  8-751   Inhalation therapy

  8-752   Laryngeal intubation inhalation

8-76   Oxygen enrichment

  8-760   Oxygen therapy

  8-761   Catalytic oxygen therapy

8-762   Hyperbaric oxygen

High pressure oxygen

8-763   Cytoreductive effect

8-764   Oxygenators

8-77   Control of atmospheric pressure and composition

  8-770   Mountain resort sanatorium

  8-771   Antigen-free air conditioning

Pollen free room

  8-772   Decompression chamber

  8-773   Helium therapy

8-78   Other respiratory procedures

  8-780   Drug prevention of further asthma attacks

  8-782   Physiotherapy for prevention of pulmonary complications
              of disease or trauma

  8-789   Other respiratory procedures

PROCEDURES AFFECTING CIRCULATORY SYSTEM

8-80   Transfusion of blodd cells

  8-800   Intravenous transfusion

  8-801   Whole blood transfusion

  8-802   Cut-down transfusion

  8-803   Replacement transfusion

Exsanguination exchange transfusion

  8-804   Injection of bone marrow

  8-805   Transfusion of packed blood cells

  8-806   Platelet transfusion

  8-809   Transfusion, unqualified

8-81   Transfusion of plasma and plasma substitutes

  8-810   Plasma transfusion

  8-811   Serum transfusion

8-812   Transfusion of blood expander

Dextran injection

8-813   Dried plasma injection

8-814   Transfusion of antihemophilic factor

8-815   Maintenance of circulation

8-82   Withdrawal of blood and body fluid

8-820   Venesection

8-821   Blood donation

8-822   Forced diuresis

8-83   Catheterization or cannulation of vessel

8-830   Arterial catheterization or cannulation

8-831   Femoral artery cannulization

8-832   Insertion of arteriovenous cannula

8-833   Catheterization of umbilical vessel

Excludes: diagnostic (1-860)

8-834   Venous catheterization or cannulation

8-835   Cut-down venous catheterization or cannulation

8-839   Other catheterization or cannulation of vessel

8-84   Injection or puncture of vessel

8-840   Intra-arterial injection, unqualified

8-841   Arterial injection for general action

8-842   Arterial injection for local action

8-843   Injection into renal artery

8-844   Arterial puncture

8-845   Cut-down intravenous injection

8-846   Venipuncture

Intravenous injection

8-849   Other injection or puncture of vessel

8-85   Extracorporeal circulation and treatment of blood

  8-850   Artificial circulation

  8-851   Operative external circulation

  8-852   Arteriovenous cannulation for blood treatment

  8-853   Hemodialysis

Renal dialysis

  8-854   Extracorporeal kidney

  8-855   Hemodialysis of vena cava

  8-856   Extracorporeal irradiation of blood

  8-857   Ultrafiltration of blood

  8-858   Hemoperfusion of liver and portal system

  8-859   Other extracorporeal circulation

Excludes: oxygenators (8-76)

8-86   Indirect blood exchange

  8-860   Peritoneal dialysis

  8-861   Intestinal dialysis

Intestinal loop lavage

8-87   Other additions to blood stream

  8-870   Arterial perfusion

  8-871   Perfusion of head and neck

  8-872   Renal perfusion

  8-873   Regional perfusion

  8-874   Intravenous perfusion

  8-875   Cut-down infusion

  8-876   Regulation of fluid and electrolyte balance

8-88   Other procedures on circulatory system

  8-880   Insertion of intravenous endocardial electrode

  8-881   Replacement of subcutaneous pulse generator or battery

  8-882   Replacement or removal of intravenous endocardial electrode

  8-884   Administration of anticoagulants

8-886   Physiotherapy for prevention of vascular complications of
         disease or trauma

8-887   Physiotherapy for maintenance of cardiovascular performance

8-889   Other circulatory procedures

PRE- AND POSTOPERATIVE PROCEDURES

8-89   Pre- and postoperative procedures

(Other available codes for use with anesthesia:
  cardiac arrest 8-660
  hypothermia 8-611
  anesthetic drugs - see Chapter 6)

8-890   Pre-anesthetic assessment

8-891   Local anesthesia for operative procedures

(Other available codes: acupuncture 8-541
                           regional 8-571
                           spinal 8-570)

8-892   General anesthesia for operative procedures

Inhalation anesthesia   Intravenous anesthesia

8-893   Anesthesia with muscle relaxant

8-894   Control of hemorrhage after operation on nose, mouth or throat

After dental extraction   After operation on tonsils

8-895   Control of hemorrhage after operation on genital organs

After operation on prostate
After operation of uterus (except obstetric hemorrhage 5-758)

8-896   Control of other postoperative hemorrhage

Excludes: post-vascular surgery (5-394)

8-897   Removal of suture or clips from skin wound

8-898   Other postoperative procedure

(Other available codes: dressing of wound 8-192
                           ligation of vessel 5-387
                           packing 8-500 to 8-509)

MONITORING OF PATIENT

8-90   Metabolic monitoring

   8-900   Monitoring metabolic crisis

   8-901   Diabetic monitoring in crisis

   8-902   Diabetic stabilization

   8-903   Monitoring, dehydration

   8-904   Monitoring, hemolysis

   8-905   Monitoring, starvation

   8-909   Other metabolic monitoring

8-91   Psychiatric monitoring

   8-910   Psychiatric observation

   8-919   Other psychiatric monitoring

8-92   Neurological monitoring

   8-920   Nursing supervision of head injury patient

   Hourly chart, 2-hourly arousal

   8-921   Screening tests for fibrinogen degradation products (FDP)

   8-922   Intracranial pressure monitoring

   Epidural transducer
   Subdural pressure transducer

   8-929   Other neurological monitoring

8-93   Monitoring of respiratory disease

   8-930   Monitoring of respiration

   8-931   Intrapleural pressure monitoring

8-94   Monitoring of heart and circulation

   8-940   Monitoring of patient in cardiac emergency

8-941   Continuous electrocardiographic monitoring

Esophageal electrode

8-942   Monitoring central venous pressure

8-943   Monitoring cardiac output

Retractable flow probe

8-944   Plethysmographic monitoring

Impedance plethysmography
Photoelectric oximeter

8-945   Continuous blood sampling

For anterior pituitary hormones

8-949   Other monitoring of heart and circulation

8-95   <u>Monitoring of renal function</u>

8-950   Monitoring of renal function

8-96   <u>Obstetric monitoring</u>

8-960   Trial labor

8-961   Monitoring of fetal heart during labor

8-969   Other obstetric monitoring

8-98   <u>Other intensive care monitoring</u>

8-980   Intensive care monitoring

8-981   Electronic monitoring

8-99   <u>Monitoring, not otherwise specified</u>

8-990   Clinical monitoring

9.   ANCILLARY PROCEDURES

9. ANCILLARY PROCEDURES

OTHER THERAPY

9-10   Emergency treatment

   9-100   Emergency dressing

9-11   Therapeutic prescription

   9-110   Drug prescription

   (See detailed list in Chapters 6, 7)

   9-111   Replacement therapy

9-12   Drug therapy

   9-120   Drug administration

   9-121   Intramuscular injection of drug

   Excludes: local action on muscle (8-585)

   9-122   Hypodermic injection of drug

   9-123   Automated drug administration

   Micro-injector

   9-124   Automated control of drug administration

   Artificial pancreas

   9-129   Chemotherapy, unqualified

9-13   Continuation of previous treatment

   9-130   Repeated prescription

   Rep.   Mist.

   9-131   Repeat of previous treatment

9-14   Dietary regime

   9-140   Nothing by mouth

   9-141   Fluid diet

   9-142   Mild diet

   9-143   Biliary stone dissolving diet

   9-144   Gluten-free diet

   9-145   Phenylalanine-free diet

   9-149   Dietary therapy

9-15   Admission to intensive care units

  9-150   Cardiac intensive care

  9-151   Respiratory intensive care

  9-152   Neurological intensive care

  Care of head injuries   Cerebrovascular attack care

  9-153   Metabolic unit

  9-154   Burns unit

  9-159   Intensive care unit, unqualified

  (Other available codes: monitoring 8-10 to 8-99)

9-16   Other hospital admission

  9-160   Emergency admission

  9-161   Detoxification centre for alcoholics

  9-169   In-patient admission

9-17   Other admission

  9-170   Night hospital care

  9-172   Day hospital care

  9-173   Psychiatric day care

  9-175   Extended care

  9-176   Domiciliary care

  9-178   Newborn

  Healthy, born in the hospital

9-18   Provision of further care

  9-180   Administrative action

  9-181   Antenatal registration

  Booking for delivery

  9-182   Booking of appointment

  For clinic attendance

  9-183   Waiting list

  9-188   Referred to another institution

9-19   Other and ill-defined therapy

   9-190   Nonoperative procedures

   9-191   Terminal care

   9-192   Shock therapy

Chemical   Insulin

   Excludes: electrical shock (8-630, 8-669)

   9-199   Therapy, unqualified

OTHER CARE

9-20   Nursing and care of patient

   9-200   Intensive nursing care

   9-201   Nursing supervision

   9-202   Intermediate nursing care

   9-203   Incontinence care

   9-204   Nursing care: dressing, irrigation

   9-205   Nursing care: injections

   9-206   Routine nursing care: aid to self-care patient

Enema administration

   9-207   Nursing care: bathing patient

   9-209   Nursing care, unqualified

9-21   Promotion of healing

   9-210   Controlled environment

Positive pressure   Amputation stump

   9-211   Oxygenation of slough

9-22   Immunological therapy

   9-220   Immunosuppression

For transplant

   9-221   Autogenous vaccine

   9-222   Rabies vaccination

   Excludes: prophylactic rabies immunization (4-342)

9-23   <u>Alimentary aid</u>

  9-230   Parenteral alimentation

  9-231   Hyperalimentation

  9-232   Prolonged intravenous feeding

  9-233   Nasal tube feeding

9-24   <u>Aids for severely handicapped persons</u>

  9-240   Provision of artificial arm

  9-241   Electrically operated typewriter

  9-249   Aids for severely handicapped, unqualified

9-25   <u>Induction of labor</u>

  9-250   Medical induction of labor

  9-251   Induction by intravenous injection or drip

  9-252   Induction by intrauterine injection

  Intra-amniotic injection

  9-253   Induction by other medical means

  9-259   Induction of labor, not otherwise specified

9-26   <u>Conduct of delivery</u>

  9-260   Routine supervision of normal delivery

  9-261   Routine manipulation for delivery

  9-262   Routine obstetric assistance, not elsewhere classified

  9-263   Routine episiotomy

  With subsequent repair

  9-269   Delivery, unqualified

9-27   <u>Treatment for infertility</u>

  9-270   Artificial insemination

  9-272   Other therapy for female infertility, not elsewhere classified

  9-274   Therapy for male infertility, not elsewhere classified

9-29   <u>Other specialized treatment</u>

  9-299   Other specialized therapy

ANATOMO-PHYSIOLOGICAL ASSISTANCE

9-30 Dental aid

  9-300   Temporary dental filling

  9-301   Provision of removable denture

  9-302   Insertion of removable denture

  9-303   Adjustment and fitting of removable denture

  9-308   Repair of denture or orthodontic aid

  9-309   Dental aid, unqualified

  Excludes: dental prophylaxis (4-53)
             scaling and polishing (4-521)

9-31 Auditory aid

  9-310   Provision of hearing aid: head worn

  9-311   Provision of hearing aid: body worn

  9-312   Provision of hearing aid: ear fitting

  9-313   Replacement of battery

  9-314   Physiological assistance to hearing

9-32 Visual aid

  9-320   Physiological assistance to vision

  9-321   Prescription of spectacles

  Facial measurements   Specification

  9-322   Provision of spectacles

  Fitting   Revision
  Adjustment   Verification

  9-323   Contact lens, mold

  9-324   Contact lens, glued

  9-325   Spectacles for aphakia

  Excludes: insertion of prosthesis for aphakia (5-147)

  9-326   Removable artificial eye

  Fitting, adjustment, insertion

9-33   Locomotory aid

  9-330   Physiological assistance for locomotion

  9-331   Surgical boots and footwear

  9-332   Surgical and supportive stockings

  9-333   Walking frame

  9-334   Appliance for lower limb

  9-335   Chiropody

  9-336   Provision of artificial leg

9-34   Other orthopedic aid

  9-340   Surgical appliance

  9-341   Maintenance of posture

  9-342   Correction of posture

  9-343   Spinal brace

  9-344   Appliance for head and neck

  9-345   Arm appliance

  9-346   Repair of appliance

  9-349   Other orthopedic aid

9-35   Excretory control

  9-350   Colostomy aid training

  9-351   Colostomy bag fitting

9-36   Urinary bladder control

  9-360   Incontinence control

  9-361   Electrical stimulation of bladder and sphincter

  9-362   Nocturnal warning system

  9-363   Indwelling urethral catheter

9-37   Other nonsurgical prosthesis

  9-370   Facial nonsurgical prosthesis

Fixed or removable

  9-371   Breast nonsurgical prosthesis

Removable replacement breast

9-379   Other cosmetic prosthesis

PHYSIOTHERAPEUTIC AND RELATED TECHNIQUES

9-40   Remedial therapy for visual defects

  9-400   Orthoptic training and exercises

9-41   Remedial therapy for speech defects and deafness

  9-410   Speech therapy

  9-411   Speech training

  9-412   Dyslexia training

  9-413   Dysphasia training

  9-414   Esophageal speech training

  9-415   Speech defect training

  9-416   Training of deaf persons in communication

  Lip reading   Finger reading

  9-417   Other deaf training

9-42   Oral rehabilitation

  9-420   Masticatory exercises

  9-421   Amelioration of swallowing defects

  9-429   Other oral rehabilitation

9-43   Muscular re-education

  9-430   Neuromuscular re-education

  9-431   Exercises for neurological disabilities

  Rigidity   Spasticity
  Paralysis

  9-432   Training of coordination

9-44   Locomotor training

  9-440   Gait training

  9-441   Training in use of lower limb prosthesis

  9-442   Fitting or adjustment of crutches

9-45   Physical exercise

   9-450   Therapeutic exercise

   9-451   Active exercise

   9-452   Assisting exercise

   9-453   Exercise for muscle strength

   9-454   Exercise for endurance

   9-455   Relaxation exercise

   9-459   Exercise, unqualified

9-46   Passive exercise

   9-460   Passive exercise

   9-461   Resistive exercise

   9-462   Joint movement and exercise

   9-463   Training in joint movements

   9-464   Mobilization of joint

   9-465   Mobilization of spine

9-47   Physical therapy for other organs

   9-470   Combined physical therapy

Without mention of the components

   9-471   Massage

   9-472   Breathing exercises

   9-473   Cardiovascular retraining

   9-474   Reduction of edema

   9-475   Training during pregnancy

   9-476   Retraining postpartum

9-48   Other physiotherapy

   9-488   Other specified physiotherapy

   9-489   Physiotherapy, unqualified

OTHER REHABILITATION

9-50   Recreational therapy

    9-500   Manual arts therapy

    9-501   Diversional therapy

    9-502   Play therapy

    9-509   Recreational therapy, unqualified

9-51   Educational rehabilitation

    9-510   Educational therapy

    9-511   Education of bed-bound children

    9-512   Special schooling for handicapped children

    9-513   Vocational schooling

    9-514   Higher education of patient

    9-519   Educational rehabilitation, unqualified

9-52   Occupational therapy

    9-520   Assessment of occupational needs

    9-521   Domestic tasks therapy

    9-522   Daily living activities therapy

    9-529   Occupational therapy, unqualified

9-53   Vocational training and rehabilitation

    9-530   Vocational retraining

    9-531   Vocational assessment

    9-532   Vocational training, general

    9-533   Work-orientated specific training

    9-534   Vocational re-education

    9-535   Change of work, same employer

Re-employment in same employment

    9-536   Change of employment

Re-employment, changed employer

    9-537   Sheltered employment

9-538   Vocational resettlement

9-539   Vocational rehabilitation, unqualified

9-54 Social rehabilitation

9-540   Rehabilitation in domestic tasks

9-541   Rehabilitation in domestic responsibilities

9-542   Organized games

9-549   Social rehabilitation, unqualified

9-55   Rehabilitation for specific disabilities

9-550   Blind rehabilitation

9-551   Blind lead dog initiation

9-552   Instruction in Braille or Moon

9-56   Daily life rehabilitation

9-560   Use of aids for daily life

9-561   Use of kitchen aids

9-562   Use of bathroom aids

9-563   Use of work aids

9-564   Use of indoor mobility aids

9-569   Daily life rehabilitation, unqualified

Excludes: daily life activities as therapy (9-522)
            psycho-social aspects (9-54)

9-59   Other and unspecified rehabilitation

9-599   Rehabilitation, unqualified

PSYCHOTHERAPY

9-60   General psychotherapy

9-609   General psychotherapy

9-61   Functional psychotherapy

9-610   Family therapy

9-619   Functional psychotherapy, unqualified

9-62   Aversion therapy

9-620   Aversion therapy for behavior correction

9-621   Aversion therapy for alcoholism

9-622   Aversion therapy for other somatic illness

9-629   Aversion therapy, unqualified

9-63   Stimulative psychotherapy

9-630   Provocative therapy

9-631   Competitive games

9-632   Rehabilitation from disabling psychological problems

9-64   Psychotherapy for daily life

9-640   Group psychotherapy

9-641   Antiphobic therapy

9-65   Anti-suicide oriented therapy

9-650   Care of potential suicidal patient

9-651   Samaritans advisory service

9-66   Anti-criminal oriented therapy

9-669   Care of potential criminal

9-67   Therapeutic hypnosis

9-679   Hypnosis for therapy

9-68   Other psychotherapy

9-680   Therapeutic psychology

9-681   Control of cardiovascular integration

Conscious control of blood pressure
Learned control of heart rate

9-689   Psychotherapy, unqualified

SOCIOPSYCHOLOGICAL AND OTHER SPECIALIZED THERAPY

9-70   Psychological nursing

9-709   Psychological nursing

9-71   Social case work

9-719   Medical social worker

9-72   Voluntary social agency

9-729   Voluntary agency

9-73   Child guidance therapy

9-739   Therapeutic child guidance

Excludes: medical guidance (4-670)

8-74   Counselling

9-740   Medical counselling of patient

9-741   Social counselling of patient

9-742   Medical counselling of family

9-743   Social counselling of family

9-744   Vocational counselling

9-745   Psychological counselling

9-746   Counselling of employer

8-75   Protective sociopsychological care

9-750   Abandoned baby care

9-751   Substitute mothering

9-752   Care of disabled

9-753   Care of aged

9-76   Other sociopsychological care

9-760   Economic rehabilitation measures

9-761   Legal measures for rehabilitation

9-762   Other socioeconomic measures

9-763   After care, unqualified

9-769   Other sociopsychological care

9-77   Other specialized treatment

9-779   Specialized treatment

LONG-TERM AND FOLLOW-UP PROCEDURES

9-80   Invalid transport facilities

   9-800   Special transport

   9-801   Wheeled chair, pedal or hand powered

   9-802   Wheeled chair, powered

   9-803   Wheeled chair, unqualified

   9-804   Tricycle, hand powered

   9-805   Three-wheeler, powered

   9-806   Invalid car

   9-807   Adaptation of motor vehicle

   9-808   Other outdoor vehicle

9-81   Provision of medical equipment

   9-810   Loan of equipment

   9-811   Loan of bedpan

   9-812   Loan of crutches

   9-819   Provision of medical equipment, unqualified

9-82   Other long-term procedures

   9-820   Recall, unqualified

   9-821   Medical follow-up

   9-822   Surgical follow-up

   9-823   Long-term assistance

ALPHABETICAL INDEX

A

Abduction
− arytenoid 5-315
Ablation - see Excision and Destruction
Abortion
− legal - see Termination, pregnancy
− therapeutic - see Termination, pregnancy
Abrasion
− epicardium 5-363
− lung 5-345
− pericardium 5-363
− pleura 5-345
− skin 8-182
Absorption
− folic acid 2-854
− iron 2-850
Acetabulectomy 5-816
Acetabuloplasty 5-816
− with prosthesis 5-816
Acetest 2-240
Achillorrhaphy 5-835
Acid
− boric
− − blood 2-156
− d-aminolevulinic
− − blood 2-153
− folic
− − absorption 2-854
− sialic
− − blood 2-134
Acid fast bacilli
− culture 2-505
− examination 2-504
Acromionectomy 5-784
Acromioplasty 5-818
ACTH stimulation 2-420
Activity
− cystic fibrosis factor 2-933
− fibrinolytic 2-865

Acupuncture 8-540
Acute phase protein
− serum 2-107
Adenectomy 5-401
Adenine
− phosphate
− − blood 2-135
Adenoidectomy 5-285
− with tonsillectomy 5-282
Adhesiolysis - see also Freeing adhesions
− joint 8-214
− middle ear 5-202
Adhesions
− joint
− − forcible breaking 8-214
Adipectomy 5-901
Adjustment
− denture
− − removable 9-303
− spectacles 9-322
Administration
− anticoagulant 8-884
− drug - see also Drug
− − automated 9-123
− − − control 9-124
Administrative measures 9-180
Admission
− alcoholic detoxification 9-161
− convalescent care 9-175
− day hospital care 9-172
− − psychiatric 9-173
− domiciliary care 9-176
− emergency 9-160
− extended care 9-175
− hospital inpatient 9-169
− inpatient 9-169
− intensive care 9-159
− − burns 9-154

Admission - *continued*
- intensive care 9-159 - *continued*
- - cardiac 9-150
- - head injury 9-152
- - metabolic 9-153
- - neurological 9-152
- - respiratory 9-151
- newborn 9-178
- - born in the hospital 9-178
- - healthy 9-178
- - sick - see Admission, inpatient
- night hospital care 9-170
Adrenal
- cortex
- - function 2-430
- - hormones 2-430
- - - estimation 2-430
- function test 2-354
- medulla hormones 2-431
- - estimation 2-431
Adrenalectomy
- bilateral 5-072
- - with oophorectomy 5-072
- partial 5-071
- total 5-072
- unilateral 5-071
Adrenalotomy 5-073
Adrenocorticotrophic stimulation 2-420
Adrenocorticotrophin 2-414
Advancement
- eye muscle 5-102
- - with resection of same muscle 5-101
- eyelid muscle 5-094
- leaflet (heart) 5-353
- ligament
- - round 5-693
- tendon 5-836
- - hand 5-825
- - thumb 5-825
Aerobic bacteria
- isolation 2-506
After care 9-763
After coming head
- delivery 5-727
- - forceps 5-726
- - manoeuvre 5-727
Agar gel precipitin technique 2-614
Agglutination
- bacterial 2-612
- latex
- - trypanosome 2-752
- rickettsial 2-613
- salmonella 2-610
- sensitized particles 2-663
- sensitized tanned red cells 2-631
- serum 2-612
Agglutinins

Agglutinins - *continued*
- irregular 2-653
Aid
- dental 9-309
- hearing 9-314
- - battery replacement 9-313
- - behind ear 9-312
- - body worn 9-311
- - head worn 9-310
- orthopedic 9-349
- severely handicapped 9-249
Aids
- bathroom 9-562
- daily life 9-560
Air
- antigen free 8-771
Airways resistance
- measurement 1-712
Alanine
- serum identification 2-100
- transaminase 2-460
Albumin
- estimation 2-104
Albumin/globulin ratio 2-103
Albustix 2-204
Alcohol
- blood 2-165
- breath 2-167
- exhaled breath 2-167
Aldosterone
- activity 2-423
Aldridge-Studdiford operation 5-594
Alimentation
- parenteral 9-230
- - partial 9-230
- - prolonged 9-232
- - total 9-231
Alkaline reserve 2-122
Allergy
- testing 1-709
Allograft (see also Graft, grafting)
- liver (orthoptic) 5-505
- nerve (freeze dried) 5-044
Alpha antitrypsin
- determination 2-689
Alpha fetoprotein 2-632
- amniotic fluid 2-632
Alpha-lipoprotein
- blood 2-144
Alpha-2 macroglobulin 2-689
Alteration
- hematological status
- - prophylactic 4-449
- immunological status
- - prophylactic 4-409
Alveolectomy 5-244
Alveoloplasty 5-244

Alveolotomy (dental) 5-240
Amebic dysentery
— fecal microscopy 2-710
Aminoacid(s)
— clearance pattern 2-340
— decarboxylase 2-482
— estimation 2-101
— — blood 2-101
— — urine 2-201
— fecal identification 2-260
— identification 2-100
— — blood 2-100
— — urine 2-200
— tolerance 2-322
Ammon's operation - see Operation,
   Ammon
Amniocentesis 5-753
Amnioscopy 1-359
Amniotic fluid
— bilirubin 2-286
— lecithin 2-286
— protein 2-286
— sphingomyelin 2-286
Amniotomy 5-730
— to induce labor 5-730
Amputation 5-859
— abdominopelvic 5-849
— above
— — elbow 5-843
— — knee 5-848
— ankle 5-847
— arm 5-843
— — through humerus 5-843
— below
— — ankle 5-846
— — knee 5-847
— breast 5-861
— cervix 5-673
— — with colporrhaphy 5-673
— Chopart 5-846
— cineplastic (see also Amputation, by site)
   5-859
— clitoris 5-713
— closed flap (see also Amputation, by site)
   5-859
— ear (external) 5-182
— elbow 5-843
— femur 5-848
— fibula 5-847
— finger 5-840
— — phalanx 5-840
— — thumb 5-841
— foot 5-846
— forearm (through radius and ulna) 5-842
— fungus cerebri 5-014
— guillotine (see also Amputation, by site)
   5-859

Amputation 5-859 - continued
— hallux 5-845
— hand 5-842
— hey 5-846
— hindquarter 5-849
— hip (disarticulation) 5-849
— humerus 5-843
— interthoracoscapular 5-844
— jaw (lower) 5-773
— kineplastic (see also Amputation, by site)
   5-859
— knee (disarticulation) 5-848
— leg (lower) (through tibia and fibula)
   5-847
— limb 5-859
— little finger 5-840
— metacarpal 5-842
— metatarsal (head) 5-782
— midtarsal 5-846
— nail 8-186
— penis 5-642
— phalanx 5-840
— — finger 5-840
— — thumb 5-841
— — toe 5-845
— pinna 5-182
— root (dental) 5-231
— shoulder 5-844
— stump, secondary operation 5-850
— supracondylar, femur 5-848
— supramalleolar 5-847
— thigh (through femur) 5-848
— thumb 5-841
— tibia 5-847
— toe (disarticulation) 5-845
— transcondylar, femur 5-848
— translumbar 5-849
— transmetatarsal 5-846
— wrist (disarticulation) 5-842
Amygdalotomy 5-012
— cerebellar 5-012
Amylase
— urinary 2-470
Analgesia
— spinal 5-037
— spinothalamic 5-032
Analysis
— chemical
— — tissue 2-952
— forensic - see Forensic, chemical analysis
Analytical methods
— other NEC 2-499
Anastomosis (see also Bypass and Shunt)
— antesternal (esophagus) 5-425
— aorta (intra-abdominal) 5-392
— — coronary 5-361
— — intrathoracic 5-392

Anastomosis - *continued*
- aorta - *continued*
- - intrathoracic 5-392 - *continued*
- - - with resection 5-382
- - systemic pulmonary 5-390
- aortocoronary 5-361
- appendix 5-479
- arteriovenous
- - intrathoracic 5-392
- - peripheral 5-392
- artery 5-392
- - abdominal 5-392
- - aorta (see also Anastomosis, aorta) 5-392
- - - abdominal 5-392
- - - thoracic 5-392
- - base of brain 5-392
- - brain 5-392
- - coronary 5-361
- - internal mammary to myocardium 5-361
- - intra-abdominal (direct) 5-392
- - intracranial 5-392
- - intrathoracic NEC 5-392
- - myocardial 5-361
- - neck 5-392
- - peripheral 5-392
- - pulmonary 5-390
- - - to systemic 5-390
- - systemic-systemic 5-392
- - thoracic NEC 5-392
- bile ducts to
- - intestine, any part 5-512
- - other bile ducts 5-512
- bladder to
- - bowel 5-578
- - ileal loop 5-567
- bronchus 5-334
- - to trachea 5-334
- caval 5-391
- cervicoesophageal 5-424
- colohypopharyngeal
- - antethoracic 5-425
- - intrathoracic 5-424
- common duct 5-512
- cystic duct 5-512
- cystocolic (bladder to colon) 5-578
- epididymis to
- - vas deferens 5-637
- esophagus 5-423
- - end to end 5-423
- - intrapleural 5-424
- - intrathoracic 5-424
- - presternal 5-425
- fallopian tube 5-666
- fascicles
- - peripheral nerve 5-046

Anastomosis - *continued*
- gallbladder to
- - intestine 5-512
- - pancreas 5-512
- - stomach 5-512
- hepatic duct 5-512
- ileal loop to
- - bladder 5-567
- ileorectal 5-458
- intestine 5-459
- - large to
- - - large 5-459
- - - small 5-458
- - small to
- - - large 5-458
- - - small 5-457
- intrahepatic duct 5-516
- jejunal 5-457
- - end to end 5-454
- lacrimal sac to
- - conjunctiva 5-088
- lymphatics 5-409
- nasolacrimal 5-087
- nerve
- - cross 5-046
- - facial to spinal accessory 5-046
- - peripheral 5-046
- oviduct 5-666
- pancreatic (duct) 5-527
- - with excision 5-524
- portal 5-391
- portocaval 5-391
- pyelonephroileovesical 5-567
- pyeloureterovesical 5-567
- rectum 5-485
- stomach 5-438
- - with
- - - bile ducts 5-512
- - - gallbladder 5-512
- subclavian-aortic 5-392
- ureter with 5-567
- - bowel (ureterocolic) 5-566
- - ileal conduit 5-564
- urethra 5-583
- - end to end 5-583
- vas deferens 5-637
- vein 5-392
- - abdominal 5-391
- - azygos 5-392
- - base of brain 5-392
- - brain 5-392
- - cava 5-391
- - - inferior 5-391
- - - superior to pulmonary artery 5-392
- - intra-abdominal 5-391
- - intracranial 5-392
- - intrathoracic 5-392

Anastomosis - *continued*
- vein 5-392 - *continued*
- - mesenteric 5-391
- - neck 5-392
- - peripheral 5-392
- - portal to inferior vena cava 5-391
- - pulmonary to 5-392
- - - azygos vein 5-392
- - - right atrium 5-392
- - renal 5-391
- - splenic and renal 5-391
- ventriculoatrial 5-023
- - for cardiac anomaly 5-355
- - for hydrocephalus 5-023
- ventriculocisternal 5-022
- ventriculopleural 5-023
- ventriculovascular 5-023
- vessels
- - peripheral 5-392
- - splenic 5-391
Anesthesia
- endotracheal 8-702
- for examination 1-901
- freezing 8-612
- inhalation 8-892
- intravenous 8-892
- local 8-891
- muscle relaxation 8-893
- nerve block 8-891
- regional block 8-891
- spinal 8-891
- whirling acupuncture 8-541
Aneurysmectomy 5-385
- arteriovenous 5-385
- brain 5-385
- heart 5-373
- intra-abdominal, except aorta 5-385
- neck 5-385
- peripheral vessel 5-385
Aneurysmorrhaphy (see also
  Aneurysmectomy) 5-385
Aneurysmotomy - see Aneurysmectomy
Angiectomy 5-385
- peripheral 5-385
Angiography
- retinal
- - fluorescein 1-802
Angioplasty 5-395
Angiorrhaphy 5-393
- peripheral 5-393
Angiotomy 5-380
Angiotripsy (peripheral) 5-399
Animal
- inoculation of fungus 2-705
- passage of protozoa 2-741
- test of chemical substance 2-573
Annuloplasty

Annuloplasty - *continued*
- mitral valve (posteromedial) 5-353
- tricuspid valve 5-353
Anodic stripping voltametry 2-491
Anoplasty 5-496
Anoscopy 1-644
- control of hemorrhage 8-502
- foreign body removal 8-113
Ansectomy 5-013
Antenatal enrolment
- for delivery 9-181
Anthropometric studies 1-950
Anti-alpha fetoprotein
- serum 2-667
Anti-D globulin
- prophylactic 4-440
Anti-DNA antibody 2-665
Antiamebic serum
- fluorescent antibody test 2-753
Antibiogram 2-530
Antibiotic
- activity of body fluid 2-624
- cover
- - prophylactic 4-379
- - prosthetic heart valve 4-371
- spectrum 2-530
Antibody, antibodies
- antireticulin 2-648
- auto-immune 2-660
- dependent toxicity 2-875
- ferritin labelled
- - detection 2-755
- heterophile 2-651
- - tissue 2-646
- meningococcal
- - assay 2-680
- mitochondrial 2-665
- to variants of normal tissue 2-644
- tumor 2-661
Anticoagulant
- administration 8-884
- prophylactic 4-441
Antidiuretic hormone
- pituitary response 2-411
Antiembolic filter 5-386
- vena cava 5-386
Antigen
- carcinoembryogenic 2-662
- elimination, by air conditioning 8-771
- separation
- - parasites 2-751
- Forssman 2-611
Antigenic reaction
- body fluid 2-689
Antihuman globulin test 2-824
Antileucocytic serum 2-640
Antinuclear factors 2-665

Antiphobic treatment 9-641
Antistreptococcal serum antibodies 2-625
Antistreptokinase 2-625
Antistreptolysin test 2-625
Antithrombin
− activity 2-863
Antitooth decay serum 4-530
Antiviral serology 2-627
− auto-immune antibodies 2-660
Antral pack for fracture 8-531
Antrectomy
− gastric 5-436
− − with vagotomy 5-436
− maxillary 5-222
− pyloric 5-436
− with vagotomy 5-436
Antrostomy
− dental 5-222
− sinus (maxillary) 5-222
Antrotomy
− exploratory 5-221
− − intranasal 5-221
− − maxillary 5-222
− − − intranasal 5-221
− mastoid 5-203
− maxillary
− − radical 5-222
− − simple 5-221
− open exploration 5-222
Aortotomy 5-380
− abdominal 5-380
Apgar scoring
− newborn 1-190
− − with other initial medical evaluation
  1-192
Apicectomy 5-237
− dental 5-237
− lung 5-323
− petrous pyramid, petrous bone 5-204
Apicolysis 5-333
Apicostomy, alveolar 5-240
Aponeurectomy 5-833
− hand 5-823
Aponeurorrhaphy 5-835
− hand 5-824
Aponeurotomy 5-830
− hand 5-820
− with finger reconstruction 5-828
Apophysectomy
− vertebral 5-784
Appendectomy (see also Appendicectomy)
  5-470
Appendicectomy 5-470
− atrial 5-373
− emergency 5-470
− optional 5-982
− prophylactic 5-982

Appendicectomy 5-470 - continued
− with drainage 5-470
Appendicocecostomy 5-479
Appendicostomy 5-479
− closure 5-479
Appendicotomy 5-471
Appliance
− arm 9-345
− head support 9-344
− neck 9-344
− orthodontic
− − insertion 5-246
− orthopedic
− − application 8-480
− − lower leg 9-334
− − repair 9-346
− surgical
− − provision 9-340
Application
− appliance
− − orthopedic 8-480
− cast
− − plaster 8-310
− caustic chemical 5-950
− − endoscopic 5-951
− cytotoxic drug
− − superficial 5-966
− fluoride
− − dental 4-532
− forceps (obstetric) - see also Delivery,
  forceps
− − failure 5-733
− irritants to pericardial sac 5-363
− plaster cast 8-310
− prosthesis 8-563
− − limb 8-564
Appointment booked 9-182
Apronectomy 5-901
Arc lamp coagulation retina 8-622
Arch bars, teeth 8-350
Argininosuccinate lysase 2-481
Arrest
− bone growth (epiphyseal) 5-789
− heart
− − cardiovascular bypass 8-660
− hemorrhage
− − anoscopy 8-502
− − nasal 8-501
− − rectal 8-502
Arterial pulse shape recording 1-252
Arteriectomy 5-385
Arterioplasty 5-395
− base of brain 5-395
− intra-abdominal 5-395
− − with bypass graft 5-392
− intracranial 5-395
− intrathoracic

Arterioplasty 5-395 - *continued*
– intrathoracic - *continued*
– – aorta 5-395
– – other 5-395
– – pulmonary artery 5-395
– neck 5-395
– peripheral 5-395
– – with bypass graft 5-392
Arteriorrhaphy 5-393
Arteriotomy 5-380
– base of brain 5-380
– head 5-380
– intra-abdominal 5-380
– – aorta 5-380
– intracranial 5-380
– intrathoracic 5-380
– neck 5-380
– peripheral vessels 5-380
Arteriovenostomy 5-392
Arthrectomy 5-809
– temporomandibular 5-774
Arthrocentesis 8-166
– diagnostic 1-854
– temporomandibular 5-774
Arthroclasis 8-214
Arthrodesis 5-812
– ankle 5-811
– finger 5-812
– foot 5-811
– hallux 5-811
– hip 5-812
– ischiofemoral 5-812
– knee 5-812
– lumbosacral 5-810
– plantar 5-811
– sacro-iliac 5-812
– shoulder 5-812
– spine 5-810
– subtalar 5-811
– tarsal 5-811
– thumb 5-812
– toe 5-811
– triple (foot) 5-811
– wrist 5-812
Arthroereisis 5-819
Arthrolysis 5-801
– jaw 5-779
– manipulative 8-214
Arthroplasty 5-819
– ankle 5-813
– elbow 5-819
– finger 5-817
– foot 5-813
– forefoot 5-813
– hallux 5-813
– hand 5-817
– hip 5-816

Arthroplasty 5-819 - *continued*
– hip 5-816 - *continued*
– – with
– – – inert implant 5-816
– – – mechanical device 5-816
– – – osteotomy 5-816
– – – total replacement 5-815
– – without mechanical device 5-816
– jaw 5-774
– knee 5-814
– – with patellectomy 5-814
– palmar shelf (wrist) 5-817
– shoulder 5-818
– spine 5-819
– sternoclavicular 5-819
– thumb 5-817
– toe 5-813
– wrist 5-817
Arthrorhisis 5-819
Arthrorrhaphy (see also Repair, joint) 5-819
– foot 5-813
– knee 5-814
Arthroscopy 1-697
Arthrostomy 5-800
Arthrotomy 5-800
– biopsy 1-504
– temporomandibular 5-774
Artificial
– anus
– – colon 5-461
– – ileum 5-462
– arm, provision 9-240
– blood vessel 5-383
– breast (removable) 9-371
– circulation 5-396
– esophagus 5-427
– eye (removable) 9-326
– foraminal valve 5-356
– heart 5-376
– insemination 9-270
– larynx 5-316
– leg, provision 9-336
– limb, fitting 8-564
– liver 8-859
– lung 5-396
– pace maker
– – implantation 5-377
– – replacement 5-378
– pancreas 9-124
– pharynx 5-293
– respiration 8-722
– rupture of membranes 5-730
– stapes 5-191
– ureter, ileal 5-568
– vagina 5-705
– valve (heart) 5-352

Arytenoidectomy (endoscopic) 5-302
Arytenoidopexy 5-315
Ascitic fluid
— chemistry 2-283
— cytology 2-917
Ascorbic acid
— in leucocytes 2-161
— saturation test 2-161
Aspartate
— transaminase 2-460
Aspiration 8-169
— abdominal cavity 8-157
— abscess 8-150
— — brain 5-010
— — extradural 5-010
— — prostate 8-162
— anterior chamber (eye) 8-152
— ascites 8-157
— biopsy - see Biopsy, non surgical
— bladder 8-161
— bone marrow 8-154
— brain substance 5-010
— breast 5-870
— — diagnostic 1-859
— bronchus 8-175
— — diagnostic 1-843
— — selective (diagnostic) 1-843
— bursa 8-167
— calculus
— — bladder 8-133
— — cranial 5-010
— craniobuccal pouch 5-076
— craniopharyngioma 5-076
— cyst 8-150
— — dermoid 8-150
— — diagnostic 1-850
— — epididymis
— — — diagnostic 1-847
— — hydatid 8-150
— — renal 8-160
— — spinal 8-151
— dermoid cyst 8-150
— diagnostic 1-859
— digestive organ 8-159
— diverticulum
— — pharynx 5-290
— endotracheal 8-175
— extradural 5-010
— hernia 5-450
— hydatid cyst 8-150
— hydrocele 8-163
— hydrocephalus 8-151
— hygroma, cystic 8-150
— intracranial 5-010
— joint 8-166
— — diagnostic 1-854
— kidney (percutaneous) 8-160

Aspiration 8-169 - continued
— kidney - continued
— — by incision (cyst) 5-550
— — diagnostic 1-846
— lens 5-146
— liver (percutaneous) 8-158
— — diagnostic 1-845
— lung 8-156
— nasal sinus 5-220
— ovary 8-164
— — diagnostic 1-851
— pericardial cavity 8-153
— pericardium 5-370
— peritoneal (fluid) 8-157
— — diagnostic 1-853
— pituitary gland 5-076
— pleura 8-155
— — diagnostic 1-844
— prostate 8-162
— — diagnostic 1-847
— Rathke's pouch 5-076
— renal (pelvis) 8-160
— skeletal structure 8-167
— spermatocele 8-163
— — diagnostic 1-847
— spinal cord
— — cyst 8-151
— subarachnoid space 5-010
— subcutaneous 8-169
— subdural space 5-010
— subperiostal 8-167
— tunica vaginalis 8-163
— — diagnostic 1-847
— uterus 8-165
— vitreous 5-157
— — for retinal reattachment 5-154
Assay
— meningococcal antibodies 2-680
— microbiological - see Microbiological
    assay
Assessment
— diagnosis 1-991
— endocrine
— — endometrial 1-352
— — vaginal cytology 1-351
— fitness to plead 4-149
— mental status 4-149
— need
— — occupational 9-520
— nutritional status 1-959
— personality 1-932
— preoperative
— — for anesthesia 8-890
— temperament 1-931
Assistance
— long term 9-823
— voluntary agency 9-729

Assisted
– delivery 8-255
– – breech 5-727
Asthma
– prevention, of further attacks, by
  medicaments 8-780
Astragalectomy 5-785
Atelectasia, controlled 8-732
Atherogenic index 2-149
Atrioseptopexy 5-357
Atrioseptoplasty 5-357
– with prosthetic device 5-356
Atrioseptostomy 5-355
– balloon 5-355
Atrioventriculostomy 5-023
Attachment
– eye muscle
– – orbicularis to eyebrow 5-094
– – rectus to frontalis 5-094
– pedicle graft 5-896
– – to hand 5-895
– – to lip 5-898
– pharyngeal flap 5-275
Attention, medical - see Medical attention
Atticoantrotomy (ear) 5-203
Atticotomy 5-202
Attitude testing 1-933
Audiological evaluation 1-233
Audiometry 1-230
– five tone 1-230
– – Bekesy 1-230
– impedance 1-231
– pure tone 1-230
– subjective 1-230
Augmentation

Augmentation - *continued*
– bladder 5-577
Augmented histamine test 2-302
Auroscopy (see also Otoscopy) 1-240
– foreign body removal 8-103
Autoanalyzer 2-495
– blood 2-495
Autogenous vaccine 9-221
– production 2-564
Autograft (see also Graft, grafting)
– heart valve 5-352
Automated
– blood count 2-807
– drug administration 9-123
– – control 9-124
– micro-injector 9-123
Autopsy - see Postmortem examination
Autotransfusion
– peritoneal 5-541
Aversion therapy 9-629
– alcoholism 9-621
– behaviour correction 9-620
– somatic illness 9-622
Avulsion
– nail
– – digit 8-186
– nerve
– – cranial 5-040
– – peripheral 5-040
– – phrenic 5-332
– – vagus 5-440
Azorubin-s
– excretion 2-324
Azostix
– blood urea test 2-112

B

Bacille, bacilli
– acid fast
– – culture 2-505
– – stain 2-504
Bacteria
– aerobic
– – culture 2-506
– – isolation 2-506
– agglutination 2-612
– anaerobic
– – culture 2-507
– – isolation 2-507
– animal virulence test 2-526
– antibiotic susceptibility 2-539
– – combinations 2-532
– – qualitative 2-530
– – quantitative 2-531
– – test NEC 2-539
– count 2-500
– culture 2-506
– – specific medium 2-510
– – type of colony 2-520
– detection 2-509
– enzyme activity 2-513
– fluorescent antibody typing 2-523
– hemolysin production 2-515
– identification 2-519
– – animal inoculation 2-516
– – strains 2-529
– isolation 2-506
– liquefaction of gelatine 2-512
– separation of antigenic components 2-527
– sugar fermentation tests 2-511
– toxin production 2-525
– – diphtheria 2-525
– – plague 2-525
– transferable resistance factor 2-533
– type of growth on culture 2-520
– typing 2-529
– – agglutinins 2-521
– – bacteriophage 2-524
– – fluorescent technique 2-523
– – phagocytosis 2-524
– – precipitins 2-522
– – toxin production 2-525
– utilization of aminoacids 2-512
– variants rough/smooth 2-520
– virulence test
– – animal inoculation 2-516

Bacteriology (see also Specific method)
– blood 2-509
– cerebrospinal fluid 2-509
– sputum 2-509
– urine 2-509
Bacteriophage typing of bacteria 2-523
Baffe's operation 5-357
Baffle intra-atrial pericardial 5-357
Bag fitting 9-351
– training 9-350
Balance (of)
– calcium 2-360
– – phosphate 2-362
– electrolytic 2-351
– nitrogen 2-350
– phosphate 2-361
– – calcium 2-362
Balanoplasty 5-643
Ballistocardiography 1-256
Balloon pump, intra-aortic 5-376
Bandage, bandaging 8-300
– elastic 8-193
Banding
– artery 5-387
– – pulmonary 5-387
– ductus (arteriosus) 5-387
– fracture 5-792
– great vessel 5-387
– – thorax 5-387
– pulmonary artery 5-387
Barr drum stick 2-922
Basal metabolic rate 1-760
Basiotripsy 5-734
Bassini's operation 5-530
Bath
– contrast 8-603
– paraffin 8-603
Bathing
– patient 9-207
Bathroom aids 9-562
Beck's operation 5-363
Bed
– cardiac 8-373
– high air loss 8-375
– special 8-373
– water 8-374
Belsey's operation 5-538
Bence-Jones protein 2-670
– urine 2-670
Benedict test 2-223

Bernheim test 2-115
Beta-galactosidase 2-645
Beta-lipoprotein
– blood 2-144
Bicarbonate
– plasma 2-122
Bicuspidisation, valve (heart) 5-353
Bicycle dynamometer 1-750
Bifurcated needle injector 8-586
Bile pigments
– serum 2-115
Biliary calculus
– analysis 2-325
Bilirubin
– direct 2-115
– indirect 2-115
– urinary 2-212
Billroth I, operation 5-436
Billroth II, operation 5-437
Binocular vision
– testing 1-216
Biochemistry (see also Specific method)
   2-289
– bacteria identification 2-511
– blood 2-189
– body fluid NEC 2-288
– cerebrospinal fluid 2-279
– feces 2-269
– screening 4-260
– – neonatal 4-215
– tissues 2-952
– urine 2-259
Biopsy
– arthrotomy 1-504
– needle - see Biopsy, non surgical
– non surgical 1-499
– – abdominal wall 1-481
– – adenoid 1-422
– – adrenal 1-400
– – anus 1-453
– – bladder 1-462
– – bone 1-484
– – bone marrow 1-425
– – brain 1-401
– – breast 1-482
– – bronchus 1-432
– – cervical smear 1-472
– – cervix uteri 1-475
– – chest 1-434
– – clitoris 1-477
– – colon 1-450
– – conjunctiva 1-413
– – duodenal capsule 1-442
– – ear 1-410
– – – auditory canal 1-410
– – – endoscopic 1-411
– – – external 1-410

Biopsy - *continued*
– non surgical 1-499 - *continued*
– – endocervical 1-473
– – endocrine structure NEC 1-409
– – endometrium 1-471
– – epididymis 1-465
– – esophagus 1-440
– – external auditory canal 1-410
– – eyebrow 1-412
– – eyelid
– – – skin 1-412
– – gastric 1-441
– – gum 1-423
– – hypopharynx 1-423
– – introitus 1-477
– – kidney 1-460
– – labia 1-477
– – larynx 1-420
– – lip 1-480
– – liver 1-454
– – lung 1-431
– – – bronchoscopy 1-432
– – – percutaneous 1-431
– – lymphatic 1-426
– – mammary gland 1-482
– – meninges 1-401
– – mouth 1-421
– – nasopharynx 1-423
– – nerve 1-402
– – nervous organ NEC 1-409
– – nose 1-415
– – – internal (by endoscopy) 1-415
– – – skin 1-414
– – oral cavity 1-421
– – oropharynx 1-423
– – ovary 1-470
– – palate 1-421
– – penis 1-466
– – perineum
– – – female 1-477
– – – male 1-483
– – periurethral tissue, male 1-466
– – pharynx 1-423
– – pleura 1-433
– – prostate 1-463
– – rectum 1-452
– – rib 1-484
– – scrotum 1-465
– – sigmoidoscopy 1-451
– – skin 1-483
– – – ear 1-410
– – – eyelid 1-412
– – – face 1-414
– – – nose 1-414
– – – vulva 1-477
– – spermatic cord 1-465
– – spleen 1-427

Biopsy - *continued*
- non surgical 1-499 - *continued*
- - sternal
- - - marrow 1-425
- - stomach 1-441
- - testis 1-465
- - tongue 1-421
- - tonsil 1-422
- - trachea 1-430
- - transvenous 1-424
- - ureter 1-461
- - urethra 1-464
- - uvula 1-423
- - vagina 1-476
- - vertebral body 1-425
- - vocal cord
- - - endoscopic 1-420
- - vulva 1-477
- - Bartholin's gland 1-477
- open operation - see Biopsy, surgical
- percutaneous - see Biopsy, non surgical
- punch - see Biopsy, non surgical
- superficial smears - see Biopsy, non
  surgical
- surgical 1-599
- - abdominal cavity 1-585
- - adrenal gland 1-584
- - anus 1-558
- - aorta
- - - abdominal 1-585
- - - thoracic 1-581
- - aponeurosis 1-502
- - - hand 1-502
- - appendix 1-556
- - artery
- - - abdominal 1-585
- - - peripheral 1-587
- - - thoracic 1-581
- - bile duct 1-552
- - biliary (tract) 1-552
- - bladder (urinary) 1-562
- - bone 1-503
- - brain (tissue) 1-510
- - - open 1-510
- - breast 1-501
- - bronchus 1-581
- - bursa 1-504
- - - hand 1-504
- - carotid body 1-583
- - cartilage 1-504
- - cervix 1-571
- - chest wall 1-589
- - choroid 1-529
- - clitoris 1-573
- - colon 1-556
- - conjunctiva 1-521
- - cornea 1-523

Biopsy - *continued*
- surgical 1-599 - *continued*
- - cul-de-sac (Douglas') 1-579
- - diaphragm (muscle) 1-550
- - ear 1-532
- - - auditory canal 1-531
- - - external 1-530
- - - skin 1-532
- - esophagus 1-559
- - external auditory canal 1-531
- - eye NEC 1-529
- - eyebrow 1-520
- - eyelid (skin) 1-520
- - fallopian tube 1-570
- - fascia 1-502
- - - hand 1-502
- - fauces 1-545
- - female genital organ NEC 1-579
- - fetus, intrauterine 5-755
- - gallbladder 1-552
- - heart 1-580
- - hepatic duct 1-552
- - hypopharynx 1-547
- - hypophysis 1-510
- - intestine 1-559
- - - large 1-556
- - - small 1-555
- - intra-abdominal organ NEC 1-585
- - intracranial tissue 1-510
- - intrathoracic organ NEC 1-581
- - joint 1-504
- - - capsule 1-504
- - kidney 1-560
- - - pelvis 1-560
- - labia (majora) (minora) 1-573
- - lacrimal
- - - apparatus 1-522
- - - gland 1-522
- - - sac 1-522
- - lens 1-529
- - ligament (joint) 1-504
- - - uterus 1-570
- - lip 1-540
- - liver 1-551
- - lung 1-581
- - lymph node (superficial) 1-586
- - male genital organ NEC 1-569
- - mammary gland 1-501
- - mediastinal organ NEC 1-581
- - mediastinum 1-581
- - meninges
- - - cerebral 1-510
- - - spinal 1-511
- - mesentery 1-559
- - mouth 1-545
- - - vestibule 1-543
- - muscle 1-502

Biopsy - *continued*
- surgical 1-599 - *continued*
- - muscle 1-502 - *continued*
- - - diaphragm 1-550
- - - eye 1-529
- - - hand 1-502
- - nasopharynx 1-548
- - neck organ NEC 1-583
- - nerve 1-519
- - - peripheral 1-512
- - nose 1-538
- - - internal 1-537
- - omentum 1-559
- - orbit 1-529
- - organ NEC 1-589
- - oropharynx 1-546
- - ovary 1-570
- - oviduct 1-570
- - palate 1-544
- - pancreas 1-553
- - parathyroid (gland) 1-582
- - pelvic mass
- - - female 1-579
- - - male 1-569
- - penis 1-564
- - pericardium 1-580
- - perineum
- - - female 1-574
- - - male 1-566
- - periosteum 1-503
- - peripheral vessel 1-587
- - perirenal tissue 1-560
- - peritoneum 1-559
- - - pelvic, female 1-579
- - periurethral tissue 1-561
- - perivesical tissue 1-562
- - pharynx 1-549
- - pineal body 1-510
- - pituitary 1-510
- - pleura 1-581
- - prostate 1-563
- - rectum 1-557
- - retina 1-529
- - retromammary tissue 1-501
- - retrosternal 1-581
- - - thyroid 1-582
- - rib 1-503
- - salivary gland or duct 1-542
- - scrotum 1-569
- - skin 1-500
- - - breast 1-501
- - - ear 1-532
- - - eyelid 1-520
- - - lip 1-540
- - - nose 1-538
- - - penis 1-564
- - - vulva 1-573

Biopsy - *continued*
- surgical 1-599 - *continued*
- - skull 1-510
- - spinal cord 1-511
- - spleen 1-585
- - sternum 1-503
- - stomach 1-554
- - sympathetic 1-519
- - synovial 1-504
- - tendon 1-502
- - - hand 1-502
- - testis 1-565
- - thorax 1-589
- - thymus 1-581
- - thyroglossal duct 1-583
- - thyroid (gland) 1-582
- - tongue 1-541
- - urethra 1-561
- - urinary organ NEC 1-562
- - uvula 1-544
- - vagina 1-572
- - vein (peripheral) 1-587
- - vertebra 1-503
- - vulva 1-573
- - - labia 1-573
- - Bartholin's gland 1-573
- unspecified type - see Biopsy, non surgical
Bisection, stapes footplate 5-191
Biuret reaction 2-102
Bjork-Shiley valve 5-352
Bladder
- diagnostic catheterization 1-332
- ileal 5-564
- injection, cytotoxic drug 5-965
- sensation evaluation 1-330
- stimulator 8-662
- washout 8-132
Blalock-Hanlon operation 5-355
Blalock-Taussig operation 5-390
Blalock's operation 5-390
Bleeding time 2-860
Blepharectomy 5-091
Blepharoplasty 5-096
Blepharopoiesis 5-096
Blepharorrhaphy 5-095
Blepharotomy 5-090
Blind
- lead dog training 9-551
- rehabilitation 9-550
Block
- ganglion
- - gasserian 5-047
- - paravertebral 5-052
- - stellate 5-052
- nerve (anesthetic) 5-047
- - cranial 5-047

Block - *continued*
- nerve - *continued*
- - paracervical 5-052
- - peripheral 5-047
- - pudendal 5-047
- - sympathetic 5-052
- - trigeminal 5-047
Block dissection 5-404
- breast 5-863
- bronchus 5-321
- larynx 5-304
- lymph nodes 5-404
- neck 5-403
- vulva 5-714
Blocking antibody 2-653
- identification 2-654
Blood (see also Plasma and Serum)
- acetaldehyde 2-172
- acetoacetic acid 2-172
- acetone 2-172
- acid
- - bile 2-171
- - boric 2-156
- - citric 2-170
- - d-aminolevulinic 2-153
- - lactic 2-170
- - organic 2-170
- - oxalic 2-170
- - pyruvic 2-170
- - sialic 2-134
- - uric 2-113
- adenine phosphate 2-135
- adrenalin 2-431
- albumin estimation 2-104
- albumin/globulin ratio 2-103
- alcohol 2-165
- - ethyl 2-165
- - isopropyl 2-166
- - methyl 2-166
- alkaline reserve 2-122
- alpha-lipoprotein 2-144
- aminoacids 2-100
- ammonia 2-111
- antibiotic assay 2-163
- anticoagulated 1-914
- autoanalyser 2-495
- bacteriostatic power 2-682
- barbiturate 2-163
- beta-hydroxybutyric acid 2-172
- beta-lipoprotein 2-144
- bile salts 2-171
- bilirubin 2-115
- biochemistry 2-189
- bromine 2-156
- calcitonin 2-439
- calcium 2-151
- carbohydrate 2-139

Blood - *continued*
- carbohydrate 2-139 - *continued*
- - metabolic intermediates 2-135
- carbon monoxide 2-123
- carotenoids 2-160
- catecholamines 2-119
- cells
- - count 2-801
- - examination method NEC 2-819
- - precursors 2-800
- centrifugation technique
- - for parasites 2-722
- cephalin flocculation 2-321
- cerebrosides 2-145
- chloride 2-155
- cholesterol 2-142
- chorionic gonadotrophin 2-433
- chromium 2-156
- chylomicrons 2-146
- coagulation test 2-869
- coagulation time 2-860
- cobalt 2-156
- copper 2-152
- count 2-801
- creatine 2-114
- creatinine 2-114
- cross matching (pretransfusion) 2-820
- cryoscopy 2-181
- cytology 2-809
- - examination method NEC 2-809
- density 2-182
- detection
- - in body fluids 2-836
- digitalis 2-163
- drug level 2-163
- electrical conductivity 2-181
- electrolytes 2-159
- epinephrine 2-431
- estrogens 2-432
- ethyl alcohol 2-165
- exogenous organic 2-169
- fatty acids
- - free 2-141
- - nonesterified 2-141
- - unsaturated 2-141
- fibrinogen 2-321
- film
- - parasites NEC 2-721
- - - malaria 2-721
- - - unstained 2-721
- flow
- - in limb 1-731
- - measurement 1-254
- - renal artery 1-730
- follicle stimulating hormone 2-412
- galactose 2-132
- gas analysis 1-714

Blood - *continued*
- gaseous constituents NEC 2-129
- globulin
- - total estimation 2-105
- glucagon 2-311
- glucocorticoids 2-422
- glucose
- - chemical estimation 2-130
- - enzymatic estimation 2-131
- - oxidase 2-131
- glycoprotein 2-133
- groups
- - antibodies 2-823
- - major 2-821
- - minor 2-822
- - salivary enzymes 2-826
- - ABO 2-821
- - Rhesus 2-821
- human growth hormone 2-413
- hydrogen ion concentration 2-180
- incubation infectivity test (BIIT) 2-739
- inorganic
- - constituents 2-159
- - phosphate 2-154
- iron 2-835
- isocitric dehydrogenase 2-458
- isopropyl alcohol 2-166
- ketoglutaric acid 2-135
- ketones 2-172
- lactose 2-132
- lead 2-153
- lipid 2-149
- - constituents 2-149
- - hexoses 2-139
- - total 2-140
- lithium 2-156
- magnesium 2-156
- malic dehydrogenase 2-458
- manganese 2-156
- mercury 2-156
- metallo-organic compounds 2-164
- methyl alcohol 2-166
- methyl mercury 2-164
- mucopolysaccharides 2-134
- mucoprotein 2-134
- nitrogen 2-119
- - constituents NEC 2-119
- - non protein, total 2-110
- organic constituents NEC 2-179
- osmolality 2-181
- oxygen 2-120
- parasites
- - centrifugation technique 2-722
- - culture 2-723
- - slide (unstained) 2-721
- parathyroid assay 2-364
- pH 2-180

Blood - *continued*
- phenylalanine assay 2-101
- phospholipids 2-145
- physico-chemical 2-188
- pituitary hormone 2-419
- - specified NEC 2-417
- porphyrin 2-834
- potassium 2-150
- pregnancy hormones 2-433
- pressure
- - arterial
- - - recording 1-253
- - measurement 1-253
- progesterone 2-433
- protein
- - bound iodine 2-400
- - chemical separation 2-103
- - examination other NEC 2-109
- - total estimation 2-102
- reaction 2-180
- red cell (see also Erythrocyte)
- - count 2-801
- - - automated 2-807
- - examination NEC 2-819
- - - for abnormal morphology 2-803
- - fragility determination 2-812
- - packed volume (hematocrit) 2-811
- - sedimentation rate 2-810
- - sickling detection 2-840
- - size determination 2-806
- - splenic pool 2-814
- - survival time 2-851
- - volume determination 2-813
- saccharose 2-139
- salicylate 2-163
- sample, sampling 1-914
- - coronary artery 1-276
- seromucoid 2-134
- serotonin 2-439
- single artery 1-731
- sodium 2-150
- specific gravity 2-182
- sphingolipids 2-145
- stains
- - identification 2-941
- - precipitin test 2-941
- steroids NEC 2-143
- sugar
- - chemical estimation 2-130
- - enzymatic estimation 2-131
- testosterone 2-439
- tests (physico-chemical) NEC 2-188
- tetraethyl lead 2-164
- thyrotrophin 2-406
- thyroxine
- - free
- - - T-4 2-404

Blood - *continued*
− thyroxine - *continued*
− − total
− − − T-4 2-402
− trace
− − elements 2-156
− tri-iodothyronine (T-3) 2-403
− triglycerides 2-141
− urea 2-112
− uric acid 2-113
− urobilinogen 2-115
− viscosity 2-183
− vitamin A 2-160
− vitamin C 2-161
− vitamin, other 2-162
− volume
− − estimation 1-737
− white cell (see also Leucocytes)
− − count 2-801
− − − differential 2-881
− − − total 2-880
− − indirect staining 2-883
− − lobulation examination 2-884
− zinc 2-156
Bodies
− Hamazaki-Wesenberg 2-876
Body
− cell mass 2-352
− densitometry 2-352
− fat balance 2-353
− fluid
− − antibiotic activity 2-624
− − chemistry (see also Specified fluid)
  2-288
− fluid NEC
− − parasites 2-726
− total water 2-352
− warming (see also Heat, heating) 8-601
− water balance 2-352
Bone
− marrow
− − examination 2-800
− − transplant 5-410
− metabolism test 2-369
Booked
− appointment 9-182
− for delivery 9-181
Boots
− orthopedic 9-331
− − prescription 9-331
Boston's operation 5-855
Bougie
− induction
− − delivery 5-731
− urethral dilation 5-585
Bouginage - see Bougie
Boyd's operation 5-847

Braille reading 9-552
− training 9-552
Brain
− examination
− − for Negri bodies 2-560
− − postmortem
− − − bacteriological 2-560
Brancher enzyme 2-463
Branchial cleft
− operation 5-291
Braunwald-Cutter valve 5-352
Breast
− artificial (removable) 9-371
Breech
− delivery (assisted) (spontaneous) 5-727
− extraction (total) 5-725
− − partial 5-727
Bricker's operation 5-564
Bridge, dental (fixed) 5-234
Brisement force, jaw 5-779
Bromcresol green
− estimation of albumin
− − serum 2-104
Bromine
− blood 2-156
Bromsulphthalein
− excretion 2-324
Bronchial challenge
− allergy 1-707
Bronchoplasty 5-334
Bronchorrhaphy 5-334
Bronchoscopy 1-620
− by tracheotomy 1-690
− foreign body removal 8-107
− with biopsy 1-432
Bronchospirometry 1-892
Bronchostomy 5-339
Bronchotomy 5-330
Brooke's operation 5-642
Buck's suspension 8-430
Buckling
− sclera 5-153
− − with vitreous implant 5-152
Bundle of His
− electrogram 1-265
Bunionectomy 5-782
Bunnell's operation
− tendon transplant 5-825
Burgess' operation 5-847
Burn
− dressing 8-194
− unit, admission 9-154
Burrholes 5-011
− for fracture 5-011
Bursectomy 5-834
− hand 5-823
Bursotomy 5-830

Bursotomy 5-830 - *continued*
– hand 5-820
By-pass (see also Anastomosis and Shunt)
– aorta
– – to carotid artery 5-392
– – to femoral artery 5-392
– aortocoronary 5-361
– – by saphenous vein 5-361
– artery 5-392
– – peripheral 5-392
– – renal 5-392
– – with excision 5-383
– atrial
– – of left ventricle 5-355
– axillary-femoral
– – prosthetic 5-392
– cardiac revascularization 5-361
– cardiopulmonary 5-396

By-pass - *continued*
– colon 5-458
– esophageal
– – prethoracic 5-425
– – retrosternal 5-424
– femoropopliteal 5-392
– gastroenterostomy 5-442
– graft 5-392
– – artery 5-392
– iliofemoral 5-392
– intestinal
– – large-large 5-459
– – small-large 5-458
– – small-small 5-457
– pharyngeal 5-293
– right heart 5-390
– stomach (witout gastric resection) 5-442
– triple aortocoronary 5-361

C

C-reactive protein 2-107
Calcium
– balance 2-360
– phosphate
– – balance 2-362
– plasma ultrafiltrate 2-151
– serum 2-151
Caldwell-Luc operation 5-222
Calibration
– colostomy 1-322
– ileal conduit 1-322
– meatal (urinary) 1-336
– urethral 5-585
Callander's operation 5-848
Caloric test
– vestibular function 1-234
Calycectomy (renal) 5-553
Calyco-ileo-neocystostomy 5-557
Calycotomy 5-551
Campimetry 1-210
Canaliculodacryocystorhinostomy 5-088
Canaliculoplasty, lacrimal 5-086
Canaliculorhinostomy 5-088
Canaloplasty
– external acoustic meatus 5-185
Cancer
– screening 4-259
– – smear (for cytology) 4-250
– – – cervix (uteri) 4-251
Cannula, cannulation (see also
  Catheterization)
– antrum 5-220
– arteriovenous 8-832
– – for blood treatment 8-852
– – for dialysis 8-852
– artery 8-830
– – femoral 8-831
– – umbilical 8-833
– bile duct 5-513
– eustachian tube 8-173
– lacrimal duct 8-141
– lymphatic NEC 5-409
– nasal sinus 8-142
– – by puncture 5-220
– pacemaker, intravenous electrode 8-880
– papilla of Vater
– – diagnostic 1-870
– peritoneal 8-144
– prosthesis, internal 8-369
– thoracic duct 5-405

Cannula - continued
– transvenous electrode 8-880
– vein, venous 8-834
– – cut-down 8-835
– – umbilical 8-833
– vessel 8-839
Canthectomy 5-092
Canthocystostomy 5-088
Canthoplasty 5-092
Canthorrhaphy 5-092
Canthotomy 5-092
Cap splint
– dental 8-335
– fracture
– – jaw 5-762
Capillary resistance test 2-860
Capsule
– carey 1-442
Capsulectomy
– joint 5-809
– – jaw 5-774
– kidney 5-559
– lens 5-149
– – with lens extraction 5-144
– ovary 5-651
Capsuloiridectomy 5-149
Capsuloplasty (see also Repair, joint) 5-819
– foot 5-813
– knee 5-814
Capsulorrhaphy 5-819
– foot 5-813
– knee 5-814
– shoulder 5-818
Capsulotomy
– joint 5-801
– – temporomandibular 5-774
– lens 5-143
Carbol fuchsin stained smear 2-504
Carbon dioxide
– partial pressure 2-121
– snow 5-949
Carbon monoxide
– blood 2-123
Carboxyhemoglobin 2-832
Carcinoembryonic antigen 2-662
Cardiac
– arrest
– – for operation 8-660
– – operation for 5-379
– function test 1-729

Cardiac - *continued*
- index 1-721
- intensive care unit 9-150
- massage
- - external 8-520
- - open 5-379
- output 1-721
- - monitoring 8-943
- pacing 8-650
- - atrial 8-656
- - - controlled 8-656
- - - fibrillation 8-656
- - - synchronous 8-654
- - demand 8-654
- - non competitive 8-654
Cardiectomy (stomach) 5-435
Cardio-ergodynamography, fetal 4-200
Cardio-omentopexy 5-363
Cardiolysis 5-372
Cardiomyotomy 5-426
Cardiopericardiopexy 5-363
Cardioplasty
- esophagus 5-427
- heart 5-374
- stomach 5-445
- - and esophagus 5-427
Cardiorrhaphy 5-374
Cardioscopy 1-691
Cardiotachyometry 8-940
Cardiotomy
- esophagus 5-426
- heart 5-371
Cardiovascular
- in-depth examination 1-250
- integration control 9-681
- stress testing 1-732
Care (of)
- abandoned baby 9-750
- aged 9-753
- disabled 9-752
- potential criminal 9-669
- potential suicide 9-650
- socioeconomic 9-762
- sociopsychological 9-769
Carey capsule 1-442
Carotid body
- operation 5-398
Carpal tunnel
- release 5-043
Carpectomy 5-785
Cast
- fixation
- - fracture 8-319
Castration
- female 5-654
- male 5-623
Catecholamines

Catecholamines - *continued*
- urine 2-442
Catheter, catheterization (see also
  Cannulation) 8-140
- adrenal venous return 1-862
- arterial
- - diagnostic 1-279
- arteriovenous 8-832
- - for blood treatment 8-852
- - for dialysis 8-852
- artery 8-830
- - cut-down 8-830
- - femoral 8-831
- - umbilical 8-833
- bile (hepatic) duct 5-514
- bladder 8-130
- - diagnostic 1-332
- - indwelling 8-134
- bronchus 8-143
- endocardial - see Catheter, heart
- esophagus 5-427
- eustachian tube 8-173
- great thoracic vessels 1-279
- heart 1-273
- - intravenous 1-273
- - left, retrograde 1-275
- - recording 1-265
- - specified NEC 1-278
- - transseptal 1-274
- inferior vena cava 1-271
- intrauterine 8-145
- jugular vein 1-270
- kidney 5-598
- lacrimal duct 8-141
- nasal sinus 8-142
- percutaneous 8-149
- renal vein 1-861
- selective organ sampling 1-860
- suprapubic 5-571
- umbilical vein 8-833
- ureter 5-598
- - urine sampling 1-654
- urethra 8-130
- - indwelling 8-134
- - - for incontinence control 9-363
- vein, venous 8-834
- - cut-down 8-835
- - umbilical 8-833
- vessel 8-839
Cauterization
- anus 5-492
- Bartholin's gland 5-711
- brain tissue adhesions 5-029
- canaliculi, lacrimal 5-085
- cervix 5-672
- chalazion 5-091
- choroid 5-155

Cauterization - *continued*
- choroid plexus 5-021
- condyloma 5-912
- - acuminata 5-912
- - anus 5-912
- corneal ulcer 5-910
- endometrial 5-681
- esophagus 5-422
- eyelid 5-091
- fallopian tubes 5-665
- - endoscopic 5-663
- - laparotomy 5-664
- hemorrhoids 5-493
- iris 5-135
- lacrimal sac 5-085
- larynx 8-789
- meibomian gland 5-091
- nose 5-911
- - epistaxis control 5-210
- - lesion 5-911
- ostium
- - uterotubal 5-665
- ovary 5-651
- pharynx 5-292
- punctum lacrimale 5-085
- rectum 5-482
- skin 5-913
- - and subcutaneous tissue 5-884
- urethra 5-582
- vocal cords 5-300
- vulva 5-712

Cavernoscopy
- renal pelvis 1-651
- thoracic 1-670

Cavernotomy (thoracic) 5-340
- kidney 5-552
Cecectomy 5-455
Ceco-ureterostomy 5-566
Cecocolostomy 5-459
Cecocystoplasty 5-577
Cecopexy 5-466
Cecoplication 5-546
Cecorrhaphy 5-467
Cecosigmoidostomy 5-459
Cecostomy 5-461
Cecotomy 5-450
Cecum
- operation 5-469
Celiotomy 5-541
- exploratory 5-541
Cells
- culture 2-925
- EAC 2-870
- LE (test) 2-872
Central venous pressure
- measurement 1-272

Cephalin-cholesterol flocculation test
  (Hanger) 2-321
Cephalocentesis 5-010
Cephalotomy, fetal 5-734
Cerclage
- anal 5-496
- cervical os 5-674
- equatorial 5-153
- patellar 5-787
Cerebrosides
- blood 2-145
Cerebrospinal fluid
- aminoacids 2-276
- betaglycuronidase 2-278
- blood detection 2-270
- calcium 2-271
- cells 2-910
- chemical 2-279
- - constituent NEC 2-278
- - examination NEC 2-279
- chloride 2-271
- colloidal gold curve 2-275
- diagnostic specimen 1-206
- electrolytes 2-271
- electrophoresis 2-275
- enzymes 2-278
- glucose 2-272
- glutamine 2-276
- homovanillic acid 2-276
- immunoglobulins 2-275
- lipoproteins 2-278
- magnesium 2-271
- parasites 2-725
- potassium 2-271
- protein 2-274
- sodium 2-271
- treponemal CF test 2-603
- turbidity 2-275
- urea 2-273
Cervical
- scrape for cytology 1-472
- smear
- - diagnostic 1-472
- - routine 4-251
Cervicectomy (uteri) 5-673
Cesarean section 5-749
- cervical 5-741
- classical 5-740
- corporeal 5-740
- extraperitoneal 5-742
- lower uterine segment 5-741
- other specified 5-748
- repeated 5-749
- specified, other 5-748
- supravesical 5-742
- transperitoneal
- - lower segment 5-741

Cesarean section 5-749 - *continued*
- transperitoneal - *continued*
- - upper segment 5-740
- transperitoneal nos 5-741
- upper uterine segment 5-740
- vaginal 5-748
Challenge
- bronchial, allergy 1-707
- nasal, allergy 1-706
Change
- cast
- - plaster 8-313
Charcoal transit time
- stomach 2-305
Charnley's operation 5-815
Cheiloplasty 5-898
Cheilorrhaphy 5-898
Cheilostomatoplasty 5-898
Cheilotomy 5-270
Chemical analysis (see also Biochemistry)
- tissues 2-952
Chemical dissection
- body 2-352
Chemistry (see also Biochemistry)
- body fluids 2-288
Chemofusion
- prolonged 8-876
Chemopallidectomy 5-013
Chemopeel 5-954
Chemosensitivity
- malignant tissue 2-934
Chemosurgery
- brain 5-014
- skin 5-904
Chemothalamectomy 5-013
Chemotherapy 9-129
- cytotoxic 5-969
Chest x-ray
- screening 4-240
Child guidance
- therapy 9-739
Chiropody 9-335
Chiropraxy 8-290
Chloride
- blood 2-155
Cholangiojejunostomy 5-512
Cholangiostomy 5-514
Cholangiotomy 5-514
Cholecystectomy 5-511
- with drainage 5-511
Cholecystocecostomy 5-512
Cholecystocolostomy 5-512
Cholecystoduodenostomy 5-512
Cholecystoenterostomy 5-512
Cholecystogastrostomy 5-512
Cholecystoileostomy 5-512
Cholecystojejunostomy 5-512

Cholecystopancreostomy 5-512
Cholecystopexy 5-519
Cholecystorrhaphy 5-519
Cholecystostomy 5-510
- with (partial) cholecystectomy 5-511
Cholecystotomy 5-510
Choledochectomy 5-515
Choledochoduodenostomy 5-512
Choledochoenterostomy 5-512
Choledochojejunostomy 5-512
Choledocholithiasis
- dietary therapy 9-143
Choledocholithotomy (transduodenal)
  5-513
Choledocholithotripsy 5-513
Choledochopancreatostomy 5-512
Choledochoplasty 5-516
Choledochorrhaphy 5-516
Choledochoscopy 5-514
- operative 1-695
Choledochostomy 5-514
Choledochotomy 5-514
Cholelithotomy 5-510
- from bile duct 5-513
- from gallbladder 5-510
Cholesterol
- blood 2-142
Cholinesterase 2-474
Chondrectomy 5-809
- costal 5-343
- ear (partial) 5-181
- - total 5-182
- intervertebral cartilage 5-803
- joint 5-809
- - temporomandibular 5-774
- nasal 5-212
- - septum 5-214
- temporomandibular 5-774
Chondroplasty 5-819
- ear
- - for prominent ear 5-184
- - other 5-186
- foot 5-813
- hip 5-816
- jaw 5-774
- larynx 5-315
- nose (septum) 5-217
- rib 5-819
- septum, nose 5-217
- soft palate 5-275
- toe 5-813
Chondrotomy (joint) 5-801
Chopart's operation 5-846
Chordectomy (laryngeal) 5-302
Chordotomy (anterolateral) (percutaneous)
  (spinal) (spinothalamic) 5-032
Choroid plexectomy 5-021

Chromatography 2-492
– gas-liquid 2-492
– ion exchange
– – serum aminoacids 2-100
– partition
– – serum pigments 2-115
– thin layer 2-492
Chromium
– blood 2-156
Chromogen
– total
– – serum 2-115
Chromosome
– aberrations determination 2-923
– banding 2-924
Chylomicrons
– blood 2-146
Ciliarectomy 5-134
Ciliarotomy 5-133
Cinching
– eye muscle 5-104
– eyelid muscle 5-094
– scleral 5-153
Cineplasty, prosthesis (limb) 5-855
Circulating anticoagulants
– control 2-861
Circulation
– artificial 8-850
– extracorporeal (see also Extracorporeal, circulation) 5-396
– – operative 8-851
– maintenance 8-815
– time 1-722
Circulatory
– function test 1-739
– output 1-721
Circumcision 5-640
– female (ritual) 5-988
– male 5-640
– surgical 5-640
Cisternal puncture 1-206
Cisterni chyli
– operation 5-405
Clamp and cautery
– hemorrhoids 5-493
Clamping
– artery 5-387
Clasis, surgical 5-789
Clavicotomy 5-781
– fetal 5-734
Cleaning
– wound 8-190
– – surgical toilet 5-883
Clearance
– aminoacids (pattern) 2-340
– creatinine 2-341
– dental 5-230

Clearance - continued
– inulin 2-342
– labelled bilirubin 2-320
– mannitol 2-342
– p-amino hippuric acid 2-341
– pelvic
– – female 5-687
– – male 5-576
– phosphate 2-341
– urea 2-341
Cleft lip
– operation 5-898
Cleidotomy
– fetal 5-734
Clinical conference 1-992
Clinical hematology 2-809
Clinistix
– glucose oxidase 2-220
Clinitest 2-223
Clipping
– aneurysm 5-395
– artery of brain 5-395
– circle of Willis 5-395
– frenulum linguae 5-258
– nails
– – fungus 2-700
– uvula 5-276
Clitoridectomy 5-713
Clitoridotomy 5-713
Closed reduction - see Reduction (closed)
Closing volume 1-710
Closure
– abdominal wound (delayed) (granulating) 5-545
– alveolar ridge
– – with palatoplasty 5-275
– appendicostomy 5-479
– artificial opening
– – bile duct 5-516
– – bladder, urinary 5-578
– – gallbladder 5-516
– – hepatic duct 5-516
– – intestine 5-465
– – larynx 5-315
– bronchostomy 5-334
– burst abdomen 5-545
– cecostomy 5-465
– colostomy 5-465
– cystostomy (urinary) 5-578
– duodenostomy 5-465
– enterostomy 5-465
– esophagostomy 5-427
– fenestration
– – aortic 5-395
– – aortic-pulmonary (valve) 5-395
– – cardiac septum 5-357
– – pulmonary 5-395

Closure - *continued*
- fistula
- - ankle 5-783
- - antrobuccal 5-226
- - anus 5-496
- - appendix 5-479
- - biliary 5-519
- - bladder, urinary 5-578
- - bone 5-783
- - branchial cleft 5-294
- - bronchus 5-334
- - cervicovesical 5-578
- - chest wall 5-346
- - cholecystojejunal 5-519
- - colo-colostomy 5-467
- - colostomy 5-465
- - cornea 5-123
- - ear, middle 5-199
- - esophagus 5-427
- - fecal 5-467
- - gallbladder 5-519
- - gastrocolic 5-445
- - gastrojejunocolic 5-445
- - heart (wall) 5-357
- - ileostomy 5-465
- - intestine 5-467
- - jaw 5-771
- - jejunum 5-467
- - joint 5-802
- - kidney 5-557
- - larynx 5-315
- - lymph 5-409
- - mastoid 5-199
- - meningeal 5-021
- - meninges spinal 5-034
- - mouth 5-274
- - - external 5-274
- - nose 5-217
- - oro-nasal 5-226
- - palate 5-275
- - pancreas 5-529
- - perineal, female 5-716
- - pharynx 5-294
- - pleura 5-346
- - rectovaginal 5-706
- - salivary 5-263
- - skin 5-884
- - stomach
- - - gastrostomy 5-445
- - thoracic duct 5-405
- - thoracic vessels 5-395
- - trachea 5-316
- - tracheoesophageal 5-427
- - ureter 5-568
- - ureterovaginal 5-706
- - urethra 5-583
- - urethrorectal 5-486

Closure - *continued*
- fistula - *continued*
- - urethrovaginal 5-706
- - uterovesical 5-578
- - vaginal 5-706
- - valve, heart 5-353
- - vesical 5-578
- - vesicocolic 5-578
- - vesicoenteric 5-578
- - vesicorectal 5-486
- - vesicouterine 5-578
- - vesicovaginal 5-706
- gastric anastomosis 5-444
- gastroenterostomy 5-444
- gastrostomy 5-445
- ileostomy 5-465
- jejunostomy 5-465
- laparotomy 5-545
- - delayed 5-545
- lid over orbit 5-167
- myelomeningocele 5-034
- nephrostomy 5-557
- perforation
- - esophagus 5-427
- - nose 5-217
- - septum (nasal) 5-217
- - tympanic 5-194
- - ulcer
- - - duodenal 5-443
- - - intestinal 5-467
- - - peptic 5-443
- proctostomy 5-486
- punctum lacrimal 5-086
- pyelostomy 5-557
- rectal stoma 5-486
- - to bladder 5-486
- rectostomy 5-486
- septal defect (heart) 5-357
- - with prosthetic device 5-356
- sigmoidostomy 5-465
- spinal meninges 5-034
- stoma - see Closure, artificial opening
- stomach opening, abnormal 5-445
- tracheostomy 5-316
- ureteroproctostomy 5-568
- urethrostomy 5-583
- vagina 5-703
Clot retraction 2-860
Clotting time
- whole blood 2-860
Coagulase test
- staphylococci 2-514
Coagulation (see also Electrocoagulation)
- cervix 5-672
- pharynx (by diathermy) 5-292
- rectal polyp 5-929
- retina

Coagulation - *continued*
- retina - *continued*
- - by arc lamp 8-622
- - for reattachment 5-154
- - other 5-155
Coagulation, blood
- defect, detection 2-863
- time 2-860
Coagulogram 2-864
Coating
- aneurysm of brain 5-395
Cobalt
- blood 2-156
Coccygectomy 5-785
Coccygotomy 5-781
Cocked hat
- thumb reconstruction 5-826
Cold agglutinins 2-650
Colectomy
- abdominoperineal
- - combined 5-455
- anterior resection for malignancy 5-455
- complete (abdominoperineal) 5-456
- left (radical) 5-455
- partial 5-455
- - in two stages 5-455
- right (radical) 5-455
- segmental 5-455
- subtotal - see Colectomy, partial
Collapse
- lung
- - non-surgical 8-730
- - surgical 5-332
- - therapy 8-739
Collar
- cervical (soft) 8-359
- - for traction of head 8-450
- stud prosthesis, cornea 5-126
Collecting bag
- fecal 9-351
Collection
- feces 1-913
- parasites
- - perianal tape 1-911
- sputum 1-912
Colloidal gold curve (CSF) 2-275
Colo-ileotomy 5-450
Colo-ureterostomy 5-566
Colocentesis 5-450
Colocholecystostomy 5-512
Colocolostomy 5-459
- end to end 5-455
- proximal to distal segment 5-455
- with excision 5-455
Colocystoplasty 5-577
Colon fiberscopy 1-641
Colonoscopy 1-641

Colonoscopy 1-641 - *continued*
- by colotomy 1-693
- operative 1-695
- via stoma 1-640
Colopexy 5-466
Coloplication 5-546
Coloproctostomy 5-459
Coloprotectomy 5-485
Color
- discrimination, testing 1-215
- fields, plotting 1-210
- lanterns, test 1-215
Colorectostomy 5-459
Colorimetry 2-490
Colorrhaphy 5-467
Coloscopy 1-641
Colosigmoidostomy 5-459
Colostomy 5-461
- closure 5-465
- colocentesis 5-461
- formation 5-461
- loop
- - excision of lesion 5-460
- - hernia 5-460
- perineal 5-481
- revision 5-464
- wet 5-566
Colotomy 5-450
Colpectomy
- partial 5-702
- total 5-703
Colpocentesis 5-700
Colpocleisis 5-703
Colpohysterectomy 5-684
Colpomicroscopy 1-663
Colpoperineoplasty (see also Colporrhaphy) 5-705
Colpoperineorrhaphy 5-706
- following delivery 5-758
Colpopexy 5-706
Colpoplasty 5-705
Colpopoiesis 5-705
Colporrhaphy 5-706
- amputation of cervix 5-673
- for cystocele 5-704
- for rectocele 5-704
- for urethrocele 5-704
- with pelvic floor repair 5-706
Colposcopy 1-663
Colpotomy 5-701
- for pelvic peritoneal drainage 5-701
Commissurotomy
- brain 5-012
- lumbosacral 5-032
- open heart 5-351
- transventricular 5-350
Compartmentalization

Compartmentalization - *continued*
− vena cava 5-386
Compatibility test
− pretransfusion
− − red cells 2-820
Competitive games
− for psychotherapy 9-631
Complement fixation
− syphilis
− − blood 2-600
− viral 2-626
Complete blood count 2-809
Completion
− graft nos 5-899
− pedicle transfer 5-896
− surgical procedure 5-999
Compliance
− respiratory 1-712
Compression
− calf
− − intermittent 8-544
− muscle
− − pneumatic 8-536
− sclerosis 5-972
− union of fracture 8-340
Computer
− assisted
− − karyotyping 2-926
− image analysis
− − tissue
− − − electron microscopy 2-906
Conchectomy 5-215
Conchotomy 5-211
Conduit
− ileal 5-564
− right ventricle
− − to pulmonary artery 5-357
Condylectomy 5-809
− jaw 5-774
Condylotomy 5-781
− femur 5-781
− jaw 5-775
Congo red method 1-737
Conization, cervix 5-671
Conjunctivodacryocystostomy 5-088
Conjunctivoplasty 5-113
Conjunctivorhinostomy 5-088
Constriction
− globe 5-153
Construction (see also Reconstruction)
 5-909
− auditory meatus 5-185
− eardrum 5-194
− esophagus - see Anastomosis, esophagus
− larynx
− − artificial 5-293
− − from trachea 5-316

Construction - *continued*
− trachea 5-316
− vagina
− − with colon graft 5-705
− − with skin graft 5-705
− venous valves, peripheral 5-395
Consultation
− inpatient 1-17-
− other patient 1-18-
− outpatient 1-16-
Consumption
− oxygen
− − bodily 1-761
Contact lens
− glued on 9-324
− mould 9-323
Continuous drip 8-876
Continuous flow analyzer 2-495
Contourograph
− cardiac 1-267
Contraceptive
− instruction 4-650
− intrauterine device
− − insertion 4-653
− − prescription 4-652
− oral 4-651
− pill 4-651
− procedure 4-659
− vaginal 4-658
Contraction velocity (heart) 1-720
Control
− bladder (sphincter)
− − test 1-335
− blood pressure
− − conscious, by patient 9-681
− heart rate
− − learned 9-681
− hemorrhage (see also Hemostasis)
− − abdominal 5-541
− − anoscopy 8-502
− − brain 5-387
− − chest 5-340
− − esophagus 5-428
− − − ligation 5-429
− − − tamponade 5-428
− − intra-abdominal 5-541
− − intracranial
− − − meninges 5-021
− − − nec 5-387
− − intrapleural 5-340
− − laparotomy site, recent 5-541
− − liver 5-505
− − nasal 5-210
− − − packing 8-501
− − packing 8-500
− − postnasal 5-210
− − postoperative 8-896

Control - *continued*
- hemorrhage - *continued*
- - postoperative 8-896 - *continued*
- - - dental 8-894
- - - genital 8-895
- - - nose 8-894
- - - prostate 8-895
- - - tonsil 8-894
- - - uterine 8-895
- - - vascular 8-896
- - postpartum 8-895
- - prostate
- - - endoscopic 5-608
- - rectal
- - - packing 8-502
- - tamponade 8-500
- - thorax 5-340
- - thyroid 5-060
- - - postoperative 5-060
- - uterine
- - - obstetric
- - - - antepartum 5-759
- - - - other 5-759
- - - postoperative 8-895
- - vaginal
- - - postoperative 8-895
- - vascular operation 5-394
Controlled atrial pacing 8-656
Controlled environment
- amputation stump 9-210
- convalescent care 9-175
- wound
- - hand 9-210
Convalescent care 9-175
Conversion
- gastric anastomosis 5-444
- to sinus rythm 8-642
Cooling
- general 8-611
- local 8-612
- stomach 8-613
Coombs test 2-824
Copper
- blood 2-152
- sulfate
- - for blood density 2-182
Copper sulfate
- application 5-950
Coprological examination - see Feces
Cordectomy
- vocal 5-302
Cordopexy
- vocal 5-315
Cordotomy
- vocal 5-313
Corelysis 5-136
Coreoplasty 5-136

Corneal tonography 1-225
Coronary artery blood sampling 1-276
Correction
- ankylosis
- - jaw 5-775
- atresia
- - meatal, ear 5-185
- - nasopharynx 5-293
- - rectum 5-480
- blepharoptosis 5-094
- breech presentation 8-251
- buccal deformity 5-274
- bulbous nose 5-217
- chalazion 5-091
- cleft palate 5-275
- club foot 5-859
- coarctation of aorta 5-382
- craniostenosis 5-020
- deformity 5-837
- - limb 5-837
- - nose 5-217
- ear 5-186
- - prominent 5-184
- ectropion 5-093
- everted punctum lacrimale 5-086
- fetal defect
- - in utero 5-755
- forcible 8-219
- - deformity 8-219
- fracture - see Reduction, fracture
- hallux valgus 5-782
- hammertoe 5-811
- hare lip 5-898
- macrostoma 5-898
- microstoma 5-898
- nose
- - saddle 5-217
- overlapping toes 5-813
- palate 5-275
- pectus carinatus 5-346
- pectus excavatum 5-346
- pelvi-ureteral junction 5-557
- posture 9-342
- ptosis
- - eyelid 5-094
- retroversion
- - by pessary 8-361
- - operative 5-695
- strabismus 5-109
- swallowing defect 9-421
- syndactyly 5-899
Corset
- medical 8-372
- trunk 8-372
Cosmetic
- operation 5-900
Costectomy 5-785

Costectomy 5-785 - *continued*
- for bone lesion 5-343
- for chest drainage 5-340
Costochondrectomy 5-809
Costotomy 5-781
Coulter
- count 2-806
Counselling
- employers 9-746
- family
- - medical 9-742
- - social 9-743
- genetic 4-660
- patient
- - medical 9-740
- - social 9-741
- psychological 9-745
- vocational 9-744
Count
- blood 2-801
- - cell 2-801
- - - automated 2-807
- - - platelets 2-802
- - - red 2-801
- - - white 2-801
- - complete 2-809
- Coulter 2-806
- leucocytes 2-801
- - differential 2-881
- - total 2-880
- platelets 2-802
- reticulocytes 2-804
- Schilling 2-881
- spermatozoids 2-915
Countershock
- heart
- - external 8-640
Cover
- antibiotic - see Antibiotic, cover
Craniectomy 5-011
- linear, strip 5-020
Cranioclasis
- fetal 5-734
Cranioplasty 5-020
Craniopuncture 5-010
Craniotomy 5-011
- biopsy, brain 1-510
- exploratory 5-011
- fetal 5-734
- open 5-011
- osteoplastic 5-020
- reopening 5-011
- with removal of blood clot NEC 5-011
- - extradural hematoma 5-011
Craterization
- bone 5-783
- - jaw 5-771

Creatine
- blood 2-114
- clearance 2-341
- kinase 2-462
Creation
- left to right shunt 5-390
Crede, placental expression 8-510
Cricoidectomy 5-302
Cricothyreotomy 5-311
Cricothyroidectomy 5-302
Cricotomy 5-311
Cricotracheotomy 5-311
Cross matching, blood 2-820
Crown, dental (ceramic) (gold) 5-234
Crurotomy
- stapes 5-190
Crushing
- bone 5-789
- - jaw 5-779
- calculus
- - biliary passages 5-513
- - bladder, urinary 5-570
- fallopian tube
- - endoscopic 5-663
- ganglion, sympathetic 5-050
- hemorrhoids 5-493
- nasal septum 5-217
- nerve
- - peripheral 5-040
- - phrenic 5-332
- - sympathetic 5-050
- - vagus 5-440
Crutches 9-442
- adjustment 9-442
- fitting 9-442
- loan 9-812
Crutchfield tongs 8-411
Cryoconization
- cervix 5-672
Cryocyclotherapy 5-133
Cryoextraction of lens 5-144
- extracapsular 5-145
Cryoglobulin 2-678
Cryohypophysectomy 5-075
Cryoleucotomy 5-012
Cryopexy, retinal 5-154
Cryoretinopexy 5-154
Cryosurgery 5-949
- bladder (transurethral) 5-573
- brain 5-014
- cataract 5-144
- cervix uteri 5-672
- ciliary body 5-133
- corneal lesion 5-123
- ear inner 5-207
- eye enucleation 5-163
- iris 5-135

Cryosurgery 5-949 - *continued*
- labyrinth 5-207
- nose 5-212
- - for epistaxis 5-210
- pituitary 5-075
- prostate 5-601
- pterygium 5-122
- retina 5-155
- skin 5-949
- stomach 5-434
- tonsil 5-281
Cryothalamotomy 5-013
Cryptectomy (anus) 5-492
Cryptorchidectomy
- bilateral 5-623
- unilateral 5-622
Cryptorchidopexy 5-624
Culdocentesis 5-700
Culdoscopy 1-696
Culdotomy 5-701
- abscess 5-701
Culture
- aerobic bacteria 2-506
- anaerobic bacteria 2-507
- arthropods 2-744
- bacteria
- - special media 2-507
- cells 2-925
- fibroblast 2-933
- fungus 2-701
- helminths
- - animal passage 2-743
- - in vitro 2-742
- lymphocyte 2-873
- malignant tissue 2-934
- miracidia 2-717
- Mycobacterium tuberculosis 2-505
- parasite 2-749
- - larva 2-717
- - ova 2-717
- protozoa
- - animal passage 2-741
- - in vitro 2-740
- stimulation of mitosis 2-925
- tissue 2-930
Curettage
- abscess
- - skin 5-883
- adenoids 5-285
- anus 5-492
- aponeurosis 5-832
- bladder 5-574
- bone 5-783
- - cavity
- - - with (chip) graft 5-783
- - jaw 5-771
- brain 5-014

Curettage - *continued*
- bursa 5-832
- cartilage (joint) 5-802
- cervical
- - diagnostic 1-475
- chalazion 5-091
- conjunctiva 5-112
- eyelids 5-091
- fascia 5-832
- jaw 5-771
- joint 5-802
- - jaw 5-771
- kidney 5-552
- lens 5-142
- lymph node 5-401
- meningeal 5-014
- mole
- - hydatidiform 5-690
- muscle 5-832
- nerve lesion 5-041
- obstetric 5-690
- skin 8-185
- socket
- - dental 5-242
- spinal 5-033
- spleen 5-413
- tendon 5-832
- ulcer
- - skin 5-883
- uterine 5-690
- - with
- - - dilation - see Dilation, cervix, and curettage
Curvature of lens
- measurement 1-224
Cut-down - see also Name of procedure
- intravenous injection 8-845
Cutter-Smeloff valve 5-352
Cutting
- ganglion, sympathetic 5-050
- nerve
- - peripheral 5-040
- - root, spinal 5-031
- - sympathetic 5-050
- pedicle (tube) graft 5-894
- pylorus (pyloromyotomy) 5-433
- ureteral meatus 5-561
- ureterovesical orifice 5-561
- urethral sphincter 5-584
CVP 1-272
Cyanocobalamin
- excretion 2-855
- metabolism 2-855
Cyclectomy 5-133
- lid margin 5-091
Cyclic adenosine 5-monophosphate 2-484
Cyclicotomy 5-133

Cycloanemization 5-133
Cyclocryotherapy 5-133
Cyclodialysis 5-133
Cyclodiathermy 5-133
Cycloelectrolysis 5-133
Cystectomy 5-575
– ovarian 5-651
– partial 5-575
– radical 5-576
– resection of lesion of bladder 5-574
– total 5-576
Cystic fibrosis factor activity 2-933
Cystine
– serum identification 2-100
Cystocolostomy 5-578
Cystolithotomy 5-571
Cystometrography 1-334
Cystometry
– continous flow 1-333
– air 1-334
Cystopexy 5-578
Cystoplasty 5-578
Cystoproctoplasty 5-578
Cystoproctostomy 5-578
Cystoprostatectomy, radical 5-576
Cystorrhaphy 5-578
Cystoscopy 1-652
– foreign body removal 8-114
– ureteric 1-650
– with destruction of lesion 5-573
Cystosigmoidostomy 5-578
Cystostomy (urinary bladder) 5-572
– suprapubic 5-572
Cystotomy 5-571
Cystoureterostomy 5-567
Cytology 2-919
– ascitic fluid 2-917

Cytology 2-919 - *continued*
– bladder 2-914
– bronchial smear 2-911
– cerebrospinal tissue 2-910
– cervical smear 2-916
– cervix uteri 2-916
– colonic washings 2-913
– duodenum
– – aspiration 1-442
– intestinal washings 2-913
– nasal smear 2-911
– papanicolaou 2-916
– peritoneal fluid 2-917
– pleural fluid 2-917
– rectal washings 2-913
– sputum 2-911
– stomach 2-912
– urine 2-914
– vagina 2-916
Cytopathic effect
– virus 2-540
Cytoreductive effect 8-763
Cytotoxic drug
– administration 5-969
– arterial injection 5-962
– – head 5-963
– bladder instillation 5-965
– injection 5-969
– peritoneal instillation 5-964
– pleural injection or instillation 5-963
– regional
– – head 5-961
– – perfusion 5-962
– subarachnoid injection 5-960
– superficial application 5-966
– therapy 5-969
– vascular injection 5-962

D

D and C - see Dilation, cervix, and curettage
D.C. shock
— brain 8-630
— heart
— — external 8-640
— — operative 8-643
D-aminolevulinic acid
— hydratase 2-478
— serum 2-153
Dacryoadenectomy 5-081
Dacryoadenotomy 5-080
Dacryocystectomy 5-085
Dacryocystorhinostomy 5-087
Dacryocystostomy 5-088
Dacryocystosyringotomy 5-084
Dacryocystotomy 5-084
Daily life aids 9-560
Daily life rehabilitation 9-569
Daily living activities therapy 9-522
Dalkon shield 4-653
Dark adaptation testing 1-214
Dark ground examination (microscopic)
  2-501
Day care
— psychiatric 9-173
Day hospital care 9-172
DCG 1-262
De-epicardialization 5-372
— with revascularization 5-372
Deaf training 9-417
Deafferentation 5-031
Deaminization
— hepatic 2-322
Debridement
— abdominal wall 5-540
— abdominal wound 5-883
— brain 5-014
— compound fracture 5-795
— dental 4-520
— skin 5-883
— — wound 5-883
— skull (fracture) 5-020
— spinal 5-030
— valve, heart (calcified) 5-351
— wound 5-883
Decapitation
— fetal 5-734
Decapsulation, kidney 5-559
Decompression
— anterior spinal 5-030

Decompression - continued
— antero-lateral, spinal 5-030
— anus, imperforate 5-480
— biliary 5-513
— brain 5-011
— carpal tunnel 5-043
— cauda equina 5-030
— chamber 8-772
— cranial 5-011
— gastric 8-121
— heart 5-370
— intestinal 8-125
— intracranial 5-011
— nerve 5-043
— orbit 5-160
— — intracranial approach 5-160
— — transantral 5-160
— pericardium 5-370
— portal 5-391
— rectum 5-480
— root sleeve
— — spinal 5-030
— sinus
— — frontal 5-223
— spinal cord 5-030
— suboccipital 5-011
— subtemporal 5-011
— subtentorial 5-011
— thoracic outlet
— — scalenus section 5-831
Decortication
— brain 5-014
— cerebral 5-014
— heart 5-372
— kidney 5-559
— lung 5-344
— nose 5-212
— periarterial 5-397
— pericardium 5-372
— pleura 5-344
— pulmonary 5-344
— ventricle, heart 5-357
Deepening
— alveolar ridge 5-244
Defatting
— pedicle graft 5-897
— skin flap 5-897
Defibrillation
— electrical 8-642
— external 8-640

Defibrillation - *continued*
- operative 8-643
- via catheter 8-641
Defibrination
- pleura 5-344
Deflation
- bulla
- - lung 8-156
Dehydrogenase 2-459
- lactic
- - serum 2-450
Delivery
- assisted 5-739
- - manually 8-255
- - suction 5-728
- breech (see also Breech, delivery) 5-727
- - extraction (see also Breech, extraction) 5-725
- destruction of fetus 5-734
- dilation of cervix 5-739
- external flexion of fetal head 9-261
- forceps
- - aftercoming head 5-726
- - failure 5-733
- - with episiotomy
- - - high 5-723
- - - low 5-720
- - - mid 5-722
- - - outlet 5-721
- - without episiotomy
- - - high 5-723
- - - low 5-720
- - - mid 5-722
- - - outlet 5-720
- - Scanzoni 5-724
- incision
- - cervix 5-739
- insertion
- - bag, pack, bougie 5-731
- instrumental 5-729
- - breech 5-725
- normal
- - supervision 9-260
- routine
- - episiotomy (with subsequent repair) 9-263
- - manipulation 9-261
- - obstetric assistance NEC 9-262
- rupture of membranes, artificial 5-730
- supervision 9-269
- surgical induction of labour 5-731
- version
- - internal 5-732
Denervation
- adrenal 5-073
- anal 5-490
- artery 5-397

Denervation - *continued*
- carotid body 5-398
- joint 5-040
- paracervical (uterus) 5-694
- periarterial 5-397
- selective
- - gastric 5-440
- ureter 5-051
- uterus 5-694
Dental
- aid 9-309
- bridge (fixed) 5-234
- crown 5-234
- filling
- - temporary 9-300
- obturator 8-561
- scaling 4-521
Dermabrasion 5-903
Dermatoglyphs 1-951
Dermatoplasty 5-899
Deroofing
- bone cavity 5-783
Desmotomy (joint) 5-801
Destruction
- brain (centres) (tissue) 5-014
- ciliary body 5-133
- ear
- - external (lesion) 5-181
- - inner 5-207
- fetal 5-734
- ganglion (wrist) 5-822
- globus pallidus 5-013
- hemorroids 5-493
- labyrinth 5-207
- lacrimal
- - gland 5-081
- - sac 5-085
- larynx 5-300
- lesion (see also Excision, lesion) 5-991
- - bronchus 5-320
- - by ultraviolet light 8-623
- - cervix 5-672
- - endoscopic 5-990
- - esophagus 5-422
- - intestine
- - - large 5-452
- - jaw 5-771
- - joint 5-802
- - kidney 5-552
- - liver 5-501
- - ovary 5-651
- - pancreas 5-521
- - pituitary 5-075
- - sclera 5-134
- - skin 5-884
- - - malignant tumor 5-885
- - testis 5-621

Destruction - *continued*
– lesion - *continued*
– – uterus 5-681
– – – cervical lesion 5-672
– – vagina 5-702
– – vulva 5-712
– liver 5-501
– lymphatics 5-409
– mediastinum 5-342
– nerve 5-041
– – cranial 5-040
– – in spine 5-037
– – sympathetic 5-051
– pituitary gland 5-075
– preauricular sinus 5-181
– prostate 5-601
– saccus endolymphaticus 5-207
– Skene's gland 5-712
– thalamic 5-013
– vestibular apparatus 5-207

Detection
– antibody
– – ferritin labelled 2-755
– antigen
– – toxocardia 2-750
– – toxoplasma 2-750
– cardiac shunt 1-723
– fungus 2-700
– hemagglutinins 2-825
– hemolysis 2-829
– micro-organisms 2-509

Determination
– fetal maturity 1-359
– threshold
– – pain 1-204
– – taste 1-200
– urinary residual volume 1-331
Detorsion
– kidney (pedicle) 5-557
– omentum 5-546
– spermatic cord 5-634
– testis 5-634
– – with orchiopexy 5-624
– volvulus 5-468
Detoxification centre
– alcoholic 9-161
Detrusor reflex
– testing 1-330
Dextran
– intravenous 8-812
Dextrin
– transglucosylase 2-463
Dextrostix
– blood sugar 2-130
Diagnex blue
– gastric secretion test 2-303

Diagnosis, diagnostic (see also Specific
  method)
– assessment 1-991
– hypnosis 1-923
– psychiatric
– – interview 1-922
– surgical technique 1-890
– syphilis
– – serologic 2-609
Dialysis
– intestinal 8-861
– peritoneal 8-860
– recirculation 8-852
– renal 8-853
Diaphragm
– resection 5-347
Diaphysectomy 5-784
Diastase
– serum 2-470
Diathermy
– medical 8-604
– surgical (see also Electrocoagulation)
  5-929
– – bladder, cystoscopic 5-921
– – choroid 5-155
– – – for reattachment of retina 5-154
– – conjunctiva (lesion) 5-112
– – esophagus 5-422
– – labyrinth 5-207
– – naevi 5-922
– – nasal 5-920
– – pharynx 5-292
– – rectum 5-482
– – retina
– – – for reattachment 5-154
– – – lesion 5-155
– – sclera 5-134
– – sinus, nasal 5-229
– – skin 5-922
– – tongue
– – – neoplasm 5-251
– – transcleral
– – – for reattachment of retina 5-154
– – turbinectomy 5-215
– – vestibule of ear 5-207
– – wart 5-922
Diet (see also Dietary prophylaxis)
– biliary stone dissolving 9-143
– diabetic 9-149
– fluid 9-141
– gluten free 9-144
– high protein 9-149
– hunger and thirst 9-140
– low calorie 9-149
– mild 9-142
– nothing to eat and drink 9-140
– phenylalanine free 9-145

Diet - *continued*
- special 9-149
- unsaturated fat 9-149
- weight reduction 9-149
- Sippy 9-142
Dietary prophylaxis 4-469
- low calory 4-461
- low carbohydrate 4-460
- low protein 4-463
- low salt 4-462
- salt free 4-462
Dietotherapy (see also Diet) 9-149
Differential white cell count 2-881
Digestion
- tissue
- - for examination of parasite 2-954
Digitalis
- blood assay 2-163
Dilatation, dilation
- achalasia 5-428
- anal sphincter 8-225
- artificial stoma
- - bowel 8-225
- bile duct 5-513
- bladder (neck) 5-579
- bronchus 5-339
- cardia (esophagus) 5-428
- cervix
- - and curettage
- - - diagnostic 5-690
- - - following abortion 5-690
- - - postpartum 5-690
- - - pregnancy 5-752
- - - termination of pregnancy 5-752
- - in labour 5-739
- - induction of abortion 5-752
- - induction of labour 5-731
- - nonobstetric 5-670
- - postpartum 5-670
- - to assist delivery 5-739
- - with cauterization 5-672
- colostomy 8-225
- duct
- - pancreatic 5-529
- - Wirsung 5-529
- endoscopic 8-220
- enterostomy 8-225
- esophagus 5-428
- frontonasal duct 8-221
- haemorrhoids 8-225
- heart valve 5-350
- introitus 8-228
- lacrimal duct 8-222
- larynx 5-319
- lymphatic channel 5-409
- meatal stricture 8-227
- nasolacrimal duct 8-222

Dilatation - *continued*
- pecten band (anal canal) 8-225
- pharynx 8-224
- punctum 8-222
- salivary duct 8-223
- sphincter
- - cardias 5-428
- - Oddi 5-518
- trachea 5-319
- ureter 5-569
- ureteral meatus 5-598
- ureterovesical orifice 5-569
- urethra 5-585
- urethrovesical junction 5-585
- vagina 8-228
Dilator
- Gerbode 5-350
- pyloric, Tubbs 5-430
Diminution
- ciliary body 5-133
Diphtheria
- immunization 4-333
- - with pertussis and tetanus 4-336
Disaccharidase activity
- intestinal 2-315
Disarticulation (see also Amputation)
- ankle 5-847
- elbow 5-843
- finger 5-840
- hip 5-849
- inter-iliac 5-849
- knee 5-848
- midtarsal 5-846
- shoulder 5-844
- tarso-metatarsal 5-846
- thumb 5-841
- toe 5-845
- wrist 5-842
Discission
- cataract 5-143
- lens 5-143
Displacement
- intertrochanteric 5-781
Dissection (see also Excision) 5-909
- aneurysm 5-385
- bronchial lesion 5-320
- larynx
- - radical 5-304
- lymph nodes (simple) 5-401
- - cervical 5-402
- - - radical 5-403
- - radical 5-404
- - regional 5-402
- mediastinum 5-342
- - with pneumonectomy 5-325
- neck
- - radical 5-304

Dissection - *continued*
- neck - *continued*
- - with thyroidectomy 5-063
- orbital fibrous bands 5-169
- pterygium 5-122
- retroperitoneal tissue 5-590
- specimen 2-950
- tonsils 5-281
- - with adenoidectomy 5-282
- vascular bundle
- - adherent 5-399
- vulva
- - block 5-714
Distension
- urinary bladder 8-226
Diuresis
- forced 8-822
Diversion
- urinary 5-566
- - cutaneous, external 5-565
- - into intestine 5-566
Diverticulectomy
- bladder
- - cystoscopic 5-573
- - suprapubic 5-574
- - transurethral 5-573
- esophageal 5-422
- intestine
- - large 5-452
- - small 5-451
- Meckel's 5-451
- pharyngeal 5-292
- urethra 5-582
Division
- adhesions - see Freeing adhesions
- angle of mandible 5-775
- aponeurosis 5-831
- artery 5-387
- bands
- - peritoneal 5-544
- - vitreous 5-157
- bladder neck 5-579
- - transurethral 5-573
- bone 5-781
- - jaw 5-775
- brain tissue 5-012
- bundle of His 5-379
- canaliculus, lacrimal 5-084
- capsule
- - joint 5-801
- - - temporomandibular 5-774
- cardiac sphincter 5-426
- cartilage (joint) 5-801
- chordae tendinae 5-351
- condyle 5-781
- - femur 5-781
- - jaw 5-775

Division - *continued*
- congenital web
- - larynx 5-319
- - pharynx 5-294
- cord tract 5-032
- ductus arteriosus 5-387
- esophageal stricture 5-422
- fallopian tube
- - bilateral 5-664
- - remaining tube 5-664
- - unilateral 5-669
- fascia 5-831
- - hand 5-821
- flexor sheath 5-831
- - hand 5-820
- ganglion, sympathetic 5-050
- intestinal adhesions 5-544
- iris
- - leucoma 5-135
- isthmus
- - horseshoe kidney 5-557
- - thyroid 5-069
- jaw 5-775
- lacrimal ductules 5-080
- laryngeal web 5-319
- ligament (joint) 5-801
- - canthal 5-092
- - carpal 5-043
- - palpebrae 5-092
- - tarsal 5-043
- - uterosacral 5-694
- - uterus 5-694
- mandible 5-775
- muscle 5-831
- - eye 5-100
- - hand 5-821
- nasolacrimal duct stricture 5-089
- nerve
- - cranial 5-040
- - - within skull 5-040
- - glossopharyngeal 5-299
- - intraspinal 5-031
- - lacrimal branch 5-050
- - opticociliary 5-133
- - peripheral 5-040
- - phrenic 5-332
- - spinal root 5-031
- - superior laryngeal 5-319
- - sympathetic 5-050
- - to adrenals 5-073
- - tracts in spinal cord 5-032
- - vagus 5-440
- otosclerotic process, middle ear 5-190
- oviducts - see Division, fallopian tube
- papillary muscle 5-351
- pharyngeal adhesion 5-294
- pylorus 5-433

Division - *continued*
- rectum 5-480
- Skene's gland 5-712
- sphincter
- - anal 5-494
- - pancreatic (oddi) 5-518
- spinal (tract) 5-032
- symblepharon 5-114
- symphysis
- - pubis 5-801
- - - obstetric 5-739
- synchondrosis 5-801
- synechia (iris) 5-136
- tendon 5-831
- - hand 5-821
- - sheath, hand 5-821
- - Achilles 5-831
- tensor fasciae latae 5-831
- thyroid 5-069
- tympanum 5-200
- ureter 5-569
- urethral stricture 5-584
- uterosacral ligament 5-694
- vas deferens (bilateral) 5-981
- - unilateral 5-636
- vein 5-387
- - varicose 5-384
- vessel 5-387
- - cornea 5-111
- vitreous bands 5-157
DL diffusing capacity 1-715
DMF
- charting 1-301
Domiciliary care 9-176
Donation
- blood 8-821
Doppler flow manometry 1-254
DPT
- immunization 4-336
Dragstedt's operation 5-440
- ileostomy 5-462
Drainage
- abdomen 5-541
- abdominal wall 5-540
- abscess (see also Drainage, by site) 5-882
- - abdominal wall 5-540
- - appendix 5-471
- - auditory canal
- - - external 5-180
- - auricle 5-180
- - Bartholin's gland 5-711
- - breast 5-871
- - buccal space 5-270
- - cornea 5-121
- - ear 5-180
- - extradural 5-011
- - extraperitoneal 5-540

Drainage - *continued*
- abscess - *continued*
- - facial region 5-270
- - groin 5-540
- - gum 5-240
- - hepatic 5-500
- - iliac fossa 5-541
- - intestine (diverticulum) 5-450
- - intracranial 5-011
- - intrahepatic 5-500
- - intranasal 5-211
- - ischiorectal 5-490
- - kidney 5-550
- - lacrimal sac 5-084
- - lip 5-270
- - lymph node 5-400
- - nose 5-211
- - omental 5-541
- - orbit 5-160
- - ovary 5-650
- - parotid gland 5-260
- - pelvic
- - - abdominal 5-541
- - - vaginal 5-701
- - pelvirectal 5-487
- - perianal 5-490
- - perigastric 5-541
- - perineum
- - - female 5-710
- - - male 5-882
- - perirectal 5-487
- - perirenal tissue 5-590
- - perisplenic 5-541
- - peritoneum, pelvic 5-701
- - peritonsillar 5-280
- - prostate 5-600
- - pulmonary 5-331
- - rectum, submucous 5-480
- - retroperitoneal 5-541
- - salivary gland 5-260
- - sclera 5-139
- - scrotum 5-610
- - Skene's gland 5-712
- - skin 5-882
- - subcutaneous 5-882
- - subdiaphragmatic 5-541
- - subhepatic 5-541
- - subphrenic 5-541
- - thyroid 5-060
- - urethra 5-580
- - vulva 5-710
- alveolus 5-240
- antrum (maxillary) 5-220
- appendix 5-471
- auditory meatus 5-180
- bile (hepatic) ducts 5-514
- bladder (urinary) 8-131

Drainage - *continued*
- bladder - *continued*
- - by anastomosis 5-578
- - incision 5-571
- bone (marrow) 5-780
- - jaw 5-770
- breast 5-871
- buccal space 5-270
- bulbourethral gland 5-589
- bursa 5-830
- - pharyngeal 5-290
- carbuncle 5-882
- cellulitis 5-882
- - teeth, supporting structures of 5-240
- cerebral cyst
- - to ventricle 5-022
- cerebrospinal fluid 5-023
- chalazion 5-090
- cisternal 5-010
- - ventricle to cisterna magnum 5-022
- communicating hydrocephalus 5-036
- conjunctiva 5-111
- continuous suction 8-179
- craniobuccal pouch by incision 5-076
- craniopharyngioma 5-076
- cyst 5-882
- - dentigerous 5-240
- - hydatid
- - - liver 5-500
- - ovary 5-650
- - pancreas 5-523
- - thyroglossal 5-060
- - thyroid 5-060
- dental condition 5-240
- diverticulum
- - bowel 5-450
- duodenal 8-126
- ear
- - air cells 5-202
- - external 5-180
- - inner 5-207
- - middle 5-200
- empyema 5-340
- endolymphatic sac 5-207
- epididymis 5-639
- epidural space
- - cerebral 5-011
- esophagus (endoscopic) 5-420
- ethmoid 5-224
- extraperitoneal 5-540
- eyelid 5-090
- facial region 5-270
- fallopian tube 5-660
- fascia 5-830
- fistula
- - anus 5-491
- floor of mouth 5-270

Drainage - *continued*
- fluid
- - middle ear 5-200
- - subretinal 5-154
- gallbladder 5-510
- gravity
- - stomach 8-122
- hematoma
- - extradural 5-011
- - nasal sinus 5-220
- hordeolum 5-090
- hydrocephalus 8-151
- - fetal 5-734
- hygroma
- - intracranial 5-011
- - intraspinal 5-030
- infratemporal fossa 5-270
- intestinal 8-126
- intracerebral 5-022
- joint 5-800
- - jaw 5-770
- kidney 5-550
- - by catheter (ureteral) 5-598
- lacrimal
- - gland 5-080
- - sac 5-084
- laryngeal 5-313
- lip 5-270
- liver 5-500
- Ludwig's angina 5-270
- lung 5-331
- - by rib resection 5-340
- - puncture 8-156
- lymph node (lymphadenitis) 5-400
- marrow
- - bone 5-780
- masticator
- - space 5-270
- mastoid antrum 5-202
- maxillary antrum
- - operative 5-222
- - puncture 5-220
- mediastinum 5-341
- meibomian gland (cyst) 5-090
- meningeal 5-011
- Moll's gland 5-090
- mucocele
- - frontal sinus
- - - incision 5-223
- - - puncture 5-220
- muscle 5-830
- nasal (septum) 5-211
- - sinus 5-220
- omentum 5-541
- orbit 5-160
- osteomyelitis 5-780
- ovary 5-650

Drainage - *continued*
- palate 5-271
- palmar whitlow 5-820
- pancreas 5-520
- - cyst 5-520
- - - with anastomosis 5-527
- - - with marsupialization 5-522
- parapharyngeal abscess 5-280
- pelvirectal 5-487
- penis 5-649
- perianal 5-490
- periapical 5-240
- pericardium 5-370
- perineal tissues 5-591
- perineum
- - female 5-710
- - male 5-882
- periprostatic tissue 5-607
- perirectal 5-487
- perirenal tissue 5-590
- perisplenic 5-541
- peritoneal (upper) 5-541
- peritonsillar 5-280
- periurethral 5-589
- perivesical 5-591
- petrous pyramid 5-204
- pharynx 5-290
- - lateral 5-290
- - oral 5-280
- pilonidal
- - sinus 5-881
- - - rectococcygeal 5-881
- pituitary gland 5-076
- pleura 5-340
- pleural 8-740
- pouch of Douglas 5-701
- prostate 5-600
- pterygopalatine 5-270
- pulp canal, teeth 5-240
- pyomyositis 5-830
- quinsy 5-280
- radicular
- - dental 5-240
- Rathke's pouch by incision 5-076
- renal pelvis 5-551
- retina 5-154
- - with retinal reattachment 5-154
- retroperitoneal 5-540
- retropharyngeal 5-280
- salivary gland 5-260
- sclera (subretineal fluid) 5-154
- scrotum (abscess) 5-610
- semicircular canal 5-207
- seminal vesicles 5-606
- sinus
- - cranial 5-011
- - ethmoidal 5-224

Drainage - *continued*
- sinus - *continued*
- - frontal 5-223
- - nasal 5-224
- - sphenoidal 5-224
- skull (bone) 5-011
- spermatic cord 5-635
- spinal (cord) 5-036
- spleen 5-412
- sty 5-090
- subarachnoid space
- - cranial 5-011
- - spinal 5-036
- subdural (brain) 5-011
- sublingual 5-270
- submandibular 5-270
- submental 5-270
- subretineal fluid 5-154
- suction
- - stomach 8-122
- suprapubic (bladder) 5-571
- suprasternal 5-341
- tendon 5-830
- testis 5-620
- thorax 5-340
- thyroid 5-060
- tongue 5-259
- tonsillar abscess 5-280
- tunica vaginalis 5-610
- urethra 5-580
- urinary NEC 5-591
- vagina 5-701
- ventriculocisternal 5-022
- vitreous 5-157
- vulva 5-710
- whitlow 5-882
- - palmar 5-820
- Zeis' gland 5-090
Drawing test 1-939
Dressing
- burn 8-194
- ulcer 8-193
- wound 8-192
- - debridement 5-883
Drilling
- bone 5-780
- jaw 5-770
Drug
- administration 9-120
- - automated 9-123
- - - control 9-124
- biological half-life 2-326
- cytotoxic - see Cytotoxic drug
- injection
- - intramuscular 9-121
- - micro-injector 9-123
- metabolizing power 2-326

Drug - *continued*
– prescription 9-110
– – repetition 9-130
– – replacement 9-111
– prophylaxis
– – anthelminthic 4-369
– – antiamebic 4-361
– – anticoagulant cover 4-441
– – antifilarial 4-363
– – antimalarial 4-360
– – antischistosomal 4-362
– – bacterial endocarditis 4-371
– – infection 4-379
– – meningococcal carrier 4-374
– – rheumatic fever 4-370
– – steroid 4-450
– – tuberculosis 4-373
– sedation
– – for diagnosis 1-924
Ductoplasty
– lacrimal 5-086
– lymphatic 5-405
– mammary 5-872
Dunn's operation 5-811
Duodenectomy 5-454
– with pancreatectomy
– – complete 5-525
– – partial 5-524
– – radical 5-526
Duodenocholecystostomy 5-512
Duodenocholedochostomy 5-512
Duodenocholedochotomy 5-514
Duodenoduodenostomy 5-457
– end to end 5-454

Duodenoduodenostomy 5-457 - *continued*
– proximal to distal segment 5-454
Duodenoesophagostomy
– intrathoracic 5-424
Duodenogastrostomy
– with partial gastrectomy 5-436
– without gastrectomy 5-442
Duodenoileostomy 5-457
Duodenojejunostomy 5-457
Duodenorrhaphy 5-467
Duodenoscopy 1-636
– fiberscopic 1-636
Duodenostomy 5-463
– closure 5-465
Duodenotomy 5-450
Duodenum, duodenal
– acidity 2-310
– aspirate
– – analysis 2-310
– – examination
– – – for giardia 2-719
– enzyme excretion 2-336
– pH 2-310
Duraplasty 5-021
Durham's operation 5-831
Dye
– fluorescence, angiography 1-801
– injection, subcutaneous (diagnostic) 1-800
– introduction diagnostic NEC 1-809
– test for toxoplasmosis 2-629
Dynamic compliance 1-712
Dynamometer test 1-750
– ECG 1-260

E

Echo track transducer 1-721

Education
– bed-bound children 9-511

Educational
– rehabilitation 9-519
– therapy 9-510

Effect
– cytophatic
– – virus 2-540

Effler's operation 5-363

Effleurage 9-471

Egot 2-460
– EGR 2-459

Eicher's operation 5-816

Ejection fraction (heart) 1-720
– EKG 1-260

Elastic hosiery 9-332

Electrical
– convulsion 8-630
– pace making - see also Pacemaker
– response
– – bladder 1-335
– – heart 1-269
– – – display 1-267
– – recording NEC 1-960
– stimulation 8-669
– – bladder 8-662
– – brain 8-630
– – carotid sinus 8-644
– – heart 8-649
– – – external 8-640
– – – intravenous (electrode) 8-641
– – – operative 8-643
– – – transvenous (electrode) 8-641
– – muscle 8-663
– – – soleus 8-663
– – specified NEC 8-668
– – spinal 8-661

Electro-anesthesia 8-630

Electrocardiography 1-260
– dynamic 1-262
– GRS stat 1-264
– operative 1-264
– report 1-266
– transvenous electrode 1-265
– vector 1-263
– with exercise test 1-262

Electrocautery (see also Cauterization) 5-914

Electrocoagulation (see also Coagulation and Diathermy, surgical)
– aneurysm
– – peripheral vessel 5-385
– brain 5-012
– – vessel 5-385
– cystoscopic 5-921
– ear
– – external (fistula) 5-181
– – inner 5-207
– fallopian tubes
– – endoscopic 5-663
– – laparotomy 5-664
– naevi 5-922
– nose 5-920
– – epistaxis 5-210
– – lesion 5-920
– ovary 5-651
– prostate 5-601
– semicircular canals 5-207
– skin 5-922
– spinal 5-032
– tracheal lesion
– – endoscopic 5-314
– turbinectomy 5-215
– urethrovesical junction, transurethral 5-573
– wart 5-922

Electrocochlearography 1-239

Electroconization
– cervix 5-672

Electroconvulsive therapy 8-630

Electrode
– anal 1-335
– esophageal 1-261
– intracardiac 8-641
– – intravenous, transvenous
– – – insertion 8-880
– – – removal 8-881
– – – replacement 8-881
– – – stimulation 8-641
– – – with subcutaneous generator 8-652
– intramural (heart), implantation 5-377

Electroencephalography 1-207

Electrogastrogram 1-321

Electrokeratotomy 5-121

Electrolysis 5-933
– eyelash 5-930
– retina 5-154

Electrolyte

Electrolyte - *continued*
- balance 2-351
- - regulation 8-876
- blood 2-159
Electromyogram 1-363
Electromyography 1-363
Electron microscopy
- bacteria 2-517
- tissue 2-906
- virus 2-541
Electronarcosis 8-630
- anesthesia 8-630
Electronic gaiter 8-544
Electrophoresis 2-496
- hemoglobin 2-841
Electroplexy 8-630
Electroresection
- see excision 5-909
Electroshock 8-630
Electrosurgery
- bladder neck transurethral 5-573
- prostate (see also Prostatectomy) 5-601
Elevation
- bone fragments 5-791
- - cranial 5-020
- - sinus
- - - frontal 5-767
- - - maxillary 5-763
- - spinal 5-034
- choroid 5-154
- cranial fracture 5-020
- depressed fragments 5-791
- - skull 5-020
- jaw fragments 5-763
- nasal (sinus) fracture 5-763
- pedicle graft 5-894
- skull fragments 5-020
- spinal facture 5-034
- sternum fragments 5-791
- tooth 5-230
Elimination
- septal defect 5-357
Elongation
- aponeurosis 5-837
- bone 5-789
- fascia 5-837
- muscle 5-837
- - eye 5-100
- tendon 5-837
- - Achilles 5-837
- - hand 5-828
- - thumb 5-828
Emasculation 5-623
Embolectomy (see also Removal, embolus)
  5-380
Embryectomy 5-744
Embryotomy 5-734

Emergency admission
- hospital inpatient 9-160
- hospital patient 9-160
Emergency dressing 9-100
Emission spectrography 2-491
Encephalopuncture 5-010
Encirclement, cervix 5-674
Endarterectomy 5-381
- coronary (with patch graft) 5-360
- with vein patch 5-381
Endoaneurysmorrhaphy 5-395
- fistula arteriovenous 5-395
Endobiopsy - see also Biopsy, non surgical
- uterus 1-471
Endocrine assessment
- endometrial 1-352
- vaginal cytology 1-351
Endocrine prophylaxis 4-459
- for psychiatric control 4-452
Endocrinology
- blood 2-439
- urine 2-449
Endometrectomy (internal) (uterine) 5-681
Endoscopy 1-689
- anus 1-644
- biopsy - see Biopsy, non surgical
- bladder 1-652
- bronchus 1-620
- cerebral ventricle 1-698
- colon 1-641
- destruction of lesion 5-990
- ear 1-240
- esophagus 1-630
- - via stoma 1-631
- intestine
- - via stoma 1-540
- larynx
- - direct 1-612
- manipulation 8-533
- nose 1-243
- operative 1-699
- peritoneum
- - culdoscopy 1-696
- pharynx 1-615
- photography 1-681
- rectum 1-643
- removal of foreign body 8-100
- specified NEC 1-679
- spinal canal 1-698
- stomach 1-633
- - via stoma 1-635
- trachea 1-621
- ureter 1-650
- urethra 1-655
- uterus 1-660
- vagina 1-663
- via enterostomy stoma 1-540

Endoscopy 1-689 - *continued*
- via orifice 1-680
- without incision 1-689
Enema 8-127
- simple 8-127
Enhancement
- immunity 4-402
Enlargement, surgical
- arterial lumen 5-381
- canthus 5-092
- intervertebral foramen 5-030
- introitus 5-710
- orbit (eye) (mechanical) (mould) 5-167
- outlet, obstetric 5-739
- palpebral fissure 5-092
- punctum lacrimale 8-222
- salivary duct
- - orifice 5-260
- septal defect 5-355
- socket (orbit) 5-167
Enterectomy 5-454
Enteroanastomosis 5-458
Enterocelectomy
- female 5-707
- male 5-539
Enterocentesis 5-450
Enterocholecystostomy 5-512
Enterocholedochostomy 5-512
Enterocolectomy NEC 5-455
Enterocolostomy 5-458
Enteroenterostomy 5-458
- proximal to distal 5-454
Enterogastrostomy
- without gastrectomy 5-442
Enterolithotomy 5-450
Enterolysis 5-544
Enteropancreatostomy 5-527
Enterorrhaphy 5-467
Enteroscopy
- by enterotomy 1-693
- by paracentesis 1-693
- operative 1-695
Enterostomy 5-463
- modification 5-464
Enterotomy 5-450
Enucleation
- cyst
- - broad ligament 5-692
- - dental 5-243
- - ovary 5-651
- - salivary gland 5-261
- eyeball 5-163
- lens 5-146
- lesion
- - dental 5-243
- - jaw 5-771
- prostate - see Prostatectomy

Enucleation - *continued*
- tumor 5-884
Enzyme(s) 2-489
- dehydrogenase 2-459
- hepatic 2-469
- histology 2-904
- hydrolase 2-479
- inhibition
- - influenza 2-623
- other 2-489
- oxidases 2-459
- reductases 2-459
- salivary test for blood groups 2-826
- transferase 2-469
Enzymology - see Enzyme
Eosinophil, eosinophilic
- reaction 2-652
- staining (in nasal secretion and sputum)
  2-882
Epicardial recording
- operative 1-264
Epididymectomy 5-633
- with orchidectomy 5-622
Epididymoplasty 5-634
Epididymostomy 5-639
Epididymotomy 5-639
Epididymovasostomy 5-637
Epiglottidectomy (endoral) (external)
  5-302
Epilation 8-180
- eyelash 8-181
- skin 8-180
Epiphysiodesis 5-787
Epiploectomy 5-543
Epiplopexy 5-546
Epiplorrhaphy 5-546
Episioperineoplasty 5-716
Episioperineorrhaphy 5-716
- during postpartum 5-758
Episioplasty 5-716
Episiorrhaphy
- during postpartum 5-758
- obstetric 5-758
Episiotomy 5-738
- nonobstetric 5-710
- routine 9-263
- - with subsequent repair 9-263
- with
- - high forceps 5-723
- - low forceps 5-721
- - mid forceps 5-722
- - outlet forceps 5-721
- - repair 5-738
Epistaxis control
- cautery 5-210
- cryosurgery 5-210
- suture 5-210

Equalization, leg 5-789
– bone fusion 5-789
– epiphyseal arrest 5-787
– ostectomy, partial 5-784
– osteotomy 5-781
Equilibration
– occlusal 5-247
Equiloudness balance 1-233
Erisiphake extraction of cataract 5-144
Erythrocyte(s) (see also Blood, red cell)
– fragility determination 2-812
– glutamate oxaloacetate transaminase
  2-460
– glutathione reductase test 2-459
– sedimentation rate 2-810
– staining for abnormal morphology 2-805
Erythrokinetics 2-859
Esophagectomy 5-423
– with reanastomosis (end to end) 5-423
Esophagocolostomy
– antesternal 5-425
– antethoracic 5-425
– intrathoracic 5-424
Esophagoduodenostomy
– intrathoracic 5-424
– with total gastrectomy 5-439
Esophagoenterostomy
– antethoracic 5-425
– intrathoracic 5-424
Esophagoesophagostomy 5-423
Esophagogastrectomy 5-423
Esophagogastromyotomy 5-426
Esophagogastroplasty
– intrathoracic 5-424
Esophagogastroscopy 1-632
Esophagogastrostomy 5-435
– antesternal 5-425
– intrathoracic 5-424
– with partial gastrectomy 5-435
Esophagoileostomy
– antethoracic 5-425
– intrathoracic 5-424
Esophagojejunoplasty
– intrathoracic 5-424
Esophagojejunostomy 5-439
– antethoracic 5-425
– intrathoracic 5-424
– with total gastrectomy 5-439
Esophagomyotomy 5-426
Esophagoplasty 5-427
Esophagorrhaphy 5-427
Esophagoscopy 1-630
– biopsy 1-440
– by gastrotomy 1-692
– dilation 5-428
– foreign body
– – extraction 8-111

Esophagoscopy 1-630 - continued
– foreign body - continued
– – removal 8-111
– intubation 5-428
– via stoma 1-631
Esophagostomy (cervical) 5-421
Esophagotomy 5-420
Esophagus
– artificial 5-427
Estrogen
– plasma 2-432
– receptor assay, breast tumor 2-439
Ethmoidectomy 5-225
Ethmoidotomy 5-224
Eugenic method NEC 4-669
Evacuation
– abscess (see also Drainage, abscess)
– – brain 5-011
– – extradural 5-011
– blood, orbital 5-160
– empyema
– – subdural 5-011
– granuloma 5-083
– – canaliculus, lacrimal 5-083
– hematoma (see also Incision, hematoma)
  5-882
– – extradural 5-011
– – orbital 5-160
– – pericardial 5-371
– – skin 8-169
– – subdural 5-011
– – temporal lobe 5-011
– – vulva
– – – postpartum 5-759
– hemorrhoids
– – thrombosed 5-499
– lacrimal duct 5-083
– lens 5-146
– – by curettage 5-142
– – by suction 5-144
– – with emulsification 5-146
– orbit 5-164
– pelvis (female) 5-687
– retained placenta 5-756
– – manual removal 5-756
– – with curettage 5-690
– streptothrix from lacrimal duct 5-083
– uterus
– – post-partum 5-756
Evaluation
– audiological 1-233
– bladder sensation 1-330
– for rehabilitation - see Rehabilitation,
  evaluation
– psychiatric
– – initial 1-921
Evans blue method 1-737

Eversion
— tunica vaginalis 5-613
Evisceration
— eyeball (with implant) 5-162
— orbit (with graft) 5-164
— pelvis
— — female 5-687
— — male 5-576
Evulsion (see also Excision) 5-909
— polyp
— — cervix 5-672
— — nasal 5-212
— — tympanic 5-204
— skin and subcutaneous tissue 5-884
Examination (see also Exploration)
— chylous fluid 2-280
— clinical
— — gynecological
— — — internal 1-350
— — in-depth
— — — heart 1-250
— — — male genital organs 1-340
— — — musculoskeletal system 1-360
— dental 1-300
— eikonometric 1-213
— eye fundus 1-220
— feces (see also Feces)
— — biochemistry 2-269
— forensic - see Forensic examinations
— gynecological 1-350
— — clinical
— — — internal 1-350
— — instrumental NEC 1-358
— health 4-199
— — administrative purpose NEC 4-169
— — adult 4-139
— — — recall 4-131
— — — self-initiative 4-130
— — after foreign travel 4-190
— — army induction 4-160
— — before employment 4-120
— — commissioned NEC 4-179
— — insurance (proposal) 4-170
— — — compensation 4-171
— — license
— — — beauticians 4-163
— — — domestic service 4-163
— — — driving (motor vehicle) 4-161
— — — food handler 4-162
— — — food vendor 4-162
— — — personal service NEC 4-163
— — occupational 4-129
— — — periodical 4-122
— — old person (geriatric) 4-110
— — police recruitment 4-160
— — prenuptial
— — — female 4-101

Examination - continued
— health 4-199 - continued
— — prenuptial - continued
— — — male 4-100
— — psychiatric
— — — determination responsibility 4-140
— — — legal purpose 4-149
— — retirement 4-125
— — specified NEC 4-190
— hematological
— — method NEC 2-889
— histological (see also Histology) 2-909
— instrumental 1-379
— — circulation NEC 1-259
— — ear NEC 1-242
— — gastrointestinal NEC 1-329
— — gynecological NEC 1-358
— — heart NEC 1-257
— — male genitals NEC 1-349
— — musculoskeletal NEC 1-369
— — neurological NEC 1-209
— — nose NEC 1-245
— — obstetric NEC 1-359
— — ophthalmological NEC 1-229
— — otorhinolaryngological NEC 1-249
— — throat NEC 1-246
— — upper digestive tract NEC 1-319
— — urinary tract NEC 1-339
— intestinal parasites 2-715
— legal purpose 4-159
— — psychiatric 4-149
— — rape victim 4-150
— — victim physical aggression 4-156
— lymph 2-280
— macroscopic
— — feces 2-714
— — organ 2-950
— — tissue 2-950
— microscopic
— — chemical identification 2-493
— — dark ground (for leptospira) (for
      treponema) 2-501
— — electronic
— — — tissue 2-906
— — — — computer image analysis 2-906
— — — feces 2-710
— — — ova concentration 2-711
— — — stained 2-713
— — — — for ova 2-712
— — forensic 2-946
— — fungus 2-700
— — polarized light 2-502
— — smear
— — — blood 2-809
— — — — for abnormal cytomorphology
           2-803
— — — bone marrow 2-800

Examination - *continued*
- microscopic - *continued*
- - smear - *continued*
- - - lymph node 2-800
- - - spleen pulp 2-800
- - tissue (see also Histology) 2-909
- - unstained slide (bacterial count)
      (hanging drop) 2-500
- naked eye
- - organ 2-950
- oral cavity
- - other NEC 1-309
- pathological 2-959
- peritoneal fluid 2-283
- pleural fluid 2-282
- post-coital plug (for infertility) 1-353
- psychiatric
- - interview 1-922
- - modified analysis 1-941
- - narcoanalysis 1-924
- - psychological tests 1-930
- screening NEC 4-279
- sensibility, topographical 1-200
- slit lamp 1-221
- stomatological
- - other NEC 1-309
- sweat 2-284
- tissue 2-939
- under anesthesia 1-901
- vagina, vaginal 1-350
- - endoscopic 1-663
- - speculum 1-350
- visual acuity 1-211
Exchange transfusion 8-803
- in utero 5-754
Excision
- abdominal wall 5-542
- abdominoperineal
- - rectum 5-484
- abscess
- - brain 5-014
- adenoid tag 5-285
- adenopathy 5-401
- adrenal (see also Adrenalectomy) 5-071
- akinetic area, heart 5-373
- ampulla of Vater 5-515
- - with reimplantation 5-515
- aneurysm 5-385
- - ventricle, heart 5-373
- - with reanastomosis 5-382
- angioma 5-385
- anus 5-495
- - crypt 5-492
- - fissure 5-492
- - fistula 5-491
- - tag 5-492
- apical

Excision - *continued*
- apical - *continued*
- - tooth 5-237
- aponeurosis 5-833
- - hand 5-823
- appendix (see also Appendicectomy)
      5-470
- artery 5-385
- arytenoid 5-302
- auricle
- - ear (lesion of) 5-181
- - heart 5-373
- bands, pharyngeal 5-294
- Bartholin's gland 5-711
- bile duct (cyst) 5-515
- bladder
- - dome 5-575
- - lesion NEC 5-574
- - partial 5-575
- - total 5-576
- - transurethral 5-573
- blood vessel 5-385
- bone
- - complete 5-785
- - facial 5-771
- - for homograft 5-784
- - jaw (lower) 5-773
- - - upper 5-772
- - lesion 5-783
- - partial 5-784
- - with fixation, prosthetic 5-784
- - with graft 5-784
- brain (lesion) (tissue) 5-014
- breast 5-860
- - aberrant tissue, supernumerary 5-869
- - lesion 5-860
- - with regional lymphadenectomy 5-862
- broad ligament 5-692
- - with ovary 5-653
- bronchiectasis 5-323
- bronchus
- - lesion 5-320
- - local 5-320
- - wide 5-321
- bubo 5-401
- bucket handle tear
- - meniscus 5-804
- bulbourethral gland 5-589
- bulla of lung 5-322
- bunion 5-782
- bunionette 5-782
- burn 5-884
- - skin graft nos 5-883
- bursa 5-834
- capsule
- - joint 5-809
- - lens 5-149

Excision - *continued*
− carbuncle 5-883
− carotid body (gland) (partial) (total) 5-398
− cartilage (joint) 5-809
− − intervertebral 5-803
− − jaw 5-774
− − knee
− − − semilunar 5-804
− − larynx 5-302
− − lumbosacral 5-803
− − nasal 5-214
− − thyroid 5-302
− caruncle, urethral 5-582
− cerebellar-pontine tumor 5-014
− cerebral tumor 5-014
− cervical rib 5-785
− cervical sinus 5-291
− cervix 5-673
− − conization 5-671
− − lesion of 5-672
− − stump 5-673
− chalazion 5-091
− chest wall
− − lesion 5-343
− − mastectomy 5-864
− − pneumonectomy 5-325
− cholesteatoma 5-204
− choroid 5-155
− choroid plexus 5-021
− cicatrix 5-884
− cilia base 5-091
− ciliary body, prolapsed 5-134
− clavicle 5-784
− − complete 5-785
− coarctation of aorta 5-382
− − with graft 5-383
− coccyx 5-784
− − complete 5-785
− cold abscess 5-883
− colon
− − complete 5-456
− − for interposition 5-453
− − lesion 5-452
− − partial 5-455
− condyle 5-809
− − jaw 5-774
− condylomata 5-712
− conjunctiva 5-112
− − for pterygium 5-122
− contracture
− − burn 5-884
− corn 8-185
− cornea 5-123
− cornual 5-665
− cortex (epileptogenous) 5-014
− cruciate ligament

Excision - *continued*
− cruciate ligament - *continued*
− − knee 5-809
− cusp, heart valve 5-351
− cyst 5-909
− − apical, tooth 5-243
− − bile duct 5-515
− − Baker 5-832
− − Bartholin's 5-711
− − brain 5-014
− − branchial 5-291
− − breast 5-860
− − conjunctiva 5-112
− − dental 5-243
− − dermoid 5-909
− − − hand 5-822
− − ear 5-181
− − eyelid 5-091
− − hydatid
− − − liver 5-501
− − involving tooth 5-243
− − kidney 5-550
− − knee
− − − meniscus 5-804
− − labia 5-712
− − ligament
− − − broad 5-692
− − − uterus 5-692
− − liver 5-501
− − lung 5-322
− − lymphatic 5-401
− − Moll's gland 5-091
− − Morgagni
− − − female 5-665
− − − male 5-621
− − nabothian 5-672
− − odontogenic 5-243
− − orbit 5-164
− − ovary 5-651
− − pancreas 5-522
− − parovarian 5-692
− − pericardial 5-372
− − periodontal 5-242
− − pilonidal 5-887
− − popliteal (synovial) 5-809
− − rectococcygeal 5-887
− − salivary 5-261
− − scrotum 5-612
− − sebaceous 5-884
− − − breast 5-860
− − − eyelid 5-091
− − − scalp 5-884
− − skin 5-884
− − spinal cord 5-033
− − subcutaneous 5-884
− − superficial 5-884
− − synovial 5-832

Excision - *continued*
- cyst 5-909 - *continued*
- - thyroglossal 5-066
- - thyroid 5-062
- - urachal 5-574
- - uterus 5-681
- - vagina 5-702
- - vallecular 5-292
- - Gartner's duct 5-702
- cystic
- - duct 5-515
- - hygroma 5-401
- - lymphangioma 5-401
- dentinoma 5-243
- diaphragm 5-347
- disc
- - articular, jaw 5-774
- - intervertebral, prolapsed 5-803
- diverticulum
- - bladder 5-574
- - - transurethral 5-573
- - duodenum 5-451
- - esophagus 5-422
- - Meckel's 5-451
- - pharyngoesophageal 5-292
- - pharynx 5-292
- - stomach 5-434
- - ventricle, heart 5-373
- duct
- - thyroglossal 5-066
- Dupuytren's contracture 5-823
- ear
- - external 5-181
- - middle 5-204
- - radical 5-182
- ependymoma 5-014
- epicanthic swelling 5-092
- epididymis 5-633
- - cyst 5-631
- - lesion 5-632
- epiglottis 5-302
- epileptogenic zone 5-014
- epithelioma 5-885
- epulis 5-242
- esophagus (local) (total) 5-423
- ethmoid cells 5-225
- extramedullary tumor 5-033
- eye (with implant) 5-163
- eyeball 5-163
- eyelid (redundant skin) 5-096
- fascia
- - for graft 5-833
- - hand 5-823
- - lesion
- - - hand 5-822
- fibroadenoma
- - breast 5-860

Excision - *continued*
- fimbria 5-665
- fissure
- - anus 5-492
- fistula 5-884
- - anal 5-491
- - appendix 5-479
- - arteriovenous 5-385
- - biliary 5-515
- - bladder, urinary 5-574
- - bone 5-783
- - - jaw 5-771
- - cervical (branchial cleft) 5-291
- - cornea 5-123
- - esophagus 5-422
- - fallopian tube 5-665
- - gallbladder 5-519
- - intestine 5-452
- - - small 5-451
- - joint 5-802
- - lacrimal
- - - gland 5-086
- - - sac 5-086
- - larynx 5-300
- - oviduct 5-665
- - pancreas 5-524
- - perirectal 5-487
- - pharynx 5-292
- - pleural 5-346
- - rectal, external 5-482
- - rectourethral 5-486
- - rectovesical 5-486
- - sacro-coccygeal 5-887
- - scrotum 5-612
- - skin 5-884
- - stomach 5-434
- - thorax 5-346
- - thyroglossal 5-066
- - ureter 5-568
- - urethral 5-582
- - vagina 5-706
- - vesicovaginal 5-706
- - vocal cord 5-300
- frenum
- - lingual (tongue) 5-250
- fundus
- - uterus 5-682
- gallbladder 5-511
- ganglion 5-822
- - joint 5-802
- - nerve
- - - cranial 5-040
- - stellate 5-051
- - sympathetic 5-051
- - tendon sheath (wrist) 5-822
- gingiva 5-242
- gland

Excision - *continued*
- gland - *continued*
- - mammary - see Mastectomy
- globe 5-163
- glomus jugulare 5-398
- goiter 5-062
- - intrathoracic, by mediastinotomy
  5-064
- granulation
- - conjunctival 5-112
- - cranial 5-020
- granuloma
- - gum 5-242
- groin
- - mass 5-404
- hemangioma
- - subcutaneous 5-884
- hematocele
- - spermatic cord 5-630
- - tunica vaginalis 5-611
- hemorrhoidal tags 5-493
- hemorrhoids 5-493
- hernia
- - cerebri 5-014
- hydatid cyst (liver) 5-501
- hydatid of Morgagni
- - female 5-665
- - male 5-621
- hydrocele 5-611
- - canal of Nuck (female) 5-692
- - female 5-692
- - round ligament 5-692
- - spermatic cord 5-630
- - tunica vaginalis 5-611
- hygroma
- - cystic 5-401
- hypophysis 5-075
- inguinal canal (lesion) 5-542
- intervertebral disc 5-803
- intestine
- - large 5-455
- - - lesion 5-452
- - small 5-454
- - - lesion 5-451
- iris 5-135
- - prolapsed 5-134
- joint 5-809
- - jaw 5-774
- - mandibular 5-774
- keloid (scar) 5-884
- kidney
- - with ureter 5-554
- lacrimal
- - gland 5-081
- - sac 5-085
- larynx
- - lesion 5-300

Excision - *continued*
- larynx - *continued*
- - radical 5-304
- - total 5-303
- lesion
- - abdominal wall 5-542
- - adenoid 5-289
- - adrenal 5-071
- - alveolus (dental) 5-243
- - ampulla of Vater 5-515
- - anus 5-492
- - aponeurosis 5-832
- - - hand 5-822
- - atrium (heart) 5-373
- - auditory canal, meatus, external 5-181
- - auricle, ear 5-181
- - bile ducts 5-515
- - bladder 5-574
- - bone 5-783
- - - antrum (nasal) 5-771
- - - facial 5-771
- - - jaw 5-771
- - - sinus
- - - - maxillary 5-771
- - brain tissue 5-014
- - breast 5-860
- - - with pectoral muscles 5-863
- - bronchus (endoscopic) 5-320
- - cerebral 5-014
- - cervix 5-672
- - - secondary excision 5-673
- - chest wall 5-343
- - - bone 5-343
- - choroid 5-155
- - colon 5-452
- - conjunctiva 5-112
- - cornea (ulcer) 5-123
- - - with lamellar graft 5-123
- - cranial 5-015
- - ear
- - - external 5-181
- - - middle 5-204
- - endometrium 5-681
- - epicardium 5-372
- - epididymis 5-632
- - esophagus 5-422
- - eye 5-164
- - eyebrow 5-884
- - eyelid 5-091
- - facial bone 5-771
- - fallopian tube 5-665
- - - with ovary 5-653
- - fascia 5-832
- - - hand 5-822
- - gallbladder 5-511
- - groin 5-542
- - - lymph nodes 5-402

Excision - *continued*
− lesion - *continued*
− − gum 5-242
− − heart 5-373
− − hepatic duct 5-515
− − inguinal canal 5-542
− − intestine
− − − large 5-452
− − − small 5-451
− − intracranial 5-014
− − intraspinal 5-033
− − intraventricular (brain) 5-014
− − jaw 5-771
− − joint 5-802
− − − jaw 5-774
− − − knee NEC 5-802
− − − − meniscus 5-804
− − kidney 5-552
− − − with partial nephrectomy 5-553
− − labia 5-712
− − lacrimal
− − − gland 5-081
− − − sac 5-085
− − larynx (endoscopic) 5-300
− − ligament
− − − broad 5-692
− − − round 5-692
− − lip 5-884
− − liver 5-501
− − lung 5-322
− − mediastinum 5-342
− − meninges
− − − cerebral 5-014
− − − spinal 5-033
− − meniscus 5-804
− − − knee 5-804
− − mesentery 5-543
− − mouth NEC 5-273
− − muscle 5-832
− − − hand 5-822
− − myocardium 5-373
− − nail 8-186
− − nasopharynx 5-292
− − nerve
− − − cranial 5-041
− − − peripheral 5-041
− − nose 5-212
− − omentum 5-543
− − orbit 5-164
− − ovary 5-651
− − oviduct 5-665
− − palate 5-272
− − pancreas 5-521
− − parathyroid gland 5-067
− − parotid gland (duct) 5-261
− − parovarian 5-692
− − penis 5-641

Excision - *continued*
− lesion - *continued*
− − pericardium 5-372
− − perineum
− − − female 5-712
− − pharynx 5-292
− − pleura 5-344
− − posterior fossa 5-014
− − rectum 5-482
− − retina 5-155
− − retroperitoneum 5-543
− − salivary gland 5-261
− − sclera 5-134
− − scrotum 5-612
− − sigmoid 5-452
− − sinus nasal 5-225
− − skin 5-884
− − − nose 5-212
− − skull 5-015
− − spermatic cord 5-632
− − spinal 5-033
− − spleen 5-413
− − stomach 5-434
− − sweat gland 5-884
− − sympathetic 5-051
− − tendon 5-832
− − − hand 5-822
− − − sheath 5-832
− − testis 5-621
− − thorax 5-343
− − thyroid gland 5-062
− − − by transternal route 5-064
− − tongue 5-250
− − − radical removal 5-253
− − tonsil 5-289
− − trachea (endoscopic) 5-314
− − ureter 5-563
− − urethra 5-582
− − uterus 5-681
− − − cervical 5-672
− − − myoma (fibroid) 5-681
− − vagina 5-702
− − vocal cords (endoscopic) 5-300
− − vulva 5-712
− − − radical excision 5-714
− ligament
− − cruciate 5-809
− lip, double 5-884
− lipoma 5-884
− − inguinal canal 5-542
− liver 5-501
− − lobectomy 5-502
− − total 5-503
− lung 5-329
− − apical 5-323
− − lobectomy 5-324
− − radical 5-325

Excision - *continued*
 - lung 5-329 - *continued*
 - - segmental 5-323
 - lymph node
 - - cervical 5-401
 - - - radical 5-403
 - - radical 5-404
 - - regional 5-402
 - - simple 5-401
 - lymphangioma 5-401
 - lymphatic
 - - channel 5-401
 - - radical 5-404
 - lymphedema 5-409
 - malleus 5-193
 - mammary
 - - duct 5-860
 - Meckel's diverticulum 5-451
 - median bar, transurethral approach
   5-573
 - mediastinum 5-342
 - meibomian gland 5-091
 - meningioma
 - - brain 5-014
 - - spinal 5-033
 - meniscus
 - - knee 5-804
 - - temporomandibular 5-774
 - mesentery 5-543
 - minimo-digital
 - - phalanx 5-784
 - mole
 - - skin 5-884
 - - uterus 5-681
 - mucosa
 - - ileostomy
 - - - redundant 5-451
 - - sinus nasal 5-225
 - muscle (see also Myectomy) 5-833
 - - eye 5-101
 - - hand 5-823
 - - levator palpebrae 5-094
 - myocardial scar 5-373
 - myositis ossificans 5-832
 - - hand 5-822
 - nabothian gland 5-672
 - naevus 5-884
 - - eyelid 5-091
 - nail 8-186
 - neck
 - - mass 5-403
 - neoplasm
 - - lung 5-322
 - nerve 5-040
 - - auditory 5-040
 - - cranial 5-040
 - - lesion 5-041

Excision - *continued*
 - nerve 5-040 - *continued*
 - - peripheral 5-040
 - - sympathetic 5-051
 - - vagus 5-440
 - neurinoma 5-041
 - neuroblastoma
 - - adrenal 5-071
 - - brain 5-014
 - - eye 5-164
 - neuroma 5-041
 - nipple 5-872
 - nodules
 - - larynx 5-300
 - - skin 5-884
 - nose
 - - wide, for tumor 5-213
 - ocular muscle segment 5-101
 - odontogenic tumor 5-243
 - omentum 5-543
 - orbital 5-164
 - - wall 5-164
 - osteochondritis dissecans 5-802
 - ovary 5-652
 - - both 5-654
 - - lesion 5-651
 - - remaining 5-654
 - - veins 5-385
 - oviduct 5-661
 - - both 5-662
 - - lesion 5-665
 - - remaining 5-662
 - - with ovary, lesion 5-653
 - pancreas (partial) 5-524
 - - total 5-525
 - pancreaticoduodenal
 - - complete 5-525
 - - partial 5-524
 - - radical 5-526
 - pannus 5-112
 - papilloma
 - - kidney 5-552
 - - rectum 5-482
 - - skin 5-884
 - parathyroid (ectopic) 5-067
 - parotid 5-262
 - - gland (duct) 5-262
 - - tumor 5-261
 - parovarian 5-692
 - patella, complete 5-785
 - pelvic
 - - mass 5-404
 - penis 5-641
 - - radical 5-642
 - perianal
 - - skin tag 5-490
 - - tissue 5-490

Excision - *continued*
- pericardial constriction 5-372
- periprostatic tissue 5-607
- perirectal tissue 5-487
- perirenal tissue 5-590
- peritoneum 5-543
- periurethral tissue 5-589
- phalanx
- – foot 5-784
- – hallux 5-782
- – hand 5-784
- – thumb 5-784
- pharyngoesophageal diverticulum 5-292
- pharynx 5-292
- – total 5-292
- – web 5-294
- piles 5-493
- pilonidal cyst (sinus) 5-887
- pineal 5-074
- pinna 5-181
- pituitary gland 5-075
- pleura 5-344
- plexus
- – brachial 5-040
- – choroid 5-021
- – sympathetic 5-051
- polyp
- – vagina 5-702
- preauricular fistula 5-181
- prolapsed
- – ciliary body 5-134
- – iris 5-134
- prostate - see Prostatectomy
- pterygium 5-122
- – with graft 5-122
- – with transposition 5-122
- ranula 5-273
- rectovaginal septum 5-487
- rectum 5-485
- – abdominoperineal 5-484
- – combined synchronous 5-484
- – local 5-482
- – mucosa 5-482
- – perineal 5-485
- – pull-through 5-483
- redundant mucosa
- – colostomy 5-452
- – urethral 5-589
- – vulva 5-712
- redundant skin
- – eyelid 5-096
- rib 5-784
- – complete 5-785
- ring of conjunctiva around cornea 5-112
- round ligament 5-692
- sac
- – lacrimal 5-085

Excision - *continued*
- salivary gland 5-262
- saphenous vein 5-385
- – for graft 5-385
- – varicose 5-384
- scalene node 5-401
- scapula 5-784
- – complete 5-785
- scar
- – burn 5-884
- scrotum 5-612
- seminal vesicle 5-606
- septum
- – nose 5-214
- – vagina 5-702
- sequestrum
- – bone NEC 5-780
- – jaw 5-770
- – nasal sinus 5-224
- – nose 5-211
- – skull 5-011
- sesamoid bone 5-833
- sigmoid 5-455
- sinus 5-884
- – branchial 5-291
- – ethmoid 5-225
- – frontal 5-223
- – nasal 5-225
- – sacro-coccygeal 5-887
- – skin 5-884
- – sphenoidal 5-225
- – spinal (dermal sinus) 5-034
- – thyroglossal 5-066
- – urachal 5-542
- Skene's gland 5-712
- skin
- – minor 8-185
- skin and subcutaneous tissue
- – for graft 5-888
- – local 5-884
- – radical 5-885
- slough 5-883
- spermatic cord NEC 5-632
- spermatocele 5-631
- spinal
- – bone 5-030
- – lesion 5-033
- spleen 5-413
- – accessory 5-419
- – lesion 5-413
- stomach - see Gastrectomy
- stricture
- – esophagus 5-422
- – ureteral 5-568
- – urethra 5-582
- subdural membranous sac 5-014
- submaxillary gland 5-262

Excision - *continued*
- sympathetic 5-051
- synovial membrane
- - tendon sheath 5-833
- - - hand 5-822
- synovioma
- - hand 5-822
- tarsal plate (lesion) 5-091
- tattoo 5-884
- tendon 5-833
- - for graft 5-833
- - - hand 5-823
- - sheath 5-833
- - - hand 5-823
- thymus 5-077
- thyroglossal (structures) (tract) 5-066
- thyroid 5-062
- - adenoma 5-062
- - lingual (subtotal) 5-065
- - partial 5-062
- - total 5-063
- - transsternal 5-064
- tongue 5-251
- - block dissection 5-253
- - Commando procedure 5-253
- - complete 5-252
- - lesion 5-250
- - partial 5-251
- - radical 5-253
- tonsil 5-281
- - lingual 5-284
- - tag 5-283
- tooth 5-231
- - apex 5-237
- - from nasal sinus 5-222
- - residual root 5-231
- torus, mandible 5-771
- tunica vaginalis 5-611
- ulcer 5-884
- - duodenum 5-451
- - peptic 5-434
- - stomach 5-434
- - varicose 5-884
- urachus 5-574
- ureter
- - with reanastomosis 5-563
- ureterocele 5-561
- urethra
- - valves (endoscopic) 5-582
- - with bladder 5-576
- uterus - see also Hysterectomy
- - supporting structures 5-692
- uvula 5-276
- vagina
- - lesion 5-702
- - septum 5-702
- - total 5-703

Excision - *continued*
- varicocele, spermatic cord 5-630
- vein 5-385
- - varicose 5-384
- ventricle
- - atrialized 5-373
- vitreous opacity 5-157
- vocal cord 5-302
- - submucous 5-302
- vulva 5-715
- - lesion NEC 5-712
- - radical 5-714
Exclusion
- colon 5-458
- pyloric 5-442
- thoracic esophagus 5-424
Excretory aids
- colostomy bag
- - fitting 9-351
Exenteration
- ethmoid cells 5-225
- orbit (with graft) 5-164
- pelvic
- - female 5-687
- - male 5-576
- petrous pyramid 5-204
Exercise 9-459
- active 9-451
- assisted
- - in pool 8-551
- assisting 9-452
- breathing 9-472
- cardiovascular 9-473
- for neurological disease 9-431
- for paralysis 9-431
- for relaxation 9-455
- for rigidity 9-431
- for spasticity 9-431
- free
- - in pool 8-552
- gymnastic 9-432
- joint 9-462
- masticatory 9-420
- passive 9-460
- relaxation 9-455
- resistive 9-461
- therapeutic 9-450
- tolerance 1-724
- vascular
- - limb 9-488
Exfoliation
- chemosurgical 5-904
Exophoria
- testing 1-216
Exostectomy 5-783
- hallux 5-782
- spinal 5-783

Expander
− blood 8-812
Expiratory flow rate 1-711
Expired breath
− alcohol 2-167
− carbondioxide 2-124
− other exogenous organic compound
  2-168
− oxygen 2-124
Exploration (see also Examination)
− abdominal
− − testis 5-624
− bone 5-780
− digital
− − buccal 1-304
− − pharynx 1-310
− − postnasal 1-310
− − rectum 1-320
− − uterus 1-350
− − vagina 1-350
− − valve, heart 5-350
− endoscopic (see also Endoscopy) 1-689
− − esophagus 1-630
− − larynx 1-610
− − mediastinum 1-691
− − rectum 1-643
− − stomach 1-633
− − urethra 1-655
− − vagina 1-663
− esophagus
− − by incision 5-420
− gastrocamera 1-634
− lacrimal
− − gland 5-080
− liver 5-500
− manual
− − uterus
− − − postpartum 5-759
− nerve
− − sympathetic 5-053
− pericardium 5-371
− petrous pyramid cells 5-204
− sinus
− − maxillary
− − − intranasal 5-221
− skull, puncture 5-010
− surgical
− − abdomen 5-541
− − abdominal
− − − wall 5-540
− − adrenal gland 5-070
− − artery 5-380
− − axilla 5-882
− − bile duct 5-514
− − bladder 5-571
− − blood vessels 5-380
− − bone 5-780

Exploration - continued
− surgical - continued
− − brain 5-012
− − breast 5-871
− − bronchus 5-330
− − burrhole 5-011
− − bursa 5-830
− − carpal tunnel 5-043
− − chest wall 5-340
− − colon (sigmoid) 5-450
− − cranial 5-011
− − disc space (intervertebral) 5-800
− − ear
− − − inner 5-207
− − − middle 5-202
− − fascia 5-830
− − fistula 5-882
− − fossa superficial 5-882
− − gallbladder 5-510
− − groin 5-540
− − inguinal ring 5-540
− − intervertebral disc 5-800
− − intestine 5-450
− − intrathoracic 5-340
− − jaw 5-770
− − joint 5-800
− − − jaw 5-770
− − kidney 5-550
− − knee 5-800
− − lacrimal
− − − duct 5-084
− − − sac 5-084
− − laparotomy 5-541
− − larynx 5-313
− − lung 5-331
− − mediastinum 5-341
− − muscle 5-830
− − neck 5-882
− − − thyroglossal tract 5-060
− − − thyroid field 5-060
− − nerve 5-043
− − − spinal root 5-030
− − nose 5-211
− − orbit 5-160
− − − intracranial approach 5-160
− − palmar 5-820
− − pancreas 5-520
− − parotid gland 5-260
− − pelvic
− − − laparotomy 5-541
− − perineum
− − − female 5-710
− − − male 5-882
− − perirenal tissue 5-590
− − perivesical tissue 5-591
− − pleura 5-340
− − popliteal space 5-882

Exploration - *continued*
- surgical - *continued*
- - rectum 5-480
- - renal pelvis 5-551
- - retropubic 5-591
- - salivary gland 5-260
- - sclera 5-139
- - sinus
- - - ethmoid 5-224
- - - frontal 5-223
- - - maxillary
- - - - external 5-222
- - - nasal 5-224
- - - pilonidal 5-881
- - - sphenoidal 5-224
- - skin 5-882
- - spermatic cord 5-639
- - spine, spinal cord 5-030
- - spleen 5-412
- - stomach 5-430
- - subcutaneous tissue 5-882
- - subdiaphragmatic space 5-541
- - tendon 5-830
- - thorax 5-340
- - thyroid 5-060
- - trachea 5-313
- - tympanum by transtympanic route 5-202
- - ureter 5-562
- - urethra 5-580
- - uterus
- - - hysterotomy 5-680
- - vagina 5-701
- - vessels 5-380
- - vulva 5-710
- uterus
- - curettage 5-690
Exposure
- abscess
- - subdural 5-011
- mastoid 5-203
- nerve 5-043
- tooth
- - orthodontic 5-245
Expression
- placenta (Crede) 8-510
- trachoma follicles 5-111
Exsanguination 8-803
- blood exchange 8-803
- transfusion 8-803
Exstrophy
- bladder
- - repair 5-578
Extended care 9-175
Extension 8-470
- spinal 8-410
Exteriorization

Exteriorization - *continued*
- colon (sigmoid) 5-460
- esophageal pouch 5-421
- intestine 5-460
External counter pulsation 8-723
Extirpation (see also Excision)
- aneurysm
- - aorta 5-385
- - intracranial 5-385
- aneurysm NEC 5-385
- larynx 5-303
- varicose veins 5-384
Extracorporeal
- circulation
- - hemodialysis 8-853
- - hepatic insufficiency 8-855
- - in open heart surgery 5-396
- - operative 8-851
- kidney 8-854
Extraction
- breech (total) 5-725
- - partial 5-727
- cataract 5-146
- - combined 5-145
- - - with iridectomy 5-145
- - erisiphake 5-144
- - extracapsular 5-145
- - intracapsular 5-144
- - linear 5-142
- comedones 8-185
- foreign body (see also Removal, foreign body)
- - abdominal cavity
- - - by incision 5-549
- - abdominal wall
- - - by incision 5-540
- - anterior chamber
- - - magnetic 5-131
- - anus
- - - by incision 5-499
- - bladder
- - - by incision 5-571
- - - endoscopic 5-570
- - bone
- - - by osteotomy 5-780
- - breast
- - - by incision 5-871
- - bronchus by incision 5-330
- - bursa
- - - by incision 5-830
- - by incision 5-909
- - cervix (vaginal approach) 5-691
- - chest wall
- - - by incision 5-340
- - choroid
- - - by incision 5-150
- - ciliary body

Extraction - *continued*
– foreign body - *continued*
– – ciliary body - *continued*
– – – by incision 5-130
– – – magnetic 5-131
– – conjunctiva
– – – by incision 5-110
– – – by magnet 5-120
– – cornea
– – – by magnet 5-120
– – – penetrating 5-130
– – eye 5-161
– – – by magnet 5-161
– – fascia
– – – by incision 5-830
– – hand
– – – by incision 5-820
– – intestine
– – – by incision 5-450
– – iris
– – – by incision 5-130
– – – by magnet 5-131
– – jaw
– – – by osteotomy 5-770
– – joint structures
– – – by incision 5-800
– – kidney
– – – by incision 5-550
– – lacrimal 5-161
– – – gland 5-161
– – – sac 5-161
– – larynx
– – – external incision 5-313
– – lens
– – – by incision 5-141
– – – by magnet 5-140
– – liver
– – – by incision 5-500
– – lung
– – – by incision 5-331
– – magnet - see also Magnet extraction
– – – conjunctiva 5-120
– – mediastinum
– – – by incision 5-341
– – muscle
– – – by incision 5-830
– – nasal sinus
– – – by incision 5-224
– – nose
– – – by incision 5-211
– – orbit 5-161
– – – by magnet 5-161
– – perineum (female)
– – – by incision 5-710
– – perirenal tissue
– – – by incision 5-590
– – pharyngotomy 5-290

Extraction - *continued*
– foreign body - *continued*
– – pleura
– – – by incision 5-340
– – – endoscopic 1-691
– – posterior eye
– – – by incision 5-150
– – – by magnet 5-151
– – rectal wall
– – – by incision 5-480
– – rectum
– – – by incision 5-480
– – retina 5-150
– – sclera
– – – by magnet 5-151
– – scrotum
– – – by incision 5-619
– – skin
– – – by incision 5-882
– – spermatic cord
– – – by incision 5-635
– – stomach
– – – by incision 5-430
– – subcutaneous tissue
– – – by incision 5-882
– – tendon
– – – by incision 5-830
– – testis
– – – by incision 5-620
– – thorax
– – – by incision 5-340
– – – endoscopic 1-691
– – trachea
– – – by tracheotomy 5-311
– – tunica vaginalis 5-619
– – – by incision 5-619
– – ureter
– – – by incision 5-562
– – – endoscopic 5-560
– – uterus (vaginal approach) 5-691
– – vagina
– – – by incision 5-709
– – vulva
– – – by incision 5-710
– lens
– – by forceps 5-144
– loose body in (knee) joint 5-800
– menstrual 8-165
– obstetric 5-739
– tooth
– – by forceps 5-230
– – impacted 5-231
– – residual roots 5-231
– – supernumerary
– – – surgical 5-231
– – surgical removal 5-231
– transfer factor 2-932

F

Face lifting 5-900
Facetectomy, spine 5-784
Failure
− forceps 5-733
False
− breast 9-371
Family counselling 9-743
− medical 9-742
− social 9-743
Family therapy 9-610
Faradism 8-631
Fascia lata
− aortic valve 5-353
Fascial sling
− tongue 5-254
Fasciectomy 5-833
− hand 5-823
Fasciodesis 5-837
− hand 5-828
Fascioplasty 5-837
− hand 5-828
Fasciorrhaphy (see also Suture, fascia)
  5-835
− hand 5-824
Fasciotomy 5-830
− hand 5-820
− orbital 5-160
− three compartment 5-831
Fasting gastric aspirate 2-300
Fat
− intestinal absorption 2-313
Feces
− aminoacids 2-260
− catalase 2-264
− chemical examination NEC 2-269
− concentration methods 2-711
− enzymes 2-264
− examination
− − biochemical 2-269
− fats 2-262
− identification of
− − helminths 2-715
− − ova 2-715
− macroscopic 2-714
− − method NEC (for parasites) 2-719
− microscopy 2-710
− − crystals 2-269
− − stained 2-713
− − − for ova 2-712
− occult blood 2-263

Feces - continued
− other nitrogen 2-261
− porphyrins 2-269
− starch detection 2-269
Feeding
− parenteral 9-230
− − prolonged 9-232
Fehling test 2-223
Fenestration
− aortic aneurysm 5-395
− cardiac valve 5-353
− chest wall 5-340
− ear 5-205
− − horizontal canal 5-205
− − inner 5-205
− − − with graft 5-205
− − oval window 5-205
− − revision 5-206
− − with graft 5-205
− fractured egg shell 5-205
− intervertebral disc 5-803
− palate 5-271
− semicircular canals 5-205
− stapes footplate 5-191
− transmeatal (ear) 5-205
− vestibule (ear) 5-205
Fermentation reactions
− fungal 2-702
Fermentation tests
− bacteria 2-511
Ferritin labelled antibody
− detection 2-755
Fetal maturity
− determination 1-359
Feto-placental products, screening 4-202
Fetoscopy
− transabdominal 5-755
Fiberscopy
− colon 1-641
− duodenum 1-636
− stomach 1-633
Fibrinogen titre 2-321
Fibrinolytic activity 2-865
Fibroidectomy, uterine 5-681
Filipuncture
− aneurysm 5-395
Filleting
− hammer toe 5-789
− pancreas 5-522
Filling

Filling - *continued*
- extrapleural 5-332
- tooth 5-232
- - temporary dressing 9-300
Filtering procedure
- eye 5-132
Filtration
- portal (extracorporeal) 8-857
Fimbriectomy 5-665
Finger reading training 9-416
Finney's operation 5-441
Fissurectomy
- anus 5-492
- skin and subcutaneous tissue 5-884
Fistulectomy (see also Excision, fistula)
- cornea 5-123
- esophagus 5-422
Fistulization
- surgical
- - appendix 5-471
- - arteriovenous 5-392
- - biliary
- - - external 5-514
- - - internal 5-514
- - bone 5-783
- - esophagus 5-421
- - fallopian tube 5-660
- - hernia 5-460
- - iris 5-132
- - lacrimal
- - - canaliculus 5-088
- - - duct 5-084
- - - sac 5-087
- - - - into nasal cavity 5-087
- - larynx 5-312
- - orbit 5-160
- - oviduct 5-660
- - salivary gland 5-260
- - thoracic duct 5-405
- - trachea 5-312
- - ureter 5-565
- - ventricle, cerebral 5-022
Fistulotomy
- anal 5-491
Fitting
- artificial limb 8-564
- prosthesis 8-562
- - limb 8-564
- spectacles 9-322
Fixation
- bone
- - external 8-331
- - - fracture 8-330
- - external cast 8-310
- - internal 5-787
- - without fracture reduction 5-787
- breast

Fixation - *continued*
- breast - *continued*
- - pendulous 5-875
- cardinal ligaments 5-693
- colon (to abdominal wall) 5-466
- device
- - internal 5-787
- - - without manipulation for reduction 5-787
- esophagus
- - posterior 5-427
- external
- - fracture 8-330
- fracture
- - bone 5-790
- - jaw wiring 5-762
- - multiple 5-797
- - skull 5-020
- hip 5-812
- internal
- - bone 5-787
- - fracture
- - - chest wall 5-792
- - - plating 5-792
- - - spine 5-792
- - joint
- - - dislocation
- - - - open reduction 5-796
- - - foot 5-811
- - - hip 5-812
- - - nec 5-812
- intestine 5-546
- - to abdominal wall 5-466
- iris 5-136
- joint (see also Repair, joint) 5-812
- kidney 5-556
- ligament
- - cardinal 5-693
- - palpebrae 5-094
- - uterus 5-693
- parametrial 5-693
- rectum (with fascia graft) 5-486
- spine with fusion 5-810
- spleen 5-419
- stapes 5-193
- tendon 5-837
- - hand 5-828
- testis 5-624
- tongue 5-254
- urethrovaginal to cooper's ligament 5-706
- uterus 5-693
- vagina 5-706
- without reduction of fracture 5-787
Fixed rate ventricular stimulator 8-653
Flail chest
- packing 8-741

Flail chest - *continued*
- plugging 8-741
Flame photometry 2-491
Flap
- advancement 5-894
- bone, cranial 5-020
- conjunctival 5-113
- cross finger 5-895
- cross leg 5-896
- dental
- - for extraction 5-231
- double pedicled 5-894
- osteoplastic (cranial) 5-020
- pocket, hand 5-895
- skin (see graft, grafting, skin) 5-894
Flexion
- fetal head (manually) 8-253
Flexorplasty 5-837
Flocculation
- cephalin-cholesterol 2-321
- thymol 2-321
- treponemal 2-601
Flowmeter cardiac catheter 1-721
Fluid
- balance regulation 8-876
Fluorescent 2-628
- antibody 2-628
- karyotyping 2-924
Fluoridated water use 4-533
Fluoride
- dentifrice 4-531
- topical dental application 4-532
Folding
- ocular muscles 5-104
Folin-Wu test 2-130
Follicle stimulating hormone 2-412
Follow-up 9-820
- medical 9-822
- surgical 9-821
Footwear
- orthopedic 9-331
- - adaptation 9-331
Forage operation
- bone 5-780
- hip 5-812
- prostate 5-601
Foraminotomy (spinal) 5-030
Forced 8-822
- diuresis 8-822
- extension
- - limb 8-212
Forceps application, obstetrical - see
  Delivery, forceps
- failure 5-733
Foreign body
- search
- - magnetometer 1-820

Foreign body - *continued*
- search - *continued*
- - means NEC 1-821
Forel field
- placement 5-013
Forensic
- chemical analysis
- - hair 2-940
- - nails 2-940
- - stomach contents 2-943
- - tissue NEC 2-944
- examinations (see also Specific method)
  2-949
Formation
- adhesions
- - pericardium and myocardium 5-363
- anus, artificial 5-461
- colostomy 5-461
- false fontanelle 5-020
- pupil 5-135
- - by iridectomy 5-135
Forssman antigen 2-611
Fouchet test 2-115
Fracture
- compression union 8-340
- fixation
- - emergency 8-331
- - without reduction 8-331
- immobilization
- - specified NEC 8-531
- manipulation - see Reduction, fracture
- support 8-303
- - sling 8-303
Fragility
- red cells 2-812
Frank's operation 5-432
Fredet-Ramstedt operation 5-433
Free fatty acids
- blood 2-141
Freeing adhesions
- abdomen 5-544
- anterior chamber (eye) 5-136
- biliary tract 5-544
- - intraluminal 5-513
- bladder (internal) 5-578
- bone 5-789
- - jaw 5-779
- bowel 5-544
- bursa 5-839
- carpal tunnel 5-043
- conjunctiva 5-114
- cornea 5-136
- - internal 5-136
- cortical, brain 5-029
- ear
- - middle 5-202
- eye muscle 5-105

Freeing adhesions - *continued*
- eyelid 5-114
- fallopian tube 5-657
- fascia 5-839
- - hand 5-829
- gallbladder 5-544
- hand 5-829
- heart 5-371
- intestines 5-544
- intracranial 5-029
- intrauterine 5-681
- iris 5-136
- joint 5-801
- - jaw 5-775
- - manipulation 8-214
- kidney 5-559
- larynx 5-319
- lung 5-333
- - for collapse 5-332
- meninges
- - spinal 5-035
- muscle 5-839
- - hand 5-829
- - ocular 5-105
- nerve 5-043
- - roots, spinal 5-035
- nose 5-219
- orbit (eye socket) 5-169
- ossicles 5-190
- ovary 5-657
- pelvic
- - female 5-544
- - male 5-544
- penis 5-649
- pericardium 5-371
- peritoneum 5-544
- pharynx 5-294
- pleura 5-333
- rectum 5-489
- retroperitoneal 5-590
- spinal cord 5-035
- spinal meninges 5-035
- spleen 5-544
- stomach 5-544
- symblepharon 5-114
- tendon 5-839
- - hand 5-829
- tongue 5-258
- trachea 5-319
- ureter 5-568
- urethra 5-584
- uterus
- - internal 5-681
- vagina 5-706
- vessels 5-399
- - peripheral 5-399
- vulva (labia) 5-716

Freezing
- basal nuclei 5-013
- tissue 5-949
Frei test
- lymphogranuloma 1-704
Frenotomy 5-258
- buccal 5-279
- labial 5-279
- - with suture 5-279
- lingual 5-258
- tongue 5-258
Frenumectomy 5-279
- tongue 5-250
Frozen section
- examination 2-900
Fructose
- diphosphate aldolase 2-480
Fulguration (see also Excision, lesion, by site)
- anus 5-492
- bladder
- - by cystotomy 5-574
- - transurethral 5-573
- eyelids 5-091
- penis 5-641
- perineum
- - female 5-712
- prostate, transurethral 5-601
- rectum 5-482
- retina 5-155
- scrotum 5-612
- skin and subcutaneous tissue 5-884
- urethra 5-582
- vulva 5-712
Fulguration
- lesion 5-932
Function tests
- adrenal 2-354
- cardiac 1-729
- endocrine NEC 2-439
- gastric 2-309
- hepatic 2-329
- intestinal 2-319
- metabolic 1-769
- - chemical 2-359
- muscular 1-759
- pancreas 2-339
- pituitary 2-419
- renal 2-349
- - chemical NEC 2-345
- thyroid 2-409
- urinary excretion 2-349
Fundectomy
- uterine 5-682
Funduscopy 1-220
Fundusectomy
- gastric 5-438

G

Gait training 9-440
Galactose
– blood 2-132
– tolerance 2-323
Galeaplasty 5-899
Games
– competitives 9-631
– organized 9-542
Gammaglutamyl transpeptidase 2-468
Ganglionectomy 5-040
– cervical
– – sympathetic 5-051
– gasserian 5-040
– nerve
– – cranial 5-040
– – peripheral 5-040
– sphenopalatine (Meckel's) 5-040
– sympathetic 5-051
– tendon sheath 5-822
– – wrist 5-822
Ganglionorrhaphy
– sympathetic 5-053
Gartners duct
– cyst excision 5-702
Gas endarterectomy
– coronary 5-360
Gas therapy
– decompression chamber 8-772
– helium 8-773
– oxygen 8-760
– – catalytic 8-761
– – hyperbaric 8-762
– – pump 8-764
Gastrectomy 5-438
– complete 5-439
– partial 5-438
– – with esophagogastrostomy 5-435
– – with gastroduodenostomy 5-436
– – with gastrojejunostomy 5-437
– – with jejunal anastomosis 5-437
– – with vagotomy 5-438
– proximal
– – with esophageal anastomosis 5-435
– radical 5-439
– subtotal - see Gastrectomy, partial
– total 5-439
Gastric
– contents
– – blood detection 2-281
– – drugs 2-281

Gastric - *continued*
– emptying time 2-305
– function test 2-309
– juice
– – basic acid output 2-300
– – edestin test 2-304
– – enzymes 2-304
– – pepsin 2-304
– – rennin 2-304
– – response to drugs 2-309
– – response to stimulation 2-302
– – trypsin 2-304
Gastrocamera 1-634
Gastrocholecystostomy 5-512
Gastrocholedochostomy 5-512
Gastroduodenectomy
– complete 5-439
– partial 5-437
– total 5-439
Gastroduodenostomy
– closure 5-444
– with gastrectomy 5-436
– with vagotomy 5-436
– without gastrectomy 5-442
Gastroduodenotomy 5-430
Gastroenterostomy
– closure 5-444
– revision 5-444
– without gastrectomy 5-442
Gastroesophagectomy 5-423
Gastroesophagoscopy 1-632
Gastrogastrostomy 5-438
– with partial gastrectomy 5-438
Gastrojejunostomy
– closure 5-444
– without gastrectomy 5-442
Gastrolysis 5-544
Gastropexy 5-445
– for hernia 5-537
Gastroplasty 5-445
Gastroplication 5-445
Gastrorrhaphy 5-445
Gastroscopy 1-633
– by gastrotomy 1-692
– foreign body removal 8-112
– operative 1-695
– via stoma 1-635
Gastrostomy
– closure 5-445
– permanent 5-432

Gastrostomy - *continued*
- temporary 5-431
- tube
- - temporary 5-431
- tubulovalvular fistula 5-432
Gastrotomy 5-430
Gavage 8-123
Genetic counselling 4-660
Genioplasty 5-775
- with bone graft 5-775
- with inert implant 5-775
Gerbode's dilator 5-350
Gerhardt test
- acetoacetic acid 2-240
Geriatric
- health care 4-119
- - medical examination 4-110
Giemsa stain 2-805
Gill's operation, shoulder 5-812
Gingivectomy 5-242
Gingivoplasty 5-241
Glacial acetic acid 5-950
- application 5-950
Globulin
- electrophoresis 2-106
- fractions estimation 2-106
- total
- - estimation 2-105
Glomectomy
- carotid body 5-398
- glomangioma (skin) 5-884
- tympanic body 5-398
Glomerular filtration rate 2-343
Glossectomy 5-251
- Commando 5-253
- complete 5-252
- partial 5-251
- radical 5-253
- total 5-252
- with neck dissection 5-253
Glossopexy 5-254
Glossoplasty 5-254
Glossorrhaphy 5-254
Glossotomy 5-259
- for tongue tie 5-258
Glucagon
- intravenous test 2-332
Glucose
- blood
- - chemical estimation 2-130
- - enzymatic estimation 2-131
- tolerance test 2-330
Glucose-6-phosphatase 2-463
Glucose-6-phosphate dehydrogenase 2-453
Glutamic oxaloacetic transaminase 2-460
Glutamic pyruvic transaminase 2-461
Glutamine

Glutamine - *continued*
- serum identification 2-100
Glycogen
- phosphorylase 2-463
- synthetase 2-463
Glycogenolytic enzyme 2-463
Glycoprotein
- blood 2-133
Goebel-Frangenheim-Stoeckel operation
  5-594
Gofman groups 2-149
Goitre prophylaxis 4-470
- iodized salt 4-471
Gold inlay
- dental 5-233
Gonadotrophin stimulation response 2-424
Goniopuncture 5-133
Gonioscopy 1-226
Goniotomy 5-133
Graft, grafting 5-893
- amnion to conjunctiva 5-113
- aneurysm 5-395
- anus 5-496
- aorta 5-395
- - bypass 5-392
- aponeurosis 5-837
- - hand 5-827
- artery
- - aorta 5-395
- - - bypass 5-392
- - aortic bifurcation (bypass) 5-392
- - aortic-femoral 5-392
- - aortic-iliac 5-392
- - aorto-iliac to popliteal 5-392
- - bypass 5-392
- - head 5-395
- arthroplasty - see Arthroplasty
- bifurcation (bypass) 5-392
- - aorta (abdominal) 5-392
- bile duct 5-516
- bladder (colon) (ileum) 5-577
- bone 5-786
- - autogenous 5-786
- - cleft palate 5-275
- - cranial (pericranial) 5-020
- - for joint repair 5-812
- - jaw (lower) 5-773
- - - upper 5-775
- - nose 5-217
- - spine with fusion 5-810
- - thumb 5-826
- - with arthroplasty
- - - foot 5-813
- - with excision
- - - intervertebral disc 5-803
- - with internal fixation 5-786
- breast

Graft - *continued*
- breast - *continued*
- - nipple 5-872
- - skin 5-875
- cartilage (see also Repair, joint) 5-819
- - nose 5-217
- - tarsal (eyelid) 5-096
- - with arthroplasty
- - - foot 5-813
- choroid
- - with amnion 5-156
- cleft palate 5-275
- columnellar 5-217
- conjunctiva 5-113
- - tarsal 5-113
- cornea 5-125
- dura 5-021
- ear
- - auricle 5-186
- - external auditory meatus 5-185
- - following stapedectomy 5-191
- - inner 5-195
- - middle (skin) (vein) 5-194
- - perforation 5-195
- - pinna 5-186
- - round window 5-195
- epicardial 5-363
- epidermal 5-893
- esophagus 5-427
- - bypass
- - - antesternal 5-425
- - intrathoracic 5-427
- eyebrow (hair-bearing skin) 5-096
- eyelid 5-096
- fallopian tube 5-666
- fascia 5-837
- - hand 5-827
- - rectal repair 5-486
- fat
- - to breast 5-873
- fenestration
- - ear 5-205
- flap - see Graft, pedicle
- gum 5-241
- hair bearing skin 5-902
- hand
- - fascia 5-827
- - free skin 5-892
- - muscle 5-827
- - pedicle (flap) 5-895
- - tendon 5-827
- hare lip 5-898
- heart
- - revascularization 5-363
- - septum 5-357
- - wall 5-374
- hernia

Graft - *continued*
- hernia - *continued*
- - epigastric 5-536
- - incisional 5-536
- - inguinofemoral 5-531
- - - bilateral 5-533
- - - unilateral 5-531
- - ventral 5-536
- intervertebral disc 5-810
- island 5-896
- jaw (lower) 5-773
- - upper 5-775
- joint (see also Arthroplasty) 5-819
- kidney 5-555
- larynx 5-315
- lip 5-898
- lymph node 5-409
- meninges
- - cerebral 5-021
- - spinal 5-034
- mouth 5-274
- - external 5-898
- - palate 5-275
- mucosal
- - buccal 5-274
- - conjunctiva 5-113
- - orbit 5-167
- - to conjunctiva 5-113
- - to eyelid 5-096
- - tongue 5-254
- muscle 5-837
- - hand 5-827
- - temporalis to orbit 5-167
- - thumb 5-827
- nasal septum 5-217
- nerve 5-044
- - cranial 5-044
- - facial 5-044
- - in ear 5-044
- nipple 5-872
- nose 5-217
- - skin 5-896
- omentum 5-546
- - to myocardium 5-363
- orbit 5-167
- ovary 5-656
- palate 5-275
- - cleft 5-275
- patch to artery 5-395
- pectoral muscle 5-363
- pedicle 5-894
- - attachment to
- - - hand 5-895
- - - site NEC 5-896
- - - thumb 5-895
- - defatting 5-897
- - delayed 5-894

Graft - *continued*
— pedicle 5-894 - *continued*
— — double 5-896
— — — hand 5-895
— — elevation 5-894
— — hand 5-895
— — larynx 5-315
— — preparation of (cutting) 5-894
— penis 5-643
— periosteal 5-786
— pinch 5-893
— — alveolus 5-244
— — anus 5-496
— — bile ducts 5-516
— — bladder 5-577
— pinna 5-186
— pocket - see Graft, pedicle
— promontory tympanic 5-195
— rotating - see Graft, pedicle
— saphenous vein (bypass) 5-392
— sclera 5-137
— scrotum 5-613
— septum
— — heart 5-357
— — nose 5-217
— skin 5-893
— — breast 5-875
— — — augmentation 5-873
— — — nipple 5-872
— — canthus 5-092
— — chin 5-893
— — dermal fat 5-893
— — ear
— — — auditory meatus 5-185
— — — middle 5-195
— — — pinna 5-186
— — eyelid 5-096
— — face NEC 5-893
— — free 5-893
— — — hand 5-892
— — — thumb 5-892
— — hand (free) 5-892
— — — pedicle 5-895
— — lip 5-898
— — — cleft 5-898
— — mouth 5-898
— — — external 5-898
— — — internal 5-274
— — pedicle - see Graft, pedicle
— — penis 5-643

Graft - *continued*
— skin 5-893 - *continued*
— — scrotum 5-613
— — vagina 5-706
— skull (bone) 5-020
— split thickness 5-893
— tendon 5-837
— — hand 5-827
— — with arthroplasty
— — — foot 5-813
— testis 5-625
— thumb 5-826
— tongue 5-254
— trachea 5-316
— tubular - see Graft, pedicle
— ureter 5-568
— vagina 5-706
— valve, heart 5-352
— vascular resection 5-383
— vein
— — arterial replacement 5-383
— — autogenous (to artery) 5-395
— — bypass 5-392
— — inner ear 5-195
— — thoracic 5-395
— — to
— — — round window 5-195
— — — tympanum 5-194
— vermilion border 5-898
Gram stain
— bacteria 2-503
Grattage
— conjunctiva 5-112
— eyelids 5-091
Grice's operation 5-811
Grip
— strength 1-751
Gritti-Stokes operation 5-848
Gross pathology 2-959
Group
— therapy 9-640
— Gofman 2-149
Growth hormone 2-413
— response to hypoglycemia 2-421
Guarinii test 2-106
Guildford's operation 5-191
Guthrie test 2-100
Guttering
— bone 5-783
— jaw 5-771

H

Hagedorn test 2-130
Hair
— metallic content 2-940
— mycological examination 2-700
Halo traction 8-411
Halometry 2-806
Hamazaki-Wesenberg bodies 2-876
Hanger test 2-321
Hanging drop
— examination (microscopic) 2-500
Haptoglobins
— serum 2-643
Harken's valve 5-352
Harrington's operation 5-810
Hartmann's operation 5-485
Haultain's operation 5-759
Hay test 2-214
Head
— appliance 9-344
Health
— examination - see Examination, health
Health care (see also Specific health care)
— geriatric 4-119
Hearing aid 9-314
— battery replacement 9-313
— behind ear 9-312
— body worn 9-311
— head worn 9-310
Hearing test 1-239
— clinical 1-232
— speech 1-232
Heart
— arrest
— — for operation 8-660
— clinical examination in-depth 1-250
— massage 8-520
— — external 8-520
— — open 5-379
— output
— — monitoring 8-943
— rate
— — learned control 9-681
— — recording 1-251
Heart-lung
— artificial 5-396
Heat, heating
— general (of body) 8-601
— hot packs 8-602
— local 8-600
— radiant 8-605

Heavy chain protein
— urine 2-671
Heavy metals
— hair 2-940
— skin 2-940
Heinecke-Mikulitz operation 5-441
Heliotherapy 8-601
— local 8-600
Helium dilution
— total lung capacity 1-710
Heller's operation 5-426
Helminths
— identification
— — feces 2-715
— intestinal ova 2-715
Hemagglutination
— indirect 2-622
— inhibition 2-621
— parasite
— — indirect 2-754
— passive 2-622
Hemagglutinins
— detection 2-825
Hematin 2-834
Hematocrit 2-811
Hemicolectomy 5-455
Hemicorporectomy 5-849
Hemicystectomy 5-575
Hemiglossectomy 5-251
Hemilaminectomy 5-030
Hemilaryngectomy 5-301
Hemimandibulectomy
— with prosthesis 5-773
Heminephrectomy 5-553
Hemipelvectomy 5-849
Hemispherectomy 5-014
Hemithyroidectomy 5-061
Hemodialysis 8-853
— vena cava 8-855
Hemofiltration
— vein
— — splenic 8-857
Hemoglobin
— analysis 2-832
— concentration 2-831
— electrophoresis 2-841
— estimation 2-830
— familial study 2-842
— fetal
— — detection in red blood cells 2-843

Hemoglobin - *continued*
– fetal - *continued*
– – electrophoresis 2-841
– genetic varieties 2-849
– mean corpuscular 2-831
– urine 2-205
Hemoglobinopathy
– blood examination 2-841
Hemogram
– Schilling 2-881
Hemolysin
– detection 2-829
Hemolytic complement level 2-655
Hemoperfusion
– liver 8-858
– – failure 8-858
Hemorrhoidectomy 5-493
Hemorrhoids
– destruction 5-493
– injection 5-973
– ligation 5-493
– manual reduction 8-243
Hemosiderin
– estimation 2-839
– urine 2-839
Hemostasis (see also Control, hemorrhage)
 8-500
– liver, suture 5-505
– nasal 8-501
– test 2-869
– uterine
– – non-obstetric 8-503
– vaginal
– – tampon 8-504
Hemostix 2-205
Henley's operation 5-438
Heparin
– assay 2-861
Hepatectomy 5-501
– anatomical 5-502
– guillotine 5-502
– lobectomy 5-502
– partial 5-501
– total 5-503
Hepatic
– detoxication 2-322
– protein dysfunction 2-321
Hepatic assistance 8-859
– extracorporeal 8-855
Hepaticodochotomy 5-514
Hepaticojejunostomy 5-512
Hepaticolithotomy 5-513
Hepaticostomy 5-514
Hepaticotomy 5-514
Hepatocholeduodenostomy 5-512
Hepatocolopexy 5-466
Hepatopexy 5-505

Hepatoplasty 5-505
Hepatopneumopexy 5-505
Hepatorrhaphy 5-505
Hepatostomy 5-505
Hepatotomy 5-500
Hernioplasty (see also Repair, hernia)
 5-530
Herniorrhaphy (see also Repair, hernia)
 5-530
Herniotomy (see also Repair, hernia) 5-530
Herzfeld test 2-115
Heterograft (see also Graft, grafting)
– artery 5-383
– heart valve 5-352
Heterophile antibodies 2-651
Hey's operation 5-846
Hibbs operation
– spinal fusion 5-810
High air loss bed 8-375
Higher education
– for patient 9-514
Hinged traction 8-475
Hinging
– mitral valve 5-353
Hippuric acid
– excretion 2-322
Histamine test 2-302
– guinea pig assay 2-573
Histidine
– decarboxylase 2-482
– serum identification 2-100
Histochemistry 2-903
Histology 2-909
– digestive tract 2-907
– enzymes 2-904
– jejunal mucosa 2-907
– organ NEC 2-909
– rectal mucosa 2-907
– unfixed section 2-900
– unstained section 2-900
HLA compatibility 2-640
Hoke's operation 5-811
Holter valve
– for hydrocephalus 5-023
– – replacement 5-024
Holth's operation 5-132
Home
– control
– – arthropods NEC 4-553
– – bedbugs 4-552
– – flies 4-550
– – mammals NEC 4-555
– – mice 4-554
– – mosquitoes 4-551
– – rats 4-554
– – rodents 4-554
– – vectors 4-559

Homogentisate oxygenase 2-451
Homogentisic acid
– serum identification 2-100
Homograft (see also Graft, grafting)
– heart valve 5-352
– tympanic membrane 5-194
Homotransplant
– renal 5-555
Hormone (see also Specific hormone)
– assay
– – tissue susceptibility 2-931
– growth 2-413
– – response to hypoglycemia 2-421
– other NEC
– – urinary 2-449
Hosiery, elastic 9-332
Hot packs 8-602
Hough's operation 5-191
House's operation 5-191
Hufnagel's operation 5-352
Hydatid
– skin test 1-704
Hydrolase 2-479
Hydrotherapy 8-550
Hymenectomy 5-702
Hymenorrhaphy 5-706
Hymenotomy 5-701
Hyperalimentation
– parenteral 9-231
Hyperbaric oxygenation 8-762
Hyperextension
– joint 8-212
Hyperventilation
– mechanical 8-710
Hypnosis
– for diagnosis 1-923
– for therapy 9-679
Hypophysectomy 5-075
– trans-sphenoidal 5-075
– transantral approach 5-075
– transethmoidal approach 5-075
– transfrontal 5-075
– transnasal approach 5-075
– transseptal approach 5-075
– transsphenoidal approach 5-075
Hypothalamic(-pituitary-adrenocortical
axis) function NEC 2-429

Hypothermia 8-610
– general 8-611
– with hypotension 8-614
Hypotympanotomy 5-202
Hysterectomy 5-683
– abdominal approach 5-683
– – with cesarean section 5-741
– extended 5-683
– for termination of pregnancy 5-744
– modified radical 5-685
– obstetric 5-683
– partial 5-682
– radical 5-685
– subtotal 5-682
– supracervical 5-682
– supravaginal 5-682
– total 5-683
– vaginal approach 5-684
– – radical 5-686
– – total (complete) 5-684
Hysterocolpectomy
– radical 5-685
Hysterolysis 5-695
– external 5-544
– internal 5-695
Hysteromyomectomy 5-681
Hysteropexy 5-693
Hysteroplasty 5-695
– postpartum 5-757
Hysterorrhaphy 5-695
– following delivery or abortion 5-757
Hysterosalpingectomy 5-683
Hysterosalpingostomy 5-666
Hysteroscopy 1-660
– operative 1-695
Hysterotomy 5-680
– abdominal 5-680
– cesarean (see also Cesarean section)
5-749
– for intrauterine transfusion 5-754
– for termination of pregnancy 5-744
– vaginal 5-680
– with removal of hydatidiform mole 5-681
Hysterotrachelectomy 5-673
Hysterotracheloplasty 5-695
Hysterotrachelorrhaphy 5-695
Hysterotrachelotomy 5-680

I

I-beam nail plate
− intertrochanteric fracture 5-792
ICCE (intracapsular cataract extraction)
 5-144
Icterus index 2-115
Ictostix 2-212
Ictotest 2-212
Identification
− antigenic determinants 2-639
− arthropods 2-737
− bacterial strains 2-529
− fungus 2-702
− parasites 2-737
− − blood 2-727
Ileal bladder 5-564
Ileectomy 5-454
Ileocecostomy 5-458
Ileocolectomy 5-455
Ileocolostomy 5-458
Ileocystoplasty 5-577
Ileoduodenotomy 5-450
Ileoesophagostomy
− intrathoracic 5-424
Ileoileostomy 5-457
− end to end 5-454
− proximal to distal segment 5-454
Ileopancreatostomy 5-527
Ileoproctostomy 5-458
Ileorrhaphy 5-467
Ileoscopy
− by ileotomy 1-693
− operative 1-695
Ileosigmoidostomy 5-458
Ileostomy 5-462
− closure 5-465
− reduction of prolapse 5-464
− repair of 5-464
− revision of 5-464
− transplantation to new site 5-462
− with plication of ileum 5-462
Ileotomy 5-450
Ileotransversostomy 5-458
Ileoureterostomy 5-566
− external 5-564
Imbrication
− right ventricle 5-357
− scleral 5-153
Immobilization
− bone 8-332
− by bandaging 8-303

Immobilization - continued
− by sling 8-303
− fracture (see also Reduction, fracture)
− − external 8-330
− − plaster 8-310
− splinting 8-329
− wound 8-333
Immunity reaction
− lymphocytic 2-640
Immunization 4-359
− bacterial 4-329
− − specified NEC 2-339
− BCG 4-330
− brucellosis 4-331
− cholera 4-320
− diphtheria 4-333
− DPT 4-336
− emergency 4-359
− epidemic parotitis 4-352
− german measles 4-351
− Haemophilus influenzae 4-339
− infancy programme 4-359
− influenza 4-343
− measles 4-350
− meningococcal 4-324
− mumps 4-352
− pertussis 4-334
− plague 4-323
− poliomyelitis 4-353
− rabies 4-342
− rubella 4-351
− salmonella 4-322
− smallpox 4-340
− staphylococcus 4-339
− TAB (C) 4-322
− tetanus 4-335
− triple vaccine 4-339
− tuberculosis 4-330
− tularemia 4-332
− typhoid-paratyphoid 4-322
− typhus 4-344
− viral NEC 4-358
− whooping cough 4-334
− yellow fever 4-341
Immunofluorescence, immunofluorescent
− histological examination 2-905
− method NEC 2-681
− parasite 2-753
− reaction
− − direct 2-615

Immunofluorescence - *continued*
- reaction - *continued*
- - virus 2-628
- tissue 2-953
Immunoglobulin
- agar gel diffusion 2-672
- complement fixation 2-676
- counter electroimmunophoresis 2-673
- detection 2-679
- estimation method NEC 2-678
- identification 2-679
- indirect hemagglutination inhibition 2-674
- membrane associated 2-871
- quantitative
- - assay 2-678
- radial immunodiffusion plate 2-672
Immunological reaction
- alteration NEC 2-659
Immunology NEC 2-629
Immunosuppression 9-220
- for transplant 9-220
Impacted tooth
- removal 5-231
Impedance pletismography monitoring 8-944
Implant, implantation (see also Insertion) 5-909
- acrylic
- - cornea 5-126
- - joint (see also Arthroplasty) 5-819
- - lens 5-147
- - nasal septum 5-217
- - orbit 5-165
- amniotic
- - artery 5-395
- artery
- - mammary, internal
- - - to coronary 5-361
- - - to myocardium 5-362
- blood vessels to myocardium 5-362
- bone 5-786
- breast 5-873
- - prosthesis 5-875
- - - for nipple-saving mastectomy 5-865
- cervix
- - irritant 5-674
- cornea 5-126
- electronic stimulator
- - bladder 5-571
- - ureter 5-562
- endosseous
- - dental 5-236
- epicardial electrodes 5-377
- eye
- - orbital 5-165
- fallopian tube in uterus 5-666

Implant - *continued*
- for retinal reattachment 5-154
- heart
- - assist system 5-376
- - septal prosthesis 5-356
- - valve
- - - prosthesis 5-352
- hip 5-816
- hormone 5-880
- inert materials
- - ureter for repair 5-568
- jaw 5-775
- kidney
- - artificial 5-559
- laryngeal plate 5-315
- limb prosthesis 5-855
- myocardium
- - aortic branches 5-362
- - internal mammary 5-362
- nerve 5-044
- nose 5-217
- orbital 5-165
- ovary 5-656
- pacemaker 5-377
- - venous route 8-880
- palate 5-275
- pancreatic duct
- - tube 5-527
- patella to tibia 5-786
- prosthetic tooth 5-236
- pulse generator 5-377
- radioactive isotope
- - bladder (requires radiology code) 5-574
- - bone marrow (requires radiology code) 5-418
- - cervix (requires radiology code) 5-679
- - pituitary (requires radiology code) 5-075
- - tongue (requires radiology code) 5-259
- - vaginal (requires radiology code) 5-702
- sclera
- - shell 5-162
- - with buckling 5-152
- septum, nasal (submucous) prosthesis 5-217
- sponge, epicardial 5-363
- stimulator
- - heart muscle 5-377
- - peripheral nerve 5-049
- - spinal 5-039
- - ureter 5-562
- subcutaneous 5-880
- subperiosteal
- - dental 5-236
- supporting fascia

Implant - *continued*
− supporting fascia - *continued*
− − mitral valve 5-352
− Tenon's capsule 5-163
− tooth 5-235
− ureter into 5-567
− − bowel 5-566
− − intestine 5-566
− − rectum 5-566
− − skin 5-565
− urethral compression 5-597
− vitreous (silicone) 5-157
− − for detached retina 5-154
Incision
− abdominal wall 5-540
− absces 5-882
− − abdominal
− − − cavity 5-541
− − − wall 5-540
− − alveolar (gum) 5-240
− − anus 5-490
− − appendix 5-471
− − auditory meatus 5-180
− − Bartholin's gland 5-711
− − bone 5-780
− − brain 5-012
− − breast 5-871
− − cerebral 5-011
− − cornea 5-121
− − ear
− − − external 5-180
− − epidural
− − − spinal 5-036
− − eyelid 5-090
− − face 5-270
− − gum 5-240
− − hand
− − − deep 5-820
− − − superficial 5-882
− − intracranial 5-011
− − ischiorectal 5-490
− − lip 5-270
− − liver 5-500
− − lung 5-331
− − meningeal 5-011
− − mouth 5-270
− − muscle 5-830
− − neck 5-882
− − nerve root 5-030
− − omental 5-541
− − orbit 5-160
− − ovary 5-650
− − palate 5-271
− − pancreas 5-520
− − pelvic
− − − female 5-701
− − − male 5-541

Incision - *continued*
− absces 5-882 - *continued*
− − pelvic - *continued*
− − − male 5-541 - *continued*
− − − − abdominal approach 5-541
− − perianal 5-490
− − perigastric 5-541
− − perirectal 5-487
− − perirenal 5-590
− − perisplenic 5-541
− − peritoneal 5-541
− − − by culdocentesis 5-701
− − peritonsillar 5-280
− − pharyngeal 5-280
− − postauricular 5-180
− − retroperitoneal 5-541
− − retropharyngeal 5-280
− − skin 5-882
− − spinal 5-030
− − − cord 5-030
− − − meninges 5-030
− − subcutaneous 5-882
− − subdiaphragmatic 5-541
− − subfascial 5-830
− − subhepatic 5-541
− − superficial 5-882
− − tonsillar 5-280
− − vulva 5-710
− alveolus, dental 5-240
− ampulla of Vater 5-514
− anal septum 5-499
− aponeurosis 5-830
− appendix 5-471
− artery - see Arteriotomy
− auditory canal, external 5-180
− auricle (ear) 5-180
− Bartholin's gland or cyst 5-711
− bile duct 5-514
− − for obstruction 5-513
− − with intubation 5-513
− bladder 5-571
− blood vessel 5-380
− bone 5-780
− − jaw 5-770
− − marrow 5-780
− brain 5-012
− breast 5-871
− bronchus 5-330
− bursa 5-830
− canaliculus, lacrimal 5-084
− capsule
− − lens 5-143
− carbuncle 5-882
− carotid gland (body) 5-398
− cellulitis 5-882
− cervix 5-680
− − obstetric 5-739

Incision - *continued*
- cervix 5-680 - *continued*
- - to assist delivery 5-739
- - to replace inverted uterus, postpartum
  5-759
- chalazion 5-090
- chest wall 5-340
- conjunctiva 5-111
- - extraction of foreign body 5-110
- cornea 5-121
- cystic hygroma 5-400
- drum (ear) 5-200
- ear
- - drum 5-200
- - external 5-180
- - inner 5-207
- - middle 5-202
- endolymphatic sac 5-207
- epididymis 5-639
- esophagus 5-420
- - web (endoscopic) 5-420
- exploratory - see Exploration, surgical
- external site 5-882
- extradural 5-011
- eyelid 5-090
- facial region 5-270
- fascia 5-830
- - hand 5-820
- fistula 5-491
- - anal 5-491
- floor of mouth 5-270
- furuncle (see also Incision, by site) 5-882
- - ear 5-180
- gallbladder 5-510
- gingival 5-240
- glands of skin (steatoma) 5-882
- hair follicles 5-882
- hematoma (removal)
- - abdominal wall 5-540
- - cerebral 5-011
- - ear 5-180
- - epidural 5-030
- - extradural 5-011
- - heart 5-371
- - intracranial 5-011
- - laparotomy site 5-540
- - ligament
- - - broad 5-692
- - meningeal 5-011
- - nerve root 5-030
- - pericardium 5-371
- - spinal
- - - cord 5-030
- - - meninges 5-030
- - subdural 5-011
- - thyroid 5-060
- hepatic duct 5-514

Incision - *continued*
- hordeolum 5-090
- hygroma
- - cerebral 5-011
- - epidural 5-030
- - intracranial 5-011
- - meningeal 5-011
- - nerve root 5-030
- - spinal
- - - cord 5-030
- - - meninges 5-030
- hypophysis 5-076
- hypopyon 5-121
- ingrown nail 5-882
- interosseous membrane 5-830
- iris
- - sphincter 5-135
- joint structures 5-800
- - jaw 5-770
- kidney 5-550
- lacrimal
- - gland 5-080
- - sac 5-084
- larynx 5-313
- - emergency tracheotomy 5-311
- liver 5-500
- lung 5-331
- lymph node 5-400
- lymphatic channels 5-400
- mediastinum 5-341
- meibomian gland 5-090
- muscle 5-830
- - hand 5-820
- nailbed or nailfold 5-882
- nasal septum (abscess) 5-211
- naso-pharynx 5-290
- neck
- - thyroid field 5-060
- nerve 5-040
- nose 5-211
- omentum 5-544
- orbit 5-160
- palate 5-271
- palmar (abscess) 5-820
- pancreas 5-520
- paronychia 5-882
- parotid gland 5-260
- penis 5-649
- perianal (abscess) 5-490
- perineum
- - male 5-882
- - non obstetrical 5-710
- peripheral vessel 5-380
- perirectal tissue 5-487
- perirenal tissue 5-590
- peritoneum
- - pelvic

Incision - *continued*
− peritoneum - *continued*
− − pelvic - *continued*
− − − female 5-701
− − peritonitis
− − localized 5-541
− periurethral (tissue) (abscess) 5-589
− perivesical tissue 5-591
− pilonidal sinus (cyst) 5-881
− pituitary gland 5-076
− postcorneal 5-139
− pouch of Douglas 5-701
− prostate 5-600
− pylorus 5-433
− quinsy 5-280
− rectum 5-480
− renal pelvis 5-551
− salivary gland 5-260
− scrotum (abscess) 5-610
− seminal vesicle (abscess) 5-606
− Skene's duct or gland 5-710
− skin 5-882
− − ear 5-180
− spermatic cord 5-639
− sphincter
− − cardia 5-426
− − oddi 5-518
− stomach 5-430
− suppurative adenitis 5-400
− tendon 5-830
− − sheath 5-830
− − − hand 5-820
− testis (abscess) 5-620
− thyroid (abscess) (field) 5-060
− tongue 5-259
− trachea NEC 5-313
− − emergency tracheotomy 5-311
− tunica vaginalis 5-610
− umbilicus 5-540
− ureter 5-562
− ureterovesical junction 5-561
− urethra 5-580
− vagina 5-701
− − for pelvic abscess 5-701
− − septum 5-701
− valve, heart 5-351
− vulva
− − nonobstetrical 5-710
− whitlow 5-882
− − palmar 5-820
− with
− − drainage - see Drainage
− − extraction of foreign body - see
    Extraction, foreign body, by site, with
    incision
Incompatibility reactions 2-649
Incomplete antibodies 2-611

Incontinence control 9-360
− bladder 9-360
− − electrical stimulation 9-361
− − indwelling (urethral) catheter 9-363
− − nocturnal warning system 9-362
− collecting bag 9-360
− prosthesis 5-597
Incudectomy 5-193
Incudopexy 5-193
− with fenestration 5-205
Indentation
− sclera 5-153
Index
− atherogenic 2-149
− opsonic 2-886
Indicator dilution flow measurement 1-721
Indirect
− antiglobulin test (IAGT) 2-824
− fluorescent antibody test 2-628
− hemagglutination test
− − malaria 2-754
Indoor mobility aids 9-564
Induction
− abortion 5-752
− − intra-amniotic injection 5-750
− labor 9-259
− − amniotomy 5-730
− − bag, bougie, pack 5-731
− − intra-amniotic injection 9-252
− − intrauterine injection 9-252
− − intravenous injection for drip 9-251
− − medical 9-250
− − − specified NEC 9-253
− − surgical 5-731
Infertility
− female
− − artificial insemination 9-270
− − treatment NEC 9-272
− male
− − treatment NEC 9-274
Inflation
− eustachian tube 8-173
− fallopian tube 5-667
Infolding
− scleral 5-153
Infraction
− nasal bone 8-210
− turbinate 8-210
Infrared physiotherapy 8-605
− ocular 8-605
Infundibulectomy
− cardiac 5-351
− hypophyseal 5-075
Infusion
− allogenic marrow 5-410
− cutdown 8-875
− intravenous 8-874

Ingleman-Sundberg operation 5-593
Inhalation therapy 8-751
Injection 8-589
– air
– – fallopian tube 5-667
– – peritoneum 8-733
– – pleural 8-731
– – vitreous 5-157
– alcohol
– – cauda equina 5-037
– – gasserian ganglion 5-047
– – nerve 5-047
– – sympathetic 5-052
– amniotic
– – for termination of pregnancy 5-750
– anterior chamber 8-572
– artery, arterial 8-840
– – cytotoxic 5-962
– – general action 8-841
– – local action 8-842
– – renal 8-843
– bladder
– – cytotoxic 5-965
– blepharospasm 5-099
– boiling water 5-955
– bone marrow 8-804
– – transplant 5-410
– breast 8-583
– – for augmentation (silicone) 5-873
– bursa 8-585
– cardiac 8-576
– caustic
– – endoscopic 5-953
– – prostate 8-581
– dye
– – fallopian tube 5-667
– endolymphatic 5-207
– epidural 5-037
– – destructive 5-037
– esophageal varices 5-429
– extra-amniotic
– – prostaglandin
– – – for termination of pregnancy 5-750
– extraocular 8-572
– ganglion
– – ciliary 5-133
– – cranial 5-047
– – Meckel's 5-047
– – sympathetic 5-052
– glacial acetic acid 5-952
– hypodermic 8-586
– – drug 9-122
– – local action 8-586
– into
– – bone marrow 8-578
– – hydrocele 8-582
– intra-amniotic

Injection 8-589 - continued
– intra-amniotic - continued
– – for termination of pregnancy 5-750
– – prostaglandin
– – – for termination of pregnancy 5-750
– intra-arterial - see Injection, artery
– intracranial abscess 5-010
– intramuscular 8-585
– – drug administration 9-121
– intraperitoneal
– – fetus 5-754
– intravenous 8-846
– – cut-down 8-845
– – dried plasma 8-813
– joint 8-584
– kidney 8-580
– larynx 5-310
– ligament 8-584
– local action 8-589
– lymphatic 8-577
– – breast 8-577
– muscle 8-585
– nerve 8-571
– – sympathetic 5-052
– opticociliary 5-133
– orbit 8-572
– pericardial 8-575
– peritoneal
– – cytotoxic 5-964
– phenol 5-952
– – epidural 5-037
– – peripheral nerve 5-047
– pleural
– – cytotoxic 5-963
– prostate 8-581
– retro-ocular 8-572
– saline
– – intrauterine
– – – for termination of pregnancy 5-750
– sclerosing agent 5-979
– – aneurysm 5-979
– – hemangioma 5-976
– – hemorrhoids 5-973
– – peritoneal 5-974
– – spinal 5-037
– – spleen (vessels) 5-411
– – varicose veins
– – – legs 5-971
– – vulval vein 5-975
– silicone
– – breast 5-873
– – subcutaneous 5-880
– specified tissue NEC 8-587
– spinal 8-570
– – destructive 5-037
– subarachnoid
– – cytotoxic 5-960

Injection 8-589 - *continued*
− subconjunctival 8-572
− subcutaneous 8-586
− − drug administration 9-122
− tendon 8-585
− tracheal 8-574
− trigger point 8-585
− tympanic 8-573
− varices
− − esophageal 5-429
− − gastric 5-429
− vessel 8-849
− vestibular 5-207
− vitreous segment 5-157
− vocal cord 5-310
Inlay
− cornea 5-125
− periosteal 5-786
− tooth 5-233
Inoculation
− animal
− − fungus 2-705
− − identification of bacteria 2-516
− − passage of protozoa 2-741
− − test of chemical substance 2-753
Inorganic salts
− supplement 4-479
Insemination, artificial 9-270
Insert
− dental (gold) 5-233
Insertion
− aphakia implant 5-147
− artificial eye 5-165
− bag
− − cervix
− − − following delivery or abortion (for
        hemorrhage control) 5-759
− − non-obstetric 8-503
− − obstetric 5-731
− − vagina
− − − following delivery or abortion (for
        hemorrhage control) 5-759
− band
− − intrathoracic artery 5-387
− bone traction 5-787
− breast implant 5-873
− − for augmentation 5-873
− cannula - see Cannulation
− catheter (tube) - see also Catheterization
− − bile (hepatic) ducts 5-514
− − chest 5-340
− − esophagus, permanent tube 5-428
− − intercostal 5-340
− denture
− − removable 9-302
− ear ring (by piercing) 5-988
− electrode

Insertion - *continued*
− electrode - *continued*
− − endocardial 8-880
− − endotracheal tube 8-700
− − epicardial electrodes 5-377
− − fascial sling (see also Sling operation)
        5-837
− − foraminal valve 5-356
− globe into eye socket (implant) 5-165
− heart valve
− − inert prosthesis 5-352
− − tissue graft 5-352
− intrauterine device 4-653
− keratoprosthesis 5-126
− laryngeal
− − keel 5-315
− − plate 5-315
− lens, artificial 5-147
− nail
− − for fracture 5-790
− − into bone 5-787
− nasal ring (by piercing) (ritual) 5-988
− neuropacemaker 5-039
− orbital graft, implant 5-167
− orthodontic appliance 5-246
− pacemaker (see also Pacemaker) 5-377
− pack - see also Packing
− − cervix
− − − following delivery or abortion (for
        hemorrhage control) 5-759
− − − to assist delivery 5-731
− − obstetric 5-759
− − vagina
− − − following delivery or abortion (for
        hemorrhage control) 5-759
− plate
− − into bone 5-787
− − laryngeal 5-315
− prosthesis
− − penis 5-649
− septum of heart (valve) 5-356
− suture cervix 5-674
− testicular prosthesis 5-626
− ureteral splint 5-562
− valve
− − Holter
− − − for hydrocephalus 5-023
− − Spitz-Holter 5-023
− wire
− − rectal 5-486
Insufflation
− eustachian tube 8-173
− fallopian tube 5-667
− therapeutic NEC 8-554
Insulin
− antibody assay 2-331
− serum 2-331

Insulin - *continued*
- test meal 2-301
- tolerance test 2-330
Intensive care (see also Admission, intensive care)
- monitoring 8-980
- unit 9-159
Intercricothyroidotomy 5-312
Intermittent positive pressure respiration 8-712
Interposition operation
- antethoracic (for esophagus) 5-425
- antiperistaltic 5-444
- colonic
- - esophagus 5-424
- - stomach 5-439
- foramen ovale 5-195
- jaw (lower) 5-773
- jejunal
- - to esophagus 5-424
- - to stomach 5-438
- pre-sternal (for esophagus) 5-425
- trichiasis 5-096
Interpretation
- electrocardiogram 1-266
Interview
- psychiatric 1-922
- - narcoanalysis 1-924
- sodium amobarbital 1-924
Intestine, intestinal
- enzyme activity 2-315
- fat absorption 2-313
- function test 2-319
- parasite examination method NEC 2-719
Intimectomy - see Endarterectomy
Intra-aortic
- balloon pump assistance 5-376
- counter pulsation 5-376
Intracardiac pressure recording 1-720
Intradermal
- antigen 1-704
- hypersensitivity reaction
- - antigen 1-704
Intrauterine pressure measurement 1-354
Intravenous
- blood expander 8-812
- endocardial electrode 8-880
- feeding 9-230
- - prolonged 9-232
- pace-maker 8-651
- - insertion 8-880
- transfusion 8-800
- - blood 8-801
Intubation
- bile duct 5-513
- cardia
- - by gastrotomy 5-430

Intubation - *continued*
- endotracheal 8-709
- - anesthetic 8-702
- esophagus 5-428
- eustachian tube 8-173
- gastric 8-120
- intestinal 8-124
- lacrimonasal duct 8-141
- larynx 8-709
- - emergency 8-701
- - for inhalation therapy 8-752
- - for respiration 8-701
- trachea 8-709
- - external 5-311
- transglottal
- - emergency 8-701
Intussusception reduction 5-468
Invagination
- diverticulum
- - pharynx 5-294
- - stomach 5-445
Invalid car
- provision 9-806
Invalid chair
- hand propelled 9-801
- pedal propelled 9-801
- powered (motor) 9-802
Inversion
- appendix 5-479
- diverticulum
- - duodenum 5-451
- - gastric 5-445
- - intestine 5-452
- tunica vaginalis 5-613
- uterus, replacement 5-759
Investigation
- biochemistry
- - other body fluids 2-289
- blood
- - biochemistry 2-189
- cerebrospinal fluid
- - biochemistry 2-279
- diagnostic 1-999
- hemolysis 2-829
- infectious disease 4-319
- - carrier 4-314
- - contact 4-313
- - new cases 4-312
- pancreas 2-339
- pituitary
- - blood 2-419
- - urine 2-419
- thyroid 2-409
Iodine
- protein bound in serum 2-400
- uptake 2-403
- urinary secretion 2-405

IOLI (intraocular lens implant) 5-147
Ionization 5-933
− nasal 5-931
Iridectomy 5-135
− for glaucoma 5-135
− optical 5-135
− with
− − capsulectomy 5-149
− − cataract extraction 5-145
Iridencleisis 5-132
Iridesis 5-136
Iridocapsulectomy 5-149
Iridocorneosclerectomy 5-132
Iridocyclectomy 5-133
Iridocystectomy 5-135
Iridodesis 5-136
Iridoplasty 5-136
Iridosclerectomy 5-132
Iridosclerostomy 5-135
Iridosclerotomy 5-135
Iridotomy 5-135
Iron
− absorption 2-850
− binding capacity 2-833
− blood estimation 2-835
− transport rate, plasma 2-853
Iron lung 8-710
Irradiation
− blood cells
− − extracorporeal 8-856
− infrared 8-600
− interstitial
− − abdominal lymph nodes (requires
   radiology code) 5-404
− − bladder (requires radiology code)
   5-574
− − cervix (requires radiology code) 5-679
− − hypophysis (requires radiology code)
   5-075
− − pituitary (requires radiology code)
   5-075
− − pleural (requires radiology code)
   5-343

Irradiation - continued
− intracavitary
− − abdominal (requires radiology code)
   5-543
− − uterine body (requires radiology code)
   5-681
− − vaginal (requires radiology code)
   5-702
− ultraviolet 8-621
Irrigation 8-179
− anterior chamber 8-152
− antrum 8-174
− bladder 8-132
− cataract 5-143
− corpus cavernosum 5-649
− nasal sinus 8-174
− rectal 8-127
− stomach 8-123
− tendon sheath 5-830
− − hand 5-820
− ventricular shunt 8-151
Irritant introduction
− pericardial 5-363
− pleural 5-345
Irving's operation 5-664
Irwin's operation 5-831
Ischiopubiotomy 5-781
Isoenzymes 2-450
Isolation 4-309
− aerobic (bacteria) 2-506
− anaerobic (bacteria) 2-507
− carrier (infectious disease) 4-302
− contact (infectious disease) 4-301
− infectious disease 4-309
− intestinal segment 5-453
− patient
− − immunosuppressed 4-303
− − infectious disease 4-300
Isoleucine
− serum identification 2-100
Isomerase 2-483
Isthmectomy, thyroid 5-062

J

Janeway's operation 5-432
Jejunectomy 5-454
Jejunocecostomy 5-458
Jejunocholecystostomy 5-512
Jejunocholedochostomy 5-512
Jejunocolostomy 5-458
Jejunoesophagostomy
– intrathoracic 5-424
Jejunogastrostomy
– without gastrectomy 5-442
Jejunoileostomy 5-457

Jejunojejunostomy 5-457
– end to end 5-454
– proximal to distal 5-454
Jejunorrhaphy 5-467
Jejunostomy 5-463
– closure 5-465
Jejunotomy 5-450
Jejunotransverse colostomy 5-458
Jet injector gun 8-586
Judet's operation 5-816

K

Kahn test 2-602
Karyotype 2-923
– computer assisted 2-926
– fluorescent method 2-924
Kates-Kessel operation 5-813
Kay-Shiley valve 5-352
Keller-Kennedy operation 5-592
Keller's operation 5-813
Kelly-Stoeckel operation 5-592
Kelotomy 5-539
– with bowel exteriorization 5-460
Keratectomy (complete) (partial)
  (superficial) 5-123
Keratomileusis 5-126
Keratoplasty 5-125
– lamellar 5-125
– penetrating 5-125
– refractive 5-126
Keratotomy 5-121

Keratotomy 5-121 - *continued*
– delimiting 5-121
– skin 5-903
Ketostix 2-240
Kidney
– erythropoietic factor 2-349
– function (see also Specific chemical
  procedure) 2-349
Kineplasty
– eye muscle 5-109
– revision of amputation stump 5-850
King-Armstrong units 2-472
– acid phosphatase 2-473
Kiotomy 5-276
Kitchen aids 9-561
Kleihauer test 2-843
Kronlein's operation 5-160
Kuhnt-Szymanowski's operation 5-093
Kustner's operation 5-759

L

Labbe's operation 5-430
Labiectomy 5-715
− bilateral 5-715
Labiorrhaphy 5-898
Labyrinthectomy 5-207
Labyrinthotomy 5-207
− transtympanic 5-207
Lactate dehydrogenase 2-450
Lactobacillus casei assay
− folic acid 2-571
Lactobacillus leichmannii assay
− vitamin B 12 2-570
Lactose absorption 2-311
Lagrange's operation 5-132
Lambrinudi's operation 5-811
Laminectomy 5-030
− opening dura 5-030
− with excision
− − intervertebral disc 5-803
Laminotomy 5-030
Lange test 2-274
Laparorrhaphy, delayed 5-545
Laparoscopy 1-694
− via pouch of Douglas 1-696
Laparotomy 5-541
− exploratory 5-541
− pelvic 5-541
− reopening of recent operative site 5-541
Laparotrachelotomy 5-741
Laryngectomy 5-302
− complete or total 5-303
− partial 5-302
− radical 5-304
− wide field 5-304
Laryngocentesis 5-310
Laryngoesophagectomy 5-304
Laryngofissure 5-313
Laryngopharyngectomy NEC 5-304
Laryngoplasty 5-315
Laryngorrhaphy 5-315
Laryngoscopy 1-610
− direct 1-612
− foreign body removal 8-105
− indirect 1-611
− suspension 1-614
Laryngostomy 5-313
Laryngotomy 5-313
Laryngotracheostomy
− permanent 5-312
Laryngotracheotomy

Laryngotracheotomy - *continued*
− emergency 5-311
− permanent opening 5-312
− temporary 5-311
Lash' operation 5-674
Latex
− agglutination 2-752
− − trypanosome 2-752
− fixation 2-663
Lavage
− bronchus 8-175
− endotracheal 8-709
− gastric 8-123
− intestinal 8-861
− − for dialysis 8-861
− maxillary antrum
− − puncture 5-220
− − wash-out 5-220
− peritoneal 8-157
− − cavity 8-157
− − dialysis 8-860
− trachea 8-175
LE cells test 2-872
Le Fort-Cleisis operation 5-703
Le Fort's operation 5-763
Lead
− blood
− − estimation 2-153
− in paintwork 2-949
Lecithin sphingomyelin ratio test 2-286
Lengthening
− bone 5-789
− fascia 5-837
− − hand 5-828
− heel cord 5-837
− ligament 5-819
− − broad 5-693
− muscle 5-837
− − eye 5-100
− − hand 5-828
− − levator palpebrae 5-094
− palate 5-275
− tendon 5-837
− − Achilles 5-837
− − hand 5-828
Lensectomy 5-146
Leucine
− serum identification 2-100
Leucocytes (see also Blood, white cell)
− agglutination 2-641

Leucocytes - *continued*
- enzyme activity 2-887
- indirect staining 2-883
- migration 2-641
- serotyping 2-641
Leucocytotoxic antiserum 2-640
Leucotomy (frontal) (subfrontal) (standard) (bimedial) 5-012
Levadopa test
- growth hormone 2-413
Levator muscle
- eyelid operation 5-094
- pelvic operation 5-593
Levulose
- tolerance 2-323
Liberation
- compressed nerve 5-043
Ligation
- adenoid 5-289
- aneurysm 5-387
- - brain 5-387
- artery 5-387
- - aberrant renal 5-557
- - adrenal 5-073
- - meningeal 5-021
- - orbit 5-169
- - thyroid 5-069
- auricle, heart 5-357
- bronchus 5-339
- coronary
- - fistula 5-369
- - sinus 5-363
- ductus arteriosus, patent 5-387
- esophageal varices 5-429
- fallopian tube
- - bilateral 5-664
- - remaining tube 5-664
- - unilateral 5-669
- fistula
- - arteriovenous 5-387
- - coronary 5-369
- funiculus (bilateral) 5-981
- - unilateral 5-636
- hemangioma
- - intracranial 5-387
- hemorrhoids 5-493
- lymphatics 5-409
- pericardium 5-374
- sinus
- - coronary 5-363
- - lateral 5-021
- - longitudinal 5-021
- spermatic cord
- - varicocele 5-630
- supernumerary digit 8-187
- thoracic duct 5-405
- thyroid (polar) 5-069

Ligation - *continued*
- tonsil 5-289
- transesophageal 5-429
- tubal 5-664
- - endoscopic 5-663
- ureter 5-569
- varicocele 5-630
- vas deferens (bilateral) 5-981
- - unilateral 5-636
- vein 5-387
- - abdominal, cava 5-386
- - cava, inferior 5-386
- - saphenous 5-387
- - scrotum
- - - varicose 5-630
- - varicose 5-384
- - - esophagus 5-429
- - with stripping 5-384
- vessel
- - esophageal 5-429
- - intra-abdominal, vena cava 5-386
- - peptic ulcer 5-443
- - splenic 5-387
- wart 8-187
Light coagulation (see also Photocoagulation)
- iris 5-135
- pupil formation 5-135
Lillehei-Kaster valve 5-352
Limb length
- measurement 1-361
Lingulectomy (lung) 5-323
Lip
- shave, leukoplakia 5-279
Lip reading training 9-416
Lipase 2-471
Lipectomy
- subcutaneous tissue 5-901
Lipids
- blood
- - total 2-140
Lipoprotein 2-144
- blood 2-144
Lithium
- blood 2-156
Litholapaxy
- bladder 5-570
- - with incision 5-571
Lithotomy
- bile duct 5-513
- bladder (urinary) 5-570
- - with incision 5-571
- gallbladder 5-510
- hepatic duct 5-513
- kidney 5-550
- pancreatic duct 5-520
- renal pelvis 5-551

Lithotomy - *continued*
- salivary gland 5-260
- ureter 5-562
- urethra 5-580
Lithotripsy 5-570
- bladder 5-570
Liver
- artificial 8-859
- profile tests 2-326
- transplant 5-504
Loan of equipment
- bedpan 9-811
- crutches 9-812
- medical 9-810
- walking frame 9-812
Lobar spirometry 1-710
Lobectomy
- brain 5-014
- liver 5-502
- lung
- - complete 5-324
- - partial 5-323
- parotid
- - superficial 5-262
- salivary gland 5-262
- thyroid 5-061
Lobotomy (brain) (prefrontal) 5-012
Localization
- placenta 1-355
Loop
- colostomy 5-460
- ileal stoma 5-462
Lorenz operation 5-781
Low protein diet
- prophylactic 4-463
LSAR test 2-286
Luc, caldwell operation 5-222
Lung
- artificial 5-396

Lung - *continued*
- compliance 1-712
- transplant 5-335
Lupus erythematosus cells, identification
  2-872
Luteinizing hormone
- release factor 2-415
- response 2-415
Lymph
- examination 2-280
- node
- - fluid, for parasites 2-724
- - smear 2-800
Lymphadenectomy 5-401
- axillary
- - regional 5-402
- - simple 5-401
- radical 5-404
- regional 5-402
Lymphadenotomy 5-400
Lymphangiectomy 5-401
Lymphangioplasty 5-409
Lymphangiorrhaphy 5-409
Lymphangiotomy 5-400
Lymphaticostomy 5-409
Lymphocyte(s)
- culture 2-873
- E binding 2-870
- reactive B 2-871
- rosette inhibition test 2-874
- thymus dependent 2-870
- transfer test 2-642
- transformation test 2-873
- types 2-879
Lymphocytotoxicity 2-640
Lymphoedema
- excision with graft 5-409
- obliteration of lymphatics 5-409
Lysozyme 2-484

M

MacDonald's operation 5-674
MacKee's operation 5-815
MacLagan units 2-321
MacReynold's operation 5-122
Macroglobulin
– estimation
– – serum 2-104
Macrophage
– mobility
– – electrophoretic 2-886
Magnesium
– balance 2-351
– blood 2-156
Magnet extraction of foreign body
– anterior chamber 5-131
– anterior eye 5-131
– choroid 5-151
– ciliary body 5-131
– cornea 5-120
– iris 5-131
– lens 5-140
– posterior eye 5-151
– retina 5-151
– vitreous 5-151
Magnetometer
– foreign body search 1-820
Maintenance
– circulation 8-815
– posture 9-341
Male genital system
– clinical examination
– – in-depth 1-340
Malleo-stapedopexy 5-193
Mammectomy - see Mastectomy
Mammilliplasty 5-872
Mammoplasty 5-875
– amputative (reduction) 5-874
– augmentation 5-873
– implant (silastic) 5-873
– reconstructive 5-875
– size-reduction 5-874
Mammotomy 5-871
Manganese
– blood 2-156
Manipulation 8-299
– abdominal 8-534
– antenatal 8-250
– bowel
– – hernia 8-241
– – prolapse 8-242

Manipulation 8-299 - *continued*
– calculus
– – salivary (parotid) (submandibular)
   8-532
– catheter
– – urinary bladder 8-133
– dislocation (joint) 8-209
– dislocation, reduction 8-209
– endoscopic 8-533
– esophagus 5-428
– external 8-530
– fracture - see Reduction, fracture
– hernia 8-241
– obstetric 8-259
– osteopathic 8-292
– temporomandibular joint 8-211
– under anesthesia 8-217
– ureteral calculus by catheter 5-560
Mannitol dehydration
– vitreous 5-157
Manometry
– esophageal 1-313
– spinal fluid 1-206
Manual arts therapy 9-500
Marshall-Marchetti-Krantz operation 5-595
Marsupialization
– abscess
– – liver 5-501
Masking
– hearing test 1-233
Massage 9-471
– heart
– – closed chest 8-520
– – external 8-520
– – open 5-379
– prostatic 8-535
– skeletal 8-536
Mast cell degradation 2-652
Mastectomy 5-869
– complete 5-861
– – simple 5-861
– extended
– – radical 5-864
– – simple (modified radical) 5-862
– for gynecomastia 5-869
– partial 5-860
– preserving nipple 5-865
– radical 5-863
– – modified 5-862
– segmental 5-860

Mastectomy 5-869 - *continued*
- simple 5-861
- subcutaneous 5-869
- - with prosthesis 5-865
Mastoidectomy 5-203
- complete 5-203
- - secondary 5-203
- conservative
- - simple 5-203
- radical (modified) 5-203
- revision 5-209
- simple 5-203
- with deep exposure 5-204
Mastoidotomy 5-202
Mastopexy 5-875
Mastoplasty - see Mammoplasty
Mastorrhaphy 5-875
Mastotomy 5-871
Maternal
- exercise in preparation for delivery 4-697
- health
- - care - see also Prenatal care and
     Postnatal care
- - education activities NEC 4-695
- instruction 4-695
- - mothercraft (to group) 4-691
- - - individual 4-690
- - nutrition 4-692
Maxillectomy 5-772
Maximum
- breathing capacity 1-711
- force exerted 1-751
- grip 1-751
McLean test 2-130
Mean corpuscular volume 2-813
Measles
- immunization 4-350
Measurement
- airways resistance 1-712
- central venous pressure 1-272
- facial
- - for spectacles 9-321
- intelligence 1-930
- limb length 1-361
- lung volume 1-710
- portal venous pressure 1-733
- pressure
- - intrauterine 1-354
- range of movements 1-362
- skin fold thickness 1-952
- skin temperature 1-370
Meatoplasty
- aural 5-185
- - correction of atresia 5-185
- urethral 5-583
Meatotomy
- aural 5-180

Meatotomy - *continued*
- ureter 5-561
- urethra 5-581
Mediastinoscopy 1-691
Mediastinotomy (anterior) 5-341
Medical attention
- initial
- - inpatient 1-11-
- - newborn 1-191
- - - with Apgar scoring 1-192
- - other patient 1-12-
- - outpatient 1-10-
- subsequent
- - inpatient 1-14-
- - other patient 1-15-
- - outpatient 1-13-
Medical social worker 9-719
Meloplasty 5-900
- auricular reconstruction 5-186
Membrane filtration concentration
- microfilaria 2-722
Membranectomy
- lens 5-149
Meningeorrhaphy, spinal 5-034
Meningococcal antibody
- assay 2-680
Meniscectomy 5-804
- temporomandibular 5-774
Menstrual extraction 8-165
Mentoplasty 5-899
- bony 5-775
Mercury
- blood 2-156
Mesopexy 5-546
Metabolic
- function test 1-769
- unit 9-153
Metallo-organic compounds
- blood 2-164
Metatarsectomy NEC 5-784
- hallux valgus 5-782
Methemoglobin 2-832
Methionine
- serum identification 2-100
Methyl mercury 2-164
- blood 2-164
Methylcrotonyl carboxylase 2-483
Methylene blue
- bladder instillation (diagnostic) 1-803
- reductase test 2-508
Metroplasty 5-695
Metyrapone test
- pituitary response 2-410
Micro-organism(s)
- antibiotic susceptibility 2-539
- culture 2-506
- detection 2-509

Micro-organism(s) - *continued*
 - dye test 2-508
 - identification 2-519
 - isolation 2-509
 - unstained microscopic examination 2-500
Microbiological assay 2-579
 - folic acid 2-571
 - vitamin
 - - other 2-572
 - vitamin b 12 2-570
Microdochectomy 5-515
Microfilarial count 2-727
Microinjector
 - automated 9-123
Microlaryngoscopy 1-613
Microscopy
 - polarizing
 - - histology 2-901
Mikulicz operation
 - for colon 5-460
Miles operation 5-484
Milk
 - serum antibody 2-631
Miller's operation 5-594
Millin-Reed operation 5-594
Millin's operation 5-603
Millon test
 - urine 2-200
Minerva 8-359
 - foam 8-359
 - plaster (of Paris) 8-312
Mist therapy 8-750
Mixed leucocyte culture 2-641
Mobilization
 - bowel 5-544
 - conjunctival flaps 5-113
 - joint
 - - operative 5-801
 - - passive 9-464
 - neostrophingic mitral valve 5-353
 - spine
 - - passive 9-465
 - stapes 5-190
 - testis 5-624
 - transcrural
 - - stapes 5-190
Monitoring 8-990
 - blood sampling, continuous (for anterior
   pituitary hormones) 8-945
 - cardiac 8-949
 - - emergency 8-940
 - central venous pressure 8-942
 - circulation (see also Monitoring, cardiac)
   8-949
 - clinical 8-990
 - dehydration 8-903
 - diabetic

Monitoring 8-990 - *continued*
 - diabetic - *continued*
 - - crisis 8-901
 - - stabilization 8-902
 - electrocardiographic, continuous 8-941
 - electronic 8-981
 - esophageal electrode (heart) 8-941
 - fetal heart during labor 8-961
 - head injury 8-920
 - heart - see Monitoring, cardiac
 - hemolysis 8-904
 - hunger strike 8-905
 - intensive care 8-980
 - intracranial pressure 8-922
 - intrapleural pressure 8-931
 - metabolic 8-909
 - - crisis 8-900
 - - - diabetes 8-901
 - neurological 8-929
 - - epidural transducer 8-922
 - - fibrinogen degradation screening
   8-921
 - - head injury 8-920
 - - intracranial pressure 8-922
 - - subdural pressure transducer 8-922
 - obstetric 8-969
 - - trial labor 8-960
 - pletismographic (impedance)
   (photoelectric oxymeter) 8-944
 - prolonged fasting 8-905
 - psychiatric 8-919
 - renal function 8-950
 - respiration 8-930
 - spinal pressure 8-922
 - starvation 8-905
Moore's operation 5-816
Morbid anatomy 2-950
Morcellement
 - femoral hernia 5-530
Morgan's operation 5-595
Moschcowitz operation 5-707
Motor vehicle
 - adaptation for invalid 9-807
Mountain resort
 - sanatorium 8-770
Mouth to mouth resuscitation 8-721
Movement
 - under anesthesia 8-217
Moxibustion 8-606
Mucopolysaccharide
 - blood 2-134
Mucoprotein
 - blood 2-134
Multiphasic screening 4-270
Muscle power
 - testing 1-205
Musculoplasty 5-837

Musculoplasty 5-837 - *continued*
— mastoid 5-199
Mustard's operation 5-357
Mycological examination 2-709
— culture 2-701
— detection 2-700
— identification 2-702
— method NEC 2-709
Myectomy (see also Excision, muscle) 5-833
— hand 5-823
— lesion 5-832
— — hand 5-822
— levator palpebrae 5-094
— ocular (oblique) (rectus) 5-101
Myelotomy
— stereotactic (longitudinal) (intermittent)
  5-032
Myocardial oxygen consumption 1-276
Myocardiectomy
— infarct 5-373
Myomectomy 5-681
— broad ligament 5-692
— uterus 5-681
Myoplasty 5-837
— hand 5-828

Myorrhaphy 5-835
— hand 5-824
Myosuture 5-835
— hand 5-824
Myotasis 5-839
— hand 5-829
Myotenoplasty 5-837
— hand 5-828
Myotenotomy 5-830
— hand 5-820
— Achilles 5-830
Myotomy 5-830
— cardia (esophagus) 5-426
— for division 5-831
— hand 5-820
— levator palpebrae 5-094
— ocular (oblique) (rectus) 5-100
Myringectomy 5-204
Myringo-malleo-labyrinthopexy 5-205
Myringodectomy 5-204
Myringoplasty 5-194
Myringostapediopexy 5-195
Myringotomy 5-200

N

Nail
– digit
– – removal 8-186
– metallic content 2-940
– mycological examination 2-700
– removal from bone 5-788
– – fracture 8-389
Nailing
– bone
– – closed fracture 8-362
– – for arthrodesis 8-362
– epiphysis 8-362
– fracture
– – blind 5-790
– – closed 5-790
– – open reduction 5-792
– intramedullary 5-787
– intramedullary (bone) 8-362
Napier test 2-629
Narcoanalysis 1-924
Narrowing
– palpebral fissure 5-092
Nasal challenge
– allergy 1-706
Nasal feeding 9-233
Needle
– biopsy - see Biopsy, non surgical
Needling
– anterior capsule (lens) 5-143
– lens 5-143
Neer's operation (humeral prosthesis)
  5-789
Nephelometry 2-494
Nephrectomy
– complete 5-554
– partial 5-553
Nephrocolopexy 5-556
Nephrocystanastomosis 5-557
Nephrolithotomy 5-550
Nephrolysis 5-559
Nephropexy 5-556
– with partial nephrectomy 5-553
Nephroplasty 5-557
Nephropyeloplasty 5-557
Nephropyeloureterostomy 5-557
Nephrorrhaphy 5-557
Nephrostomy 5-550
– closure 5-557
Nephrotomy 5-550
Nephroureterectomy 5-554

Nephroureterocystectomy 5-554
Nerve
– block (peripheral) 5-047
– – anesthesia 8-891
– – sympathetic 5-052
– conduction testing 1-203
Neuraminidase
– inhibition 2-623
Neurectasis (peripheral) 5-049
Neurectomy (selective) (sacral) (presacral)
  5-040
– intraspinal root 5-031
– opticociliary 5-133
– paracervical 5-694
– sympathetic 5-051
– tympanic 5-209
Neurexeresis - see Neurectomy
Neuroanastomosis 5-046
– hypoglossal facial 5-044
Neurological unit 9-152
Neurolysis
– carpal tunnel 5-043
– peripheral 5-043
Neuromuscular re-education 9-430
Neuroplasty (peripheral) 5-046
Neuropraxy 5-040
Neurorrhaphy 5-042
Neurosurgery 5-029
Neurotomy 5-040
– lacrimal branch (parasympathetic) 5-050
Neurotripsy (peripheral) 5-040
Neutralization
– virus 2-620
Neutralizing antibodies
– serum 2-624
Newborn
– Apgar scoring 1-190
– – with other initial medical evaluation
  1-192
– birthweight recording 1-193
– crown-heel length recording 1-194
– in hospital care 1-199
– initial medical evaluation 1-191
– – with apgar scoring 1-192
– measurement NEC 1-195
– subsequent care 1-198
Night hospital care 9-170
Nitro blue tetrazolium test 2-885
Nitrogen
– balance 2-350

Nitrogen - *continued*
− nonprotein in blood 2-110
− washout 1-710
Noble's operation 5-446
Nocturnal warning system
− for urinary incontinence 9-362
Nodulectomy
− thyroid 5-062
Nonne-Apelt test 2-274
Nonprotein nitrogen
− total
− − blood 2-110
Notched lip operation 5-898
Nothing by mouth 9-140
Notification
− infectious disease 4-312
− local disease 4-509
− ophthalmia 4-500
Nucleus-cytoplasm ratio 2-920
Nursing
− care 9-209
− − intensive level 9-200

Nursing - *continued*
− care 9-209 - *continued*
− − intermediate level 9-202
− − − dressings 9-204
− − − incontinence care 9-203
− − − injections 9-205
− − − irrigation 9-204
− − routine level
− − − aid to self-care patients 9-207
− − − bathing patient 9-207
− − − enema 9-206
− psychological 9-709
− services
− − drug administration 9-120
− − massage 8-539
− supervision 9-201
Nutrition
− assessment 1-959
− parenteral 9-230
− − prolonged 9-232
Nylon strap fixation
− fracture 5-792

O

Obliteration
- aneurysm 5-387
- bone cavity 5-789
- cavity
- - bone 5-789
- - mandible 5-773
- cul-de-sac 5-707
- ductus arteriosus 5-387
- lung cavity 5-332
- lymphatics 5-409
- orbit 5-167
- pleura 5-345
- pouch of Douglas 5-707
- skene's gland 5-712
- vagina 5-703
- - cul-de-sac 5-707
Observation
- psychiatric 8-910
Obturator
- dental 8-561
- - introduction 8-561
- palatal 8-560
Occlusal moulds
- diagnostic 1-302
Occlusion
- oviducts
- - endoscopic 5-663
- - laparotomy 5-664
- patent ductus arteriosus 5-387
Occult blood
- feces 2-263
Occupational therapy 9-529
Ocular
- muscle function testing 1-216
- tissues
- - examination
- - - for parasites 2-730
Odontectomy 5-231
Odontotomy (prophylactic) 5-245
- with removal of tooth 5-231
Oleothorax 5-332
Omentectomy 5-543
Omentofixation 5-546
Omentopexy 5-546
Omentoplasty 5-546
Omentorrhaphy 5-546
Omentotomy 5-544
Omphalectomy 5-542
Onychectomy 8-186
Onychotomy 5-882

Oophorectomy 5-652
- bilateral 5-654
- partial 5-651
- unilateral 5-652
- with
- - hysterectomy 5-683
- - removal
- - - tube (fallopian) 5-653
- - salpingectomy 5-653
Oophorocystectomy 5-651
Oophorohysterectomy 5-683
Oophoropexy 5-656
Oophoroplasty 5-656
Oophororrhaphy 5-656
Oophorostomy 5-656
Oophorotomy 5-650
Open heart 5-359
- massage 5-379
- technique
- - valve 5-354
- - with
- - - coronary perfusion 5-379
- - - hypothermia 5-379
Open reduction
- dislocation 5-796
- - jaw 5-779
- - with bone graft 5-796
- fracture 5-791
- - alveolar 5-764
- - facial NEC 5-767
- - jaw 5-763
- - limb 5-791
- - - multiple 5-797
- - limb with internal fixation 5-792
- - multiple 5-797
- - multiple limbs 5-797
- - nasal bone 5-216
- - orbital 5-765
- - - with graft or implant 5-765
- - pelvis
- - - with internal injuries 5-797
- - - with limb bones 5-797
- - skull 5-020
- - - with limb bones 5-797
- - thorax
- - - with internal injuries 5-797
- - - with limb bones 5-797
- - with internal fixation 5-792
- - zygoma, zygomatic 5-761
- separated epiphysis 5-794

Open reduction - *continued*
- separated epiphysis 5-794 - *continued*
- - with nailing 5-794
- skull 5-020
Opening
- bony labyrinth 5-207
- cranial suture 5-020
- dura
- - spinal 5-030
- mitral valve
- - closed technique 5-350
- - open heart technique 5-354
- saccus endolymphaticus 5-207
- valve, heart (manual) 5-350
Operation (of)
- abandoned before onset 5-994
- abdomen 5-549
- abdominal wall 5-549
- adrenal 5-073
- antenatal 5-759
- antepartum 5-759
- anterior chamber 5-139
- antrum
- - maxillary 5-229
- anus 5-499
- aorta 5-399
- aponeurosis 5-839
- - hand 5-829
- appendix 5-479
- artery 5-399
- arytenoid 5-319
- atrium (heart) 5-379
- auricle
- - ear 5-189
- - heart 5-379
- biliary tract 5-519
- bladder 5-579
- bone 5-789
- - marrow 5-418
- brain 5-029
- breast 5-879
- bronchus 5-339
- buccal cavity 5-279
- bursa 5-839
- - hand 5-829
- canthus 5-092
- capsule
- - joint 5-809
- carotid body 5-398
- cecum 5-469
- cervix 5-679
- chest wall 5-349
- chorda tympani 5-209
- chordae tendinae 5-354
- choroid 5-156
- cilia
- - eyelash 5-096

Operation - *continued*
- ciliary body 5-139
- cochlea 5-209
- colon 5-469
- completion 5-999
- conjunctiva 5-119
- cord
- - vocal 5-319
- cornea 5-129
- cricoid 5-319
- dental 5-249
- ear 5-209
- - external 5-189
- - inner 5-209
- - middle 5-209
- endocrine 5-079
- epididymis NEC 5-639
- esophagus 5-429
- eyeball 5-169
- eyelid 5-099
- fallopian tube 5-669
- fascia 5-839
- - hand 5-829
- fetus
- - intrauterine 5-755
- gallbladder 5-519
- genital system
- - male 5-649
- globus pallidus 5-013
- glomus coccygeum 5-884
- glomus jugulare 5-398
- gum 5-242
- heart 5-379
- - mitral valve 5-359
- - open 5-379
- - septum 5-359
- - valve 5-359
- - wall 5-379
- hydrocele 5-619
- incus 5-193
- intervertebral disc 5-803
- intestine 5-469
- iris 5-139
- jaw 5-779
- joint 5-859
- kidney 5-559
- lacrimal apparatus 5-089
- lacrimal gland 5-082
- larynx 5-319
- later stages 5-999
- lens 5-149
- lip 5-279
- liver 5-509
- lung 5-339
- lymphatic system 5-409
- mediastinum 5-349
- meninges

Operation - *continued*
- meninges - *continued*
- - cerebral 5-029
- - spinal 5-039
- mouth 5-279
- multiple systems 5-859
- muscle 5-839
- - hand 5-829
- - ocular 5-109
- musculoskeletal 5-859
- nasopharyngeal 5-299
- nerve 5-049
- nervous system 5-059
- nose 5-219
- not completed 5-995
- not elsewhere classified 5-909
- obstetric 5-759
- orbit 5-169
- orthopedic 5-859
- ortodontic 5-247
- ossicular chain 5-193
- ovary 5-659
- palate 5-279
- pancreas 5-529
- parathyroid 5-069
- penis 5-649
- pericardium 5-379
- perineum
- - female 5-719
- periodontium 5-242
- pharynx 5-299
- pleura 5-349
- plexus
- - brachial 5-049
- - cervical 5-049
- - choroid 5-029
- - tympanic 5-209
- postpartum 5-759
- prostate 5-608
- rectum 5-489
- - sphincter saving 5-485
- renal pelvis 5-559
- retina 5-156
- salivary gland 5-269
- sclera 5-139
- scrotum 5-619
- second stage 5-999
- sinus
- - nasal 5-229
- skin 5-908
- small intestine 5-469
- specified NEC 5-909
- spermatic cord 5-639
- spleen 5-419
- stomach 5-449
- subcutaneous tissue 5-908
- suprarenal gland 5-073

Operation - *continued*
- surgical
- - before foreign travel (preventive) 5-982
- - preventive 5-982
- - - appendectomy 5-982
- - prophylactic 5-982
- sympathetic 5-053
- tendon 5-839
- - hand 5-829
- testis 5-629
- thoracic duct 5-405
- thymus 5-079
- thyroid 5-069
- tongue 5-259
- tonsil 5-289
- tooth 5-249
- trachea 5-319
- tunica vaginalis 5-619
- umbilical cord, to assist delivery 5-739
- ureter 5-569
- urethra 5-589
- urinary tract 5-599
- uterine supports 5-699
- uterus 5-699
- uvula 5-276
- vagina 5-709
- vas deferens 5-639
- vessel 5-399
- vitreous 5-157
- vulva 5-719
Operation
- Aldridge-Studdiford 5-594
- Ammon
- - blepharoplasty 5-096
- - dacriocystotomy 5-084
- - ectropion correction 5-093
- - enlargement palpebral fissure 5-092
- - epicanthus correction 5-092
- Baffe 5-357
- Bassini 5-530
- Beck 5-363
- Belsey 5-538
- Billroth I 5-436
- Billroth II 5-437
- Blalock 5-390
- Blalock-Hanlon 5-355
- Blalock-Taussig 5-390
- Boston 5-855
- Boyd 5-847
- Bricker 5-564
- Brooke 5-462
- Bunnell
- - tendon transplant 5-825
- Burgess 5-847
- Caldwell-Luc 5-222
- Callander 5-848

Operation - *continued*
- Charnley 5-815
- Chopart 5-846
- Dragstedt
- - ileostomy 5-462
- - vagotomy 5-440
- Dunn 5-811
- Durham 5-831
- Effler 5-363
- Eicher 5-816
- Finney 5-441
- Frank 5-432
- Fredt-Ramstedt 5-433
- Gill, shoulder 5-812
- Goebel-Frangenheim-Stoeckel 5-594
- Grice 5-811
- Gritti-Stokes 5-848
- Guildford 5-191
- Harrington 5-810
- Hartmann 5-485
- Haultain 5-759
- Heinecke-Mikulicz 5-441
- Heller 5-426
- Henley 5-438
- Hey 5-846
- Hibbs, spinal fusion 5-810
- Hoke 5-811
- Holth 5-132
- Hough 5-191
- House 5-191
- Hufnagel 5-352
- Ingleman-Sundberg 5-593
- Irving 5-664
- Irwin 5-831
- Janeway 5-432
- Judet 5-816
- Kates-Kessel 5-813
- Keller 5-813
- Keller-Kennedy 5-592
- Keller-Stoeckel 5-592
- Kronlein 5-160
- Kuhnt-Szymanowski 5-093
- Kustner 5-759
- Labbe 5-430
- Lagrange 5-132
- Lambrinudi 5-811
- Lash 5-674
- Le Fort 5-763
- Le Fort-Cleisis 5-703
- Lorenz 5-781
- Luc-Caldwell 5-222
- MacDonald 5-674
- MacKee 5-815
- MacReynold 5-122
- Marshall-Marchetti-Krantz 5-595
- Mikulicz
- - for colon 5-460

Operation - *continued*
- Miles 5-484
- Miller 5-594
- Millin 5-603
- Millin-Reed 5-594
- Moore 5-816
- Morgan 5-595
- Moschcowitz 5-707
- Mustard 5-357
- Neer 5-789
- Noble 5-546
- Paul-Mikulicz 5-460
- Pereyra 5-596
- Pirogoff 5-847
- Polya 5-437
- Pomeroy 5-664
- Potts-Smith 5-390
- Rankin 5-484
- Rashkind 5-355
- Ring 5-815
- Roux-Herzen-Judine 5-425
- Rubin 5-667
- Rush 5-787
- Saemisch 5-121
- Scanzoni 5-724
- Schanz
- - osteotomy 5-781
- Schauta-Amreich 5-686
- Scheie 5-132
- Schlatter 5-439
- Schukneckt 5-191
- Sengstaken 5-428
- Shea 5-191
- Shirodkar, suture 5-674
- Slocum 5-848
- Smith 5-493
- Sondergaard 5-357
- Spinelli 5-759
- Spivack
- - gastrostomy 5-432
- Ssabanejev-Frank 5-432
- Stamm-Kader 5-432
- Stanmore, hip 5-815
- Steinberg 5-444
- Strayer 5-831
- Stromeyer-Little 5-500
- Summerskill 5-087
- Swenson 5-483
- - cystoplasty 5-577
- Syme 5-847
- Thompson, hip 5-816
- Torek 5-624
- Torkildsen 5-022
- Toti 5-087
- Trendelenburg
- - pulmonary embolism 5-380
- - varicose veins 5-384

Operation - *continued*
− Urban 5-864
− Vineberg 5-362
− von Kraske 5-485
− Waterston 5-390
− Weir 5-479
− Wertheim 5-685
− West 5-087
− Wharton-Jones 5-096
− Wheeler 5-093
− Whipple 5-526
− Whitehead 5-493
− Yount 5-831
− Ziegler 5-135
Operculectomy 5-242
Ophrioplasty 5-096
Ophthalmectomy 5-163
Ophthalmodynamometry 1-225
Ophthalmoscopy 1-220
Opponens plasty 5-827
Opsonic index 2-886
Orbitotomy 5-160
− intracranial approach 5-160
− transfrontal 5-160
Orchidectomy 5-622
− bilateral 5-623
− − for sterilization 5-981
− remaining testis 5-623
− unilateral 5-622
Orchidopexy 5-624
Orchidoplasty 5-625
Orchidorrhaphy 5-625
Orchidotomy 5-620
Orchiochalasia 5-624
Orchiopexy 5-624
Organ puncture
− for parasites 2-735
Organized games 9-542
Orthopedic procedure 8-489
− compensation for deformity 8-231
Orthoptic
− examination 1-216
− exercises 9-400
− training 9-400
Osmotic fragility
− red blood cells 2-812
Ossiculectomy (partial) 5-193
− stapes 5-191
− with fenestration 5-205
Ossiculotomy 5-193
Ostectomy 5-784
− complete 5-785
− jaw (lower)
− − ramisection 5-775
− − upper
− − − with reconstruction 5-775
− − with reconstruction 5-773

Ostectomy 5-784 - *continued*
− partial 5-784
− − jaw (lower) 5-773
− − − upper 5-772
− − nasal sinus 5-772
− − premandibular 5-773
− wedge - see Ostectomy, partial
Osteoarthrotomy 5-781
− jaw 5-774
Osteoclasis 5-789
Osteolysis 5-789
− jaw 5-779
Osteopathy, manipulation 8-291
Osteoplasty 5-789
− jaw (lower) 5-773
− − upper 5-775
− mandible 5-773
− nasal bones 5-226
− skull 5-020
Osteorrhaphy 5-789
− jaw 5-775
Osteosynthesis 5-789
− bone graft 5-786
− metallic 5-787
− patellar cerclage 5-787
− pertrochanteric 5-787
Osteotomy 5-781
− derotational 5-781
− displacement 5-781
− jaw 5-770
− metatarse 5-781
− pseudoarthrosis 5-781
− rhinoplasty 5-217
− rotational 5-781
− stapedovestibular 5-190
− triple
− − with hamstring transfer 5-781
− vertebral 5-781
− with muscle transfer 5-781
Otonecrectomy 5-204
Otoplasty 5-186
− auditory meatus 5-185
− auricle 5-186
− ear pinning 5-184
Otoscopy 1-240
− foreign body removal 8-103
− magnifying 1-241
− routine 1-240
Ouchterlony reaction 2-614
Outdoor chair
− powered (motor) 9-802
Outdoor vehicle
− adaptation for invalid 9-808
Outfolding
− scleral 5-153
Output
− cardiac 1-721

P

P.K. 1-705
Pacemaker (heart) 8-650
– asynchronous 8-653
– atrial synchronous 8-654
– bladder 8-662
– – insertion 5-579
– emergency 8-651
– evaluation of function 8-658
– external
– – insertion of electrodes 5-377
– insertion 5-377
– noncompetitive 8-654
– permanent 8-652
– spinal 8-661
– – insertion 5-039
– transvenous 8-651
– triggered 8-654
– ureter 8-668
– – insertion 5-569
Packed cell volume 2-811
Packing 8-500
– flail chest 8-741
– liver 8-500
– – with hepatotomy 5-500
– nasal 8-501
– postpartum 5-759
– rectum 8-502
– uterus
– – non-obstetric 8-503
– vaginal 8-504
– wound, thorax 5-340
Pain threshold
– determination 1-204
Paired serum samples 1-914
Palatoplasty 5-275
Palatorrhaphy 5-275
Pallidectomy 5-013
Pallidoansectomy 5-013
Pallidotomy 5-013
Palmar shelf
– wrist arthroplasty 5-817
Pancreas
– artificial 9-124
– aspirate (of secretion) 2-336
– function test 2-339
Pancreatectomy 5-524
– complete 5-525
– distal 5-524
– partial 5-524
– proximal 5-524

Pancreatectomy 5-524 - *continued*
– radical 5-526
– total 5-525
Pancreaticocystoenterostomy 5-523
Pancreaticocystogastrostomy 5-523
Pancreaticocystojejunostomy 5-523
Pancreaticoduodenectomy 5-524
– complete 5-525
– partial 5-524
– radical 5-526
– with anastomosis 5-526
Pancreaticoduodenostomy 5-527
Pancreaticoenterostomy 5-527
Pancreaticogastrostomy 5-527
Pancreaticoileostomy 5-527
Pancreaticojejunostomy (caudal) 5-527
Pancreatotomy 5-520
Pancreolithotomy 5-520
Pandy test 2-274
Panendoscopy 1-653
– urinary 1-653
Panhysterectomy 5-683
Panniculectomy
– abdominal 5-901
Panniculotomy 5-901
Panproctocolpectomy 5-714
Pantaloon operation 5-444
Papanicolaou stained smear (uterine cervix)
  2-916
Papillectomy
– anus 5-492
Papillotomy
– Wirsung 5-518
Paracentesis
– abdominal 8-157
– tympanum 5-200
Parasites
– examination method NEC 2-739
– identification
– – blood 2-727
– postmortem search 2-736
Parathyroid
– hormone 2-364
– response to calcium 2-364
Parathyroidectomy 5-067
– partial 5-067
– total 5-068
– with complete thyroidectomy 5-063
Parotidectomy 5-262
– superficial 5-262

Parotidectomy 5-262 - *continued*
- total 5-262
Pars plana approach
- cataract 5-146
Partial prothromboplastin time 2-862
Partial punch
- cataract extraction 5-146
Passage
- catheter - see Catheterization
Passive transfer test 1-705
Patch graft
- heart valve 5-353
- vessel 5-395
Patellapexy 5-837
Patellaplasty 5-789
Patellectomy (complete) 5-785
- partial 5-784
- with knee arthroplasty 5-814
Patent ductus arteriosus
- occlusion 5-387
Paul-Bunnell test 2-651
Paul-Mikulitz operation 5-460
Pectenotomy 5-494
Pedicle implant (see also Graft, pedicle)
- myocardial revascularization 5-363
Pelvimetry
- external 1-359
Pelviolithotomy 5-551
Pelvioplasty, kidney 5-557
Pelviotomy (bone) 5-781
Pelviureteroplasty 5-557
Percussion
- rhythmic
- - for neuroma 8-542
Percutaneous
- biopsy - see Biopsy, non surgical
Pereyra's operation 5-596
Perforation
- stapes footplate 5-190
Perfusion
- artery 8-870
- - carotid 8-871
- - head 8-871
- - - cytotoxic 5-961
- - renal 8-872
- carotid 8-871
- cytotoxic 5-969
- diagnostic 1-870
- - other 1-879
- head 8-871
- parenteral alimentation 9-230
- regional 8-873
- renal 8-872
- whole body 8-874
Pericardiectomy 5-372
Pericardiocentesis 5-370
- diagnostic 1-842

Pericardiolysis 5-372
Pericardioplasty 5-374
Pericardiorrhaphy 5-374
Pericardiotomy 5-371
Perilimbal suction 1-225
Perimetry 1-210
Perinectomy NEC 5-715
Perineoplasty (non obstetric) 5-716
Perineorrhaphy 5-716
- obstetric 5-758
- - third degree 5-758
Perineotomy 5-710
Periosteorrhaphy 5-789
Periosteotomy 5-780
- jaw 5-770
Peripheral vascular resistance 1-735
Peritectomy 5-112
Peritomy 5-111
Peritoneal fluid
- examination 2-283
Peritoneoscopy 1-694
Peritoneotomy 5-541
Personality assessment 1-932
Pertussis
- immunization 4-334
- - with diphtheria and tetanus 4-336
Pessary
- insertion (postpartum) 8-361
Petrosectomy 5-204
Phacoeresis 5-144
Phakoemulsification 5-146
Phalangectomy 5-784
- for hallux valgus 5-782
Phalangisation
- metacarpus 5-828
Pharyngeal flap
- palatoplasty 5-275
Pharyngectomy 5-292
- with laryngectomy 5-304
Pharyngoplasty 5-293
- for cleft palate 5-275
Pharyngorrhaphy 5-294
Pharyngoscopy 1-615
Pharyngotomy 5-290
Phase contrast
- micro-organisms 2-502
Phenistix 4-212
Phenol sympathectomy 5-052
Phenosulfonphthalein
- clearance 2-342
Phenylalanine-4-hydroxylase 2-454
Phenylketonuria
- screening 4-212
- test 2-240
Phlebectomy 5-385
- varicose veins 5-384
Phleborrhaphy

Phleborrhaphy - *continued*
- cranial sinus 5-021
- peripheral 5-393
Phlebotomy 5-380
Phonocardiography 1-255
- intracardiac 1-255
Phosphatase
- acid (formol stable) (of prostatic origin) (tartrate labile) (tartrate resistant) (total) 2-473
- alkaline 2-472
Phosphate
- balance 2-361
- inorganic
- - blood 2-154
Phospholipids
- blood 2-145
Photocoagulation (see also Light coagulation) 8-624
- iris 5-135
- macular hole 8-622
- orbital lesion 5-164
- pupil formation 5-135
- retinal detachment 8-622
Photographic recording 1-961
Photography
- fiberscopic 1-681
- fundus oculi 1-222
- medical 1-961
Photonystagmography 1-223
Phototherapy 8-620
Phrenemphraxis 5-332
Phrenicotomy 5-332
Phrenicotripsy 5-332
Physical
- agent
- - therapeutic 8-699
- - - specified NEC 8-690
- medicine (see also Physiotherapy) 9-489
- therapy - see Physiotherapy
Physiological assistance
- hearing 9-314
- locomotion 9-330
- vision 9-320
Physiotherapy 9-489
- combined (unspecified procedures) 9-470
- during disease
- - maintenance of cardiovascular performance 8-887
- - prevention complications
- - - cardiovascular 8-886
- - - pulmonary 8-782
- infrared 8-605
- - ocular 8-605
- post-traumatic
- - maintenance of cardiovascular performance 8-887

Physiotherapy 9-489 - *continued*
- post-traumatic - *continued*
- - prevention complications
- - - cardiovascular 8-886
- - - pulmonary 8-782
- prevention
- - cardiovascular complications (of disease or trauma) 8-886
- - pulmonary complications (of disease or trauma) 8-782
- specified NEC 9-488
Phytohemagglutination, lymphocytes 2-873
Piercing
- ear lobe 5-988
- nasal septum (ritual) 5-988
Pigmentation
- skin
- - therapeutic 5-880
Pinealectomy 5-074
Pinning
- ear, pinna 5-184
- fracture 5-790
Pirogoff's operation 5-847
Pituitary
- lactogen hormone 2-417
- response to
- - antidiuretic hormone 2-411
- - metyrapone 2-410
Pituitectomy 5-075
Placed on waiting list 9-183
Placement
- intra-atrial baffle 5-357
Placenta
- localization 1-355
- - acoustic 1-355
Planing, skin 5-903
Plaque reduction neutralization test 2-620
Plasma (see also Blood and Serum)
- angiotensin 2-345
- bicarbonate 2-122
- chorionic gonadotrophin 2-433
- cortisol 2-422
- iron
- - transport rate 2-853
- lignocaine half-life 2-326
- renin 2-206
- turbidity 2-146
Plaster (of Paris) 8-310
- application of cast 8-310
- collar support 8-312
- jacket
- - application 8-311
- minerva 8-312
Plastic repair
- alveolar ridge 5-244
- amputation stump 5-850
- aponeurosis 5-837

Plastic repair - *continued*
— aponeurosis 5-837 - *continued*
— — hand 5-828
— auricle of ear 5-186
— bladder 5-578
— — exstrophy 5-578
— — reconstruction 5-577
— bone 5-789
— breast - see Mammoplasty
— bronchus 5-334
— canaliculus
— — lacrimal 5-086
— canthus 5-092
— chin 5-773
— cleft lip 5-898
— cleft palate 5-275
— cystocele 5-704
— dental supporting structures 5-244
— ear (external) 5-186
— — canal 5-185
— — pinning 5-184
— enterostomy 5-464
— esophagus 5-427
— external auditory meatus 5-185
— eyelid 5-096
— face 5-899
— fallopian tube 5-666
— fascia 5-837
— — hand 5-828
— gingiva (gums) 5-241
— hand 5-828
— hip 5-816
— — total replacement 5-815
— jaw (lower) 5-773
— — upper
— — — with resection and bone graft 5-775
— — with prosthesis (inert) 5-773
— — with resection and bone graft 5-773
— joint 5-819
— — foot 5-813
— kidney 5-557
— knee 5-814
— lacrimonasal duct 5-087
— larynx nos 5-315
— ligament NEC 5-819
— lip 5-898
— — with excision 5-898
— mouth 5-898
— — internal 5-274
— — skin 5-898
— muscles 5-837
— — hand 5-828
— nasal sinus 5-226
— nipple 5-872
— nose (external) 5-217
— orbit (socket) 5-167
— ovary 5-656

Plastic repair - *continued*
— penis 5-643
— peritoneum 5-546
— pharynx 5-293
— — diverticulum 5-293
— pinna NEC 5-186
— pinning 5-184
— rectocele 5-704
— rectum 5-486
— renal (pelvis) 5-557
— retina 5-154
— salivary gland 5-263
— scrotum 5-613
— shoulder 5-818
— sinus, nasal 5-226
— size reduction 5-901
— skin 5-899
— spinal 5-034
— spleen 5-419
— stomach 5-445
— tendon 5-837
— — hand 5-828
— — thumb 5-828
— tooth 5-234
— trachea 5-316
— tympanum 5-194
— ureter 5-568
— urethra 5-583
— uterine ligaments 5-693
— uterus 5-695
— vagina 5-706
— vulva 5-716
— with pedicle graft 5-896
— with skin graft 5-893
Platelet
— aggregation time 2-866
— count 2-802
— life span 2-863
Platinectomy 5-191
Plating
— fracture 5-792
— — skull 5-020
Play therapy 9-502
Pleating
— muscle
— — ocular 5-104
Pleoptic evaluation 1-216
Plethysmography
— body 1-712
— impedance
— — monitoring 8-944
— monitoring 8-944
— total lung capacity 1-710
— whole limb 1-734
Pleuracentesis 8-155
Pleural fluid
— chemistry 2-282

Pleurectomy 5-344
Pleurodesis 5-345
Pleurolysis 5-333
Pleuropexy 5-349
Pleuropneumonectomy 5-344
Pleurotomy 5-340
Plexectomy
– choroid 5-021
Plication
– annulus
– – heart valve 5-351
– bladder neck 5-592
– bowel 5-546
– diaphragm 5-538
– eye muscle 5-104
– fascia 5-837
– – hand 5-828
– heart
– – thinned wall 5-374
– intestine 5-546
– joint capsule 5-819
– ligament
– – broad 5-693
– – joint 5-819
– – sacrouterine 5-693
– muscle 5-837
– sphincter, urinary 5-578
– tendon 5-837
– – hand 5-828
– ureter 5-568
– urethra 5-592
– urethrovesical junction 5-592
– vena cava 5-386
Plicotomy (middle ear) 5-202
Plombage
– choroid 5-152
– episcleral 5-152
– lung 5-332
Plugging
– bone 5-786
– ductus arteriosus 5-387
– flail chest 8-741
– uterus 8-503
– – obstetric 5-759
Pneumocentesis 8-156
Pneumonectomy
– complete 5-325
– extended 5-325
– partial 5-324
– radical 5-325
Pneumonolysis 5-333
Pneumonotomy 5-331
Pneumoperitoneum 8-733
Pneumothorax
– artificial 8-731
– therapeutic 8-731
Polarised light

Polarised light - continued
– biochemistry 2-494
– micro-organisms 2-502
Polarography 2-499
Poliomyelitis
– immunization 4-353
Polishing
– teeth 4-521
Politzerization 8-173
Pollen
– antibodies 2-630
– skin test 1-702
Pollen free room 8-771
Pollicization
– finger 5-828
– thumb 5-826
Polya's operation 5-437
Polychromasia
– staining 2-805
Polymorphonuclear
– lobulation classification 2-884
– migration inhibition 2-886
Polypectomy
– anal 5-492
– aural (tympanic) 5-204
– cervix 5-672
– colon 5-452
– gastric 5-434
– intestinal
– – small 5-451
– intestine
– – large 5-452
– laryngeal (vocal cord) 5-300
– nasal 5-212
– rectal 5-482
– tracheal 5-314
Pomeroy's operation 5-664
Pool
– therapeutic 8-551
Porphyrin
– blood 2-834
Portal venous pressure
– measurement 1-733
Positive pressure respiration 8-712
Posterior pituitary hormone 2-417
Postmortem examination 2-979
– bacteriological 2-562
– brain 2-971
– chest 2-972
– complete 2-970
– for parasites 2-736
– limited
– – abdomen 2-973
– – chest 2-972
– – region NEC 2-973
– – skull 2-971
– microbiologic 2-562

Postmortem examination 2-979 - *continued*
— microbiologic 2-562 - *continued*
— — brain 2-562
— — organ NEC 2-562
— — respiratory 2-561
— tissue (microscopy) 2-909
Postmortem isolation
— fungus 2-706
Postnatal care
— by midwife - see Postnatal care, by nurse
— by nurse 4-633
— — home visit 4-636
— — initial 4-631
— — subsequent 4-633
— by other health personnel 4-783
— — home visit 4-790
— — initial 4-782
— — subsequent 4-783
— medical 4-622
— — initial
— — — did not have prenatal care 4-620
— — — had prenatal care 4-610
— — subsequent 4-622
Potassium
— balance 2-351
— plasma 2-150
Potts-Smith operation 5-390
Poudrage
— intrapericardial 5-363
— pleura 5-345
Precipitating antibodies
— foodstuffs 2-630
— pigeons 2-630
Precipitin
— agar gel diffusion technique 2-614
— reaction
— — bacterial typing 2-522
— — serum 2-614
Pregnancy
— current
— — ambulatory care - see Prenatal care
— hormones
— — blood 2-433
— — urine 2-444
— stress tests 4-201
— termination - see Termination, pregnancy
— test
— — immunological 2-666
Premature care
— at home 4-702
— — incubator 4-700
Prenatal care
— by midwife - see Prenatal care, by nurse
— by nurse 4-632
— — home visit 4-635
— — initial 4-630
— — subsequent 4-632

Prenatal care - *continued*
— by other health personnel 4-781
— — home visit 4-790
— — initial 4-780
— — subsequent 4-781
— medical 4-620
— — initial
— — — in first trimester 4-601
— — — in second trimester 4-602
— — — in third trimester 4-603
— — subsequent 4-620
— screening examination 4-209
Preoperative assessment 8-890
Preparation
— pedicle skin graft 5-894
— skin flap 5-894
Preschool child care
— by nurse 4-726
— — conference (with parent) 4-726
— — — first 4-725
— — — subsequent 4-726
— — home visit 4-728
— — — first 4-727
— — — subsequent 4-728
— by other health personnel 4-787
— — first attention 4-786
— — subsequent 4-787
— medical 4-721
— — initial 4-720
— — subsequent 4-721
Prescription
— lenses
— — anisoeikonic 1-213
— spectacles 9-321
— — for aphakia 9-325
Prevention
— collapse of lung 8-749
Probing
— bone 1-832
— canaliculus
— — lacrimal 1-830
— joint 1-833
— — with incision 5-800
— lacrimal passage 1-830
— nasolacrimal duct 1-831
Procedure
— cardiovascular (system)
— — therapeutic 8-889
— diagnostic 1-999
— — specified NEC 1-990
— — surgical 1-890
— — — minor 1-891
— non-operative 9-190
— obstetric 5-759
— orthopedic 8-489
— physiotherapeutic 9-489
— postoperative 8-898

Procedure - *continued*
- respiratory (system)
- - therapeutic 8-789
- surgical 5-999
- - before foreign travel (preventive)
    5-982
- - preventive 5-982
- - - appendectomy 5-982
- - second stage 5-999
- therapeutic
- - cardiovascular (system) 8-889
- - physical agent 8-699
- - respiratory (system) 8-789
Proctectomy (see also Excision, rectum)
    5-485
Proctocecostomy 5-459
Proctocolectomy 5-485
Proctocolpectomy 5-714
Proctolysis 5-489
Proctopexy 5-486
Proctoplasty 5-486
Proctoproctostomy (end to end) 5-485
Proctorrhaphy 5-486
Proctoscopy 1-643
- biopsy 1-452
- diagnostic 1-643
- foreign body removal 8-113
- surgical 1-695
Proctosigmoidectomy 5-485
Proctosigmoidopexy 5-486
Proctosigmoidoscopy 1-642
Proctosigmoidostomy 5-459
Proctostomy 5-481
- closure 5-486
Proctotomy 5-480
- for pelvic peritoneal drainage 5-480
Proctovalvotomy 5-480
Production
- adhesions
- - pericardium 5-363
- - pleura 5-345
- ankylosis (see also Arthrodesis) 5-812
- ankylosis
- - ankle, foot 5-811
- - spine 5-810
- defect of septum (heart) 5-355
Profile
- enzymes 2-489
- liver 2-326
Profundoplasty, vessel 5-383
Projective test 1-934
Prolactin 2-417
Prophylaxis 4-499
- administration
- - anti-D globulin 4-400
- - anticoagulant 4-441
- - gammaglobulin 4-400

Prophylaxis 4-499 - *continued*
- administration - *continued*
- - inorganic salt NEC 4-479
- - iodine 4-470
- - iodized salt 4-471
- - steroid 4-450
- - vitamin supplements NEC 4-473
- - vitamin D supplements 4-472
- against infection 4-389
- alteration
- - hematological status 4-449
- - immunological status 4-409
- dental 4-539
- - extraction 4-430
- - surgical 4-529
- diet 4-469
- - low calory 4-461
- - low carbohydrate 4-460
- - low protein 4-463
- - low salt 4-462
- - salt free 4-462
- - unsaturated fat 4-464
- endocrine 4-459
- - psychiatric control 4-452
- general disease 4-499
- goitre 4-470
- - with iodine 4-470
- - with iodized salt 4-471
- pellagra 4-473
- removal
- - potential source of infection 4-439
- - tooth 4-430
- ricketts 4-472
- scurvy 4-473
- specific anomalies 4-661
- - specified NEC 4-480
Prostatectomy 5-605
- cutting loop 5-601
- endoscopic 5-601
- perineal 5-605
- perurethral 5-601
- radical 5-604
- retropubic 5-603
- suprapubic 5-602
- transcapsular 5-605
- - perineal 5-605
- - retropubic 5-603
- transurethral 5-601
- transvesical 5-602
Prostatocystectomy (see also
    Prostatectomy) 5-576
Prostatocystotomy 5-600
Prostatolithotomy 5-600
Prostatotomy 5-600
Prostatovesiculectomy 5-604
Prosthesis
- application 8-563

Prosthesis - *continued*
- artery
- - peripheral 5-383
- - with repair of heart 5-356
- atrium (heart) 5-356
- bifurcation 5-392
- - aorta (abdominal) 5-392
- bioelectric (limb) 5-855
- breast 5-873
- cardiac (valve) 5-352
- chin, receding 5-773
- cineplastic (limb) 5-855
- cosmetic NEC 9-379
- dental
- - fixed 5-236
- eye (after enucleation) 5-163
- finger 5-817
- fitting 8-562
- for absent ear 5-186
- internal
- - insertion 8-369
- jaw (lower) 5-773
- - upper 5-775
- joint
- - hip 5-816
- - - total replacement 5-815
- - nec 5-819
- limb 8-565
- - application 8-565
- - bioelectric 5-855
- - fitting 8-564
- - implantation 5-855
- middle ear 5-191
- non surgical
- - breast (removable) 9-371
- - face (fixed) (removable) 9-370
- outflow (heart) 5-356
- palate 5-275
- penile 5-649
- septum
- - heart
- - - foraminal valve 5-356
- skull 5-020
- stapes replacement 5-191
- testicular 5-626
- vessel, after resection 5-383
- - bypass NEC 5-392
Protamine neutralization 2-861
Protein
- acute phase, serum 2-107
- antigen, reiter 2-600
- Bence-Jones 2-670
- chemical separation, in blood 2-103
- immunoassay 2-679
- total
- - plasma estimation 2-102
- urinary

Protein - *continued*
- urinary - *continued*
- - clinical test 2-202
Prothrombin
- consumption test 2-863
- test 2-862
Protozoa
- examination of blood 2-721
Provision
- artificial arm 9-240
- artificial leg 9-336
- denture
- - removable 9-301
- medical equipment 9-819
- spectacles 9-322
- - for aphakia 9-325
- supportive stockings 9-332
Provocation test 1-709
- skin 1-704
Provocative therapy 9-630
Pseudoisochromatic plates 1-215
Psittacosis
- xenodiagnosis 2-563
Psychiatric
- diagnosis 1-920
Psychoanalysis 1-940
Psychogalvanic reflex 1-925
Psychology, psychological
- analysis 1-940
- - modified 1-941
- - specified NEC 1-949
- diagnostic 1-920
- - interview 1-921
- - other techniques 1-929
- test NEC 1-939
- - psychometric 1-930
- therapeutic 9-680
Psychometric test 1-930
Psychotherapy 9-689
- antiphobic 9-641
- competitive games 9-631
- couples 9-640
- encounter 9-630
- family 9-610
- functional 9-619
- general 9-609
- group 9-640
- multiple family 9-640
- multiple impact 9-630
Psychotropic drug
- for examination 1-902
Pterygium operation 5-122
Pubiotomy
- nonobstetric 5-781
- obstetric 5-739
Pubococcygeoplasty 5-593
Puerperium

Puerperium - *continued*
- current
- - ambulatory care - see Postnatal care
Pull-through
- abdomino-anal 5-483
- resection
- - rectum 5-483
Pulmonary blood flow measurement 1-714
Pulmonary resistance 1-712
- vascular 1-714
Pulpectomy 5-237
Pulpotomy 5-237
Pump
- balloon
- - intra-aortic 5-376
- oxygenator 8-764
Punch autograft
- hair follicles 5-902
Punch biopsy - see Biopsy, non surgical
Punch operation
- bladder neck 5-573
- resection
- - larynx 5-302
- - prostate 5-601
Punch sclerectomy 5-132
Puncture
- abscess
- - subdural 5-011
- anterior
- - chamber
- - - diagnostic 1-840
- antrum (highmore) 5-220
- artery, arterial 8-844
- bladder 8-161
- bone 5-780
- bone marrow
- - diagnostic 1-425
- - for transplant 5-410
- brain 5-010
- bursa 5-830
- cisternal
- - diagnostic 1-206
- cranial 5-010
- cul-de-sac 5-700
- fontanel, anterior 5-010
- four-point abdominal
- - diagnostic 1-853
- hydrocele 8-163
- iris 5-135
- joint
- - diagnostic 1-854
- - aspiration 8-166

Puncture - *continued*
- larynx 5-310
- lumbar
- - diagnostic 1-206
- - for drainage 5-036
- lung 8-156
- nasal
- - sinus 5-220
- orbit
- - diagnostic 1-841
- pericardium 5-370
- peritoneal
- - diagnostic 1-853
- pleura 8-155
- - diagnostic 1-844
- sinus, nasal 5-220
- spinal
- - diagnostic 1-206
- - drainage 5-036
- spleen 5-411
- - for biopsy 1-427
- subdural abscess 5-010
- tunica vaginalis 8-163
- vein 8-846
- - diagnostic 1-869
- ventricle
- - brain 5-010
- - - drainage 5-010
- vessel 8-849
Pupillotomy
- by light coagulation 5-135
Pure tone
- audiometry 1-230
Pyelolithotomy 5-551
Pyeloplasty 5-557
Pyelorrhaphy 5-557
Pyeloscopy 1-651
- operative 1-695
Pyelostomy 5-551
- closure 5-557
Pyelotomy 5-551
- with removal of tumor 5-552
Pylon
- walking 9-333
Pylorectomy 5-436
Pyloromyotomy 5-433
Pyloroplasty 5-441
- with vagotomy 5-441
Pylorostomy 5-441
Pylorotomy 5-433

Q

Quadruple therapy 5-969
— cytotoxic drugs 5-969
Quantitative
— assay
— — antibiotic susceptibility 2-531

Quantitative - *continued*
— Khan test 2-602
— VDRL test 2-602
Quotient
— respiratory 1-762

R

Rachitomy 5-030
Radiant heat 8-605
Radiation
— infrared 8-600
— ultraviolet 8-621
Radicotomy 5-031
Radiculectomy 5-031
Radiculotomy 5-031
— for disc lesion 5-031
Ramisection 5-781
— jaw 5-775
— nerve 5-040
— — spinal root 5-031
— — sympathetic 5-050
— sympathetic 5-050
Range of mobility
— measurement 1-362
Rankin's operation 5-484
Rapid screening test
— blood coagulation 2-860
Rashkind's operation 5-355
Ratio
— albumin/globulin 2-103
— dead space/tidal volume 1-715
Re-education
— neuromuscular 9-430
— vocational 9-534
Re-employment
— changed employer 9-536
— same employer 9-535
Re-entry operation
— thoracic aorta 5-395
Re-exploration
— stapedectomy 5-192
Reaction (of) (see also Test)
— biuret 2-102
— incompatibility 2-649
— Ouchterlony 2-614

Reaction - *continued*
— Takata-Ara 2-321
— Wassermann 2-600
— Weil-Felix 2-613
Reading
— test
— — for visual acuity 1-211
Readjustment
— pacemaker 5-378
— prosthesis 8-566
Reamputation
— stump 5-850
Reanastomosis
— intestines 5-458
— nerve 5-042
Reattachment
— arm 5-852
— choroid 5-156
— finger 5-851
— foot 5-853
— hand 5-852
— joint capsule nos 5-819
— leg 5-854
— ligament (see also Repair, joint) 5-819
— — patellar 5-814
— — uterosacral 5-693
— muscle
— — eye 5-103
— — — for ptosis 5-094
— — hand 5-825
— — papillary 5-354
— patellar tendon
— — dovetail operation 5-781
— retina 5-154
— — photocoagulation 8-622
— tendon 5-836
— — hand 5-825
— thumb 5-851

Reattachment - *continued*
- toe 5-853
- tooth 8-240
Reboring
- artery 5-381
Recall
- follow-up 9-820
Recession
- ocular muscle 5-102
- - with resection 5-101
- tendon 5-836
- - hand 5-825
- - thumb 5-825
Reclination
- lens 5-149
Reconstruction (see also Repair and graph, by site)
- alveolar ridge 5-244
- annulus
- - cardiac 5-353
- anterior segment
- - eye 5-129
- artery NEC 5-395
- auricle (ear) 5-186
- bladder 5-577
- - with ileum 5-577
- - with sigmoid 5-577
- bone 5-789
- bronchus 5-334
- cleft lip 5-898
- colostomy 5-464
- cruciate ligaments 5-814
- diaphragm 5-347
- ear
- - auricle 5-186
- - external auditory meatus 5-185
- - pinning 5-184
- esophagus 5-427
- eyebrow 5-096
- eyelid 5-096
- fallopian tube 5-666
- foot
- - joint 5-813
- hip 5-816
- - with prosthesis 5-816
- jaw (lower) 5-773
- - upper 5-775
- joint (see also Arthroplasty) 5-819
- - spine 5-819
- knee 5-814
- ligaments
- - knee 5-819
- lip 5-898
- lymphatic by transplantation 5-409
- mandible
- - with bone graft 5-773
- maxilla

Reconstruction - *continued*
- maxilla - *continued*
- - with bone graft 5-775
- mouth 5-898
- - external 5-898
- - internal 5-274
- nose (bone) (cartilage) 5-217
- - septum 5-217
- operation 5-899
- ossicles 5-193
- palate 5-275
- pelvic floor 5-693
- penis 5-643
- pharynx 5-293
- scrotum 5-613
- shoulder 5-818
- skull 5-020
- socket of eye 5-167
- spine 5-810
- tendon 5-836
- - hand 5-827
- thumb 5-826
- toe
- - joint 5-813
- trachea 5-316
- tunica albuginea
- - penis 5-643
- tympanic cavity 5-195
- urethra 5-583
- vagina 5-705
- vas deferens, divided 5-637
Recording
- electric 1-960
- intracardiac pressure 1-720
- photographic 1-961
Recreational therapy 9-509
Rectal scraping
- for ova 2-716
Rectopexy 5-486
Rectoplasty 5-486
Rectosigmoidectomy 5-485
Rectostomy 5-481
Red cell(s) (see also Blood red cell and Erythrocyte)
- count 2-801
- life span 2-851
- site of destruction 2-852
- volume 2-813
Reductase 2-459
Reduction (closed)
- adipose tissue 5-901
- batwing arms 5-901
- breast 5-874
- buttocks 5-901
- dislocation 8-209
- - jaw 5-779
- - manipulation 8-209

Reduction - *continued*
— dislocation 8-209 - *continued*
— — with traction 8-474
— displacement (organ) 8-249
— — nasal septum 8-201
— edema 9-474
— elephantiasis
— — scrotum 5-612
— fracture 8-208
— — alveolus (of jaw) 5-762
— — ankle 8-205
— — arm 8-202
— — — upper 8-202
— — elbow 8-202
— — facial bone NEC 5-766
— — femur 8-204
— — finger 8-203
— — foot 8-205
— — forearm 8-203
— — hand 8-203
— — hip 8-204
— — humerus 8-202
— — intertrochanteric (femur) 8-204
— — jaw 5-762
— — leg 8-205
— — — lower 8-205
— — — upper 8-204
— — malar 5-760
— — mandible 5-762
— — maxilla 5-762
— — metacarpus 8-203
— — metatarsus 8-205
— — multiple 5-797
— — multiple limbs 5-797
— — nasal bone 8-200
— — nose (septum) 8-200
— — orbital 5-766
— — pelvis
— — — with internal injuries 5-797
— — — with limb bones 5-797
— — radius 8-203
— — shoulder 8-202
— — skull 5-020
— — — with limb bones 5-797
— — specified site NEC 8-208
— — thorax
— — — with internal injuries 5-797
— — — with limb bones 5-797
— — thumb 8-203
— — toe 8-205
— — ulna 8-203
— — with internal fixation 5-790
— — wrist 8-203
— — zygoma, zygomatic arch 5-760
— hemorrhoids
— — manually 8-243
— hernia (see also Repair, hernia) 5-530

Reduction - *continued*
— hernia - *continued*
— — manually 8-241
— intussusception 5-468
— inverted uterus
— — surgical 5-759
— malrotation
— — intestine 5-468
— mucocele
— — lacrimal 5-084
— open - see Open reduction
— prolapse 8-242
— — bowel 8-242
— — colostomy 5-464
— — enterostomy 5-464
— — ileostomy 5-464
— — rectum 8-242
— separated epiphysis 5-793
— — with nailing 5-793
— tooth
— — forcible 8-219
— torsion
— — kidney pedicle 5-557
— — omentum 5-546
— — spermatic cord 5-634
— — testis 5-634
— — — with orchidopexy 5-634
— — volvulus
— — — intestine 5-468
— — — stomach 5-449
— trochanteric lipomatosis 5-901
— volvulus 5-468
— — stomach 5-449
Reduction
— eosinophilia by acth 2-420
Reefing
— joint capsule 5-819
— — foot 5-813
— — hand 5-817
— — jaw 5-774
— — knee 5-814
— — shoulder 5-818
Reference
— other clinic 9-188
Reflex testing 1-201
Refraction
— with contact lens 1-224
Refracture
— bone 5-789
— — nasal 8-210
— — with wrench 5-789
— callus 5-789
— jaw 5-779
— turbinate 8-210
Refrigeration
— brain 5-014
— — globus pallidus 5-013

Refrigeration - *continued*
− brain 5-014 - *continued*
− − thalamus 5-013
Regulation
− body temperature
− − cooling
− − − local 8-612
− − warming
− − − general 8-601
− − − local 8-600
− electrolyte balance 8-876
− fluid balance 8-876
Rehabilitation 9-599
− blind 9-550
− by economic methods 9-760
− by legal measures 9-761
− daily life activities 9-569
− domestic responsibilities 9-541
− domestic tasks 9-540
− educational 9-519
− oral 9-429
− psychological disability 9-632
− social 9-549
− vocational 9-539
Rehabilitation evaluation 1-979
− disability
− − current 1-975
− − longterm 1-976
− medical 1-970
− occupational therapist 1-976
− other 1-978
− physiotherapist 1-975
− psychiatric 1-971
− psychological 1-972
− social 1-973
− vocational 1-974
Reimplantation
− eye muscle 5-103
− muscle 5-836
− severed limb 5-859
− tooth 8-240
− ureter into
− − bladder 5-567
− − pelvis 5-557
Reinsertion
− extruded orbital implant 5-165
− pacemaker 5-378
Reiter, protein antigen 2-600
Relaxation
− exercises 9-455
− scar 5-891
Release
− carpal tunnel nerve for decompression 5-043
− chordee 5-643
− colostomy
− − scar tissue 5-464

Release - *continued*
− contracture 5-831
− − Dupuytren's
− − − fasciotomy 5-821
− − joint 5-837
− − Volkmann's 5-823
− − − fasciotomy 5-831
− fascia 5-831
− intrinsic hand contracture
− − muscle advancement 5-825
− − tenotomy 5-821
− joint 5-801
− − capsule, adherent 5-801
− − structure 5-801
− muscle division 5-831
− − hand 5-821
− nerve 5-043
− psoas 5-837
− retinaculum of finger 5-821
− retracted nipple 5-872
− scar 5-891
− syndactyly 5-899
Relief
− chordee 5-643
− hernia
− − strangulated (inguinal) 5-530
− ileus 5-469
− intestinal obstruction NEC 5-469
− intraocular tension 5-132
− nerve 5-043
− tension pneumothorax 8-742
Relocation
− prostate (after injury) 5-608
Remobilization
− stapes 5-190
Remodelling
− cardiac annulus
− − on ring frame 5-353
Removal
− anal tags 5-492
− appliance
− − orthopedic 8-481
− biliary tube, cannula 5-517
− blood clot
− − after vascular operation 5-394
− − bladder 5-570
− − − by cystotomy 5-571
− − − without incision 5-570
− − ureter
− − − transurethral 5-560
− bone
− − fixation (internal) 5-788
− − fragments
− − − fracture 5-795
− − − jaw 5-770
− − − open reduction
− − − − fracture 5-791

Removal - *continued*
- bone - *continued*
- - fragments - *continued*
- - - skull 5-020
- - graft 5-789
- - spicules, spinal canal 5-034
- bone marrow 8-154
- brace 8-382
- bursa
- - calcareous deposit 5-832
- - contents 5-830
- calcification
- - valve cusps (heart) 5-353
- calculus
- - bile duct 5-513
- - bladder 5-570
- - - perurethral 5-570
- - - with incision 5-571
- - - without incision 5-570
- - gallbladder 5-510
- - hepatic duct 5-513
- - kidney 5-550
- - - by incision 5-550
- - - without incision 5-560
- - lacrimal gland 5-083
- - pancreas 5-520
- - perirenal tissue 5-590
- - pharynx 5-290
- - prostate 5-600
- - - by incision 5-600
- - renal pelvis 5-551
- - salivary
- - - by incision 5-260
- - - without incision 8-110
- - ureter
- - - by incision 5-562
- - - cystoscopic 5-560
- - urethra
- - - by cystoscopy 5-589
- - - by incision 5-580
- - urinary 5-570
- - vesical 8-133
- - vesical (urinary) 5-570
- callosity 8-185
- cartilage
- - larynx 5-302
- cast 8-380
- cerumen 8-171
- chalazion 5-091
- clip
- - from wound 8-897
- conjunctiva for pterygium 5-122
- cusps, valve (heart) 5-351
- cyst
- - dental 5-243
- - lung 5-322
- - ovarian 5-651

Removal - *continued*
- cyst - *continued*
- - stomach 5-434
- debris
- - wound (without incision) 8-191
- decidua
- - manual 5-756
- - with curettage 5-690
- disc, intervertebral 5-803
- ectopic fetus 5-743
- ectopic pregnancy 5-743
- electrode
- - endocardial 8-882
- embolus 5-380
- - with endarterectomy 5-381
- encircling tube (retinal detachment)
  5-150
- epulis 5-242
- excess mucosa
- - cleft lip 5-898
- - urethra
- - - female 5-702
- - vulva 5-702
- extradural hematoma 5-011
- extrauterine embryo NEC 5-743
- eyeball 5-163
- fetus
- - extrauterine 5-743
- fixation 8-389
- - device 8-389
- fixation device
- - internal 5-788
- foreign body (see also Extraction, foreign
  body) 8-119
- - adenoid (without incision) 8-110
- - anoscopy 8-113
- - anus 8-118
- - bladder
- - - cystoscopy 8-114
- - brain 5-011
- - breast 8-119
- - bronchoscopy 8-107
- - bronchus
- - - by bronchoscopy 8-107
- - buttock (without incision) 8-116
- - cerebral meninges 5-011
- - conjunctiva 8-101
- - cornea
- - - superficial 8-101
- - cystoscopy 8-114
- - ear 8-103
- - - by auroscopy 8-103
- - ear, external 5-189
- - endoscopic 8-100
- - esophagoscopy 8-111
- - esophagus 8-111
- - - by incision 5-420

Removal - *continued*
- foreign body - *continued*
- -- eyelid 8-102
- -- finger (without incision) 8-116
- -- foot 8-119
- -- from orifice 8-100
- -- hand (without incision) 8-116
- -- heart 5-371
- -- in orifice 8-100
- -- laryngoscopy 8-105
- -- leg 8-119
- -- nerve 5-043
- -- - root 5-030
- -- nose 8-104
- -- - by rhinoscopy 8-104
- -- orbit 8-102
- -- pericardium 5-371
- -- perineum (without incision) 8-116
- -- pharyngoscopy 8-111
- -- pharynx (without incision) 8-110
- -- - endoscopic 8-111
- -- proctoscopy 8-113
- -- rectum
- -- - endoscopic 8-113
- -- - proctoscopic 8-113
- -- salivary duct (without incision) 8-110
- -- sigmoidoscopy 8-113
- -- skin (without incision) 8-116
- -- skull, except plate 5-011
- -- spinal cord 5-030
- -- spinal meninges 5-030
- -- stomach
- -- - gastroscopy 8-112
- -- subcutaneous tissues 8-119
- -- superficial tissues 8-119
- -- thigh 8-119
- -- thoracoscopy 8-108
- -- tonsil (without incision) 8-110
- -- trachea
- -- - endoscopic 8-106
- -- tracheoscopy 8-106
- -- vagina (without incision) 8-115
- -- vulva 8-115
- -- without incision 8-119
- gallbladder 5-511
- with
- -- - drainage 5-511
- -- - gallstones 5-511
- glioma 5-014
- granulation tissue
- -- cranial 5-020
- -- spinal canal 5-034
- -- spinal process 5-783
- grommet 5-201
- guinea worm 8-117
- -- bronchoscopy 8-107
- hair follicle 5-882

Removal - *continued*
- helminth larva 8-117
- hemangioma
- -- intracranial 5-385
- hydatidiform mole
- -- by curettage 5-690
- -- by hysterotomy 5-681
- -- with hysterectomy 5-683
- impacted feces 8-127
- implant
- -- orbital 5-166
- infixed pin in bone 8-460
- internal fixation device (of bone) 5-788
- intrauterine contraceptive device 5-691
- intravenous electrode 8-882
- laryngeal plate 5-319
- lens implant 5-148
- ligature
- -- ureter 5-568
- -- vas deferens 5-637
- marrow
- -- bone 8-154
- meconium 8-127
- missed abortion 5-690
- mucous membranous labyrinth 5-207
- myringotomy device 5-201
- nail
- -- bed or fold 8-186
- -- digit 8-186
- -- fixation of bone (fracture) 8-389
- -- from bone 8-389
- -- metalic 5-788
- nasal polyp 5-212
- necrotic tissue (without incision) 8-191
- obliteration
- -- artery 5-381
- -- - coronary 5-360
- ocular implant 5-166
- odontoma 5-243
- outer attic wall 5-204
- ovarian pregnancy 5-743
- ovary
- -- bilateral 5-654
- -- remaining 5-654
- -- unilateral 5-652
- -- with tube
- -- - bilateral 5-655
- -- - remaining 5-655
- -- - unilateral 5-653
- ovo-testis 5-623
- pacemaker (cardiac) (implanted) 5-378
- pancreatic tube 5-529
- patella - see Patellectomy
- pessary 8-115
- phlebolith (see also Removal, embolus) 5-380
- placenta

Removal - *continued*
- placenta - *continued*
- - operative 5-690
- plaque 4-520
- plaster 8-380
- plate
- - skull 5-020
- plating
- - from fractured bone 5-788
- polyp
- - cervix 5-672
- potential source of infection 4-439
- prosthesis
- - joint cavity 5-800
- redundant
- - mucosa, vulva 5-712
- - skin
- - - canthus 5-092
- - - eyelids 5-096
- retained placenta
- - manual 5-756
- - with curettage 5-690
- retained poducts of conception 5-690
- rhinolith 5-211
- rib
- - cervical 5-785
- rice bodies, tendon sheath 5-830
- - hand 5-820
- roof of orbit 5-160
- secundines
- - manual 5-756
- - with curettage 5-690
- septum
- - anal 5-499
- sequestrum 5-770
- - facial (bone) 5-770
- - nose 5-211
- - skull 5-011
- skin blemish
- - minor 8-185
- splint 8-381
- - intraurethral 8-389
- - ureter 5-569
- support 8-382
- suture
- - cervix, encircling 5-699
- - eye muscle 5-109
- - from wound 8-897
- symblepharon 5-114
- tags
- - hemorrhoidal 5-492
- tattoo mark 8-184
- testis (see also Orchidectomy) 5-622
- - remaining 5-623
- thrombus 5-380
- tonsil NEC 5-281
- tooth 5-230

Removal - *continued*
- tooth 5-230 - *continued*
- - forceps extraction 5-230
- - impacted 5-231
- - surgical 5-231
- tracheostomy tube 8-109
- tubal pregnancy 5-743
- tube, encircling, eye 5-150
- tympanostomy tube 5-201
- valve
- - vas deferens 5-637
- ventricular shunt 5-024
- vitreous
- - opaque flake of 5-157
Renal
- clearance (see also Clearance)
- - beta-alanine 2-341
- - beta-aminoisobutyric acid 2-341
- - creatinine 2-341
- - glycine 2-341
- - inulin 2-342
- - mannitol 2-342
- - para-aminohippuric acid 2-341
- - phenol red 2-342
- - phosphate 2-341
- function test NEC 2-349
Reopening
- abdominal wound 5-541
- bone 5-780
- craniotomy 5-011
- - for examination 5-011
- - for ventriculostomy 5-024
- laminectomy site for examination 5-030
- osteotomy site 5-780
- - facial 5-770
- oval window nos 5-206
- recent laparotomy site 5-541
- recent operation site, liver 5-500
- thyroid field wound 5-060
- vas deferens 5-637
- wound
- - abdominal 5-541
Reoperation
- arteriovenous fistula 5-394
- vascular graft 5-394
Rep. mist. 9-130
Repair (see also Reconstruction, Suture, Plastic repair) 5-909
- abdominal wall (muscles) 5-546
- - resuture 5-545
- alveolus (dental) 5-244
- anal sphincter 5-496
- - postpartum 5-758
- aneurysm 5-395
- - coronary fistula 5-369
- - endoaneurysmorrhaphy 5-395
- - femoral 5-395

Repair - *continued*
- aneurysm 5-395 - *continued*
- - heart
- - - ligation 5-369
- - - ruptured 5-374
- - - sinus of Valsalva 5-354
- - wiring 5-395
- anus 5-496
- - imperforate 5-496
- - postpartum 5-758
- aorta
- - abdominal
- - - bypass 5-392
- - - replacement 5-383
- - coarctation, by resection 5-382
- - thoracic 5-395
- appliance
- - orthopedic 9-346
- - prosthetic 8-566
- artery 5-395
- - banding 5-387
- - bypass graft 5-392
- - ligation 5-387
- - occlusion 5-387
- - patch graft 5-395
- - resection with reanastomosis 5-382
- - resection with replacement 5-383
- - revision of anastomosis 5-394
- - suture 5-393
- artificial opening
- - intestine 5-464
- atrial septal defect 5-357
- bile duct 5-516
- bladder (neck) 5-578
- - obstetric 5-758
- - sphincter 5-578
- blepharoptosis 5-094
- bone 5-789
- - flap, cranial 5-020
- - jaw (lower) 5-773
- - - upper 5-775
- breast 5-875
- broad ligament 5-693
- bronchus 5-334
- canaliculus, lacrimal 5-086
- cancrum oris 5-274
- canthus 5-092
- cartilage (joint) (see also Arthroplasty) 5-819
- cerebral meninges 5-021
- cerebrospinal fistula (intracranial) 5-021
- cervix 5-675
- - following delivery or abortion 5-757
- - internal os 5-674
- chest wall 5-346
- choroid 5-156
- cleft lip 5-898

Repair - *continued*
- cleft palate 5-275
- coarctation
- - with graft 5-383
- - with prosthesis 5-383
- colostomy 5-464
- colpocele 5-704
- conjunctiva
- - plasty 5-113
- - suture 5-115
- cornea
- - other plasty 5-126
- - suture 5-124
- - transplant 5-125
- cranial 5-020
- - suture (premature closure) 5-020
- - with plate or graft 5-020
- cryptorchidism 5-624
- - replacement in abdomen 5-624
- cuff
- - rotator 5-837
- cusp
- - valve (heart) 5-353
- cystocele
- - female 5-704
- - male 5-530
- defect
- - lip
- - - upper 5-898
- dental arch 5-247
- denture 9-308
- diaphragm 5-347
- diastasis recti 5-835
- diastematomyelia 5-034
- dura mater 5-021
- ear drum only 5-194
- ectropion 5-093
- encephalocele 5-021
- endocardial cushion defect 5-357
- endolymph fistula
- - inner ear 5-209
- - poststapedectomy 5-192
- enterocele
- - female 5-707
- - male 5-539
- enterostomy 5-464
- entropion 5-093
- epicanthus 5-092
- epiglottis 5-315
- episiotomy 5-758
- - routine 9-263
- - secondary 5-758
- epispadias
- - female 5-583
- - male 5-643
- esophagus 5-427

Repair - *continued*
- esophagus 5-427 - *continued*
- - hiatus - see Repair, hernia, diaphragmatic
- eye socket 5-167
- eyebrow 5-096
- eyelid 5-096
- fallopian tube 5-666
- fascia
- - hand
- - - suture 5-828
- - other plasty 5-837
- fimbriae 5-666
- fistula
- - arteriovenous NEC 5-395
- - - coronary 5-369
- - - ligation 5-387
- - - occlusion 5-387
- - cerebrospinal fluid 5-021
- - coronary 5-369
- - lacrimal 5-086
- - mastoid antrum 5-199
- - perineal 5-716
- - rectourethral 5-486
- - sinus
- - - cavernous 5-021
- - - nasal 5-226
- - ureterovaginal 5-706
- - vaginal 5-706
- fracture (see also Reduction, fracture)
- - larynx 5-315
- funnel chest 5-346
- gallbladder 5-519
- gastric ulcer 5-443
- gastroschisis 5-535
- - with plastic sheet 5-536
- hand 5-824
- hare lip 5-898
- heart NEC 5-374
- - cusp (with patch) 5-353
- hematocele 5-611
- hepatic duct 5-516
- hernia 5-535
- - abdominal (wall) (anterior) 5-535
- - - with prosthesis 5-536
- - crural - see Repair, hernia, inguinofemoral
- - diaphragmatic 5-537
- - - abdominal route 5-537
- - - thoracic route 5-538
- - - thoracoabdominal route 5-538
- - epigastric - see Repair, hernia, abdominal wall
- - hiatus - see Repair, hernia, diaphragmatic
- - incisional - see Repair, hernia, abdominal wall

Repair - *continued*
- hernia 5-535 - *continued*
- - inguinal - see Repair, hernia, inguinofemoral
- - inguinofemoral
- - - bilateral 5-532
- - - - with graft 5-533
- - - - with prosthesis 5-533
- - - recurrent 5-530
- - - unilateral 5-530
- - - - with graft 5-531
- - - - with mesh fabric 5-531
- - - - with prosthesis 5-531
- - internal 5-539
- - intervertebral disc 5-803
- - ischiatic 5-539
- - ischiorectal 5-539
- - lumbar 5-539
- - muscle 5-837
- - obturator 5-539
- - parasternal 5-538
- - paraumbilical 5-534
- - perineal 5-539
- - pudendal 5-539
- - recurrent 5-535
- - retroperitoneal 5-539
- - sciatic 5-539
- - sliding (inguinal) 5-530
- - umbilical 5-534
- - uveal 5-136
- - ventral - see Repair, hernia, abdominal wall
- hydrocele 5-611
- - of spermatic cord 5-630
- hypospadias
- - male 5-643
- ileostomy 5-464
- ingrown toenail 8-186
- intestinal trauma 5-467
- joint (capsule) (see also Arthroplasty) 5-819
- - finger 5-817
- - hand 5-817
- - jaw 5-774
- - shoulder 5-818
- - toe(s) 5-813
- kidney 5-557
- laceration
- - cervix 5-675
- - - internal os 5-674
- - - obstetrical 5-757
- - obstetrical
- - - nos 5-758
- - - perineal 5-716
- - - obstetrical 5-758
- - skin 5-890
- - urethra 5-583

Repair - *continued*
- laceration - *continued*
- - urethra 5-583 - *continued*
- - - obstetrical 5-758
- - uterus
- - - nonobstetric 5-695
- - - obstetrical 5-757
- - vagina
- - - obstetrical 5-758
- lacrimal apparatus 5-086
- lamina cribrosa (intracranial) 5-021
- laryngostomy 5-315
- larynx 5-315
- leaflet
- - cardiac valve 5-353
- ligament
- - broad 5-693
- - cardinal 5-693
- - joint 5-819
- - - foot 5-813
- lip 5-898
- liver 5-505
- lop ear 5-186
- lung
- - hernia 5-334
- lymphatic channels 5-409
- macrostoma 5-898
- mastoid 5-199
- meninges
- - cerebral 5-021
- - spinal 5-034
- meningocele
- - cranial 5-021
- - spinal 5-034
- meningoencephalocele 5-021
- meningomyelocele 5-034
- microstoma 5-898
- mouth
- - external 5-898
- - internal 5-274
- multiple injuries
- - abdominal organs 5-549
- muscle
- - rectus (abdominal) 5-546
- - - secondary 5-545
- musculotendinous cuff 5-835
- myelocele 5-034
- nasopharynx atresia 5-293
- nerve
- - old injury 5-046
- - suture 5-042
- - transplant 5-044
- nose 5-217
- omentum 5-546
- omphalocele 5-534
- open wound 5-890
- orbit 5-167

Repair - *continued*
- ovary 5-656
- pacemaker, heart 5-378
- palate 5-275
- palpebral fissure 5-092
- pancreas 5-529
- pancreatic duct 5-529
- pelvic floor
- - male 5-489
- - obstetric 5-758
- pelvis
- - renal 5-557
- penis 5-643
- perforation 5-443
- - duodenal ulcer 5-443
- - gastric ulcer 5-443
- - intestinal 5-467
- - peptic ulcer 5-443
- - tympanic 5-194
- pericardium 5-374
- perineum 5-716
- - male 5-890
- - obstetric 5-758
- peripheral nerve (see also Repair, nerve) 5-042
- peritoneum 5-546
- pharynx NEC 5-294
- - plastic 5-293
- - suture 5-294
- postpuerperal 5-716
- pouch of Douglas 5-707
- - male 5-486
- prolapse
- - rectal mucosa 5-486
- - rectum 5-486
- - uterine 5-693
- - uterovaginal 5-693
- ptosis
- - eyelid 5-094
- rectocele (female) (with colporraphy) 5-704
- rectum 5-486
- retina 5-154
- rupture
- - bladder 5-578
- - uterus
- - - obstetric 5-757
- salivary gland or duct 5-263
- sclera 5-137
- - with graft 5-137
- scrotum 5-613
- septum
- - heart 5-357
- - - with prosthesis 5-356
- - nasal 5-217
- - - with graft 5-217
- sinus, nasal 5-226

Repair - *continued*
– skin 5-890
– skull 5-020
– socket (orbit) 5-167
– spermatic cord 5-634
– sphincter
– – anus 5-496
– – – obstetric 5-758
– spina bifida 5-034
– spinal cord 5-034
– spleen 5-419
– sternum
– – defect 5-346
– stoma, artificial, intestines 5-464
– stomach 5-445
– symblepharon 5-114
– synovial membrane 5-819
– tendon 5-837
– – hand 5-828
– – – pulley reconstruction 5-827
– – – reattachment 5-825
– – – suture 5-824
– – – transfer 5-825
– – other plasty 5-837
– – reconstruction 5-836
– – suture 5-835
– testis 5-625
– tetralogy of Fallot
– – anastomosis aortopulmonary 5-390
– – correction of septal defect 5-357
– – valvulotomy, pulmonary 5-351
– thymus gland 5-079
– tongue 5-254
– tooth 5-232
– trachea 5-316
– tunica vaginalis 5-613
– tympanum 5-194
– ureter 5-568
– ureterostomy opening 5-568
– urethra 5-583
– – obstetric 5-758
– urethrocele (female) 5-704
– urinary injuries 5-578
– uterus 5-695
– – following delivery or abortion 5-757
– – prolapsed 5-693
– – supports 5-693
– uvula 5-276
– vagina 5-706
– – for
– – – cystocele 5-704
– – – hernia 5-704
– – – rectocele 5-704
– – – urethrocele 5-704
– – postpartum 5-758
– – prolapse 5-704
– – wall 5-706

Repair - *continued*
– valves
– – heart NEC 5-354
– – – with graft 5-352
– – – with prosthesis 5-352
– varicocele 5-630
– vas deferens 5-637
– vein NEC 5-395
– – angioplasty 5-395
– – suture 5-393
– – venovenostomy 5-392
– ventricular septal defect 5-357
– vermilion border 5-898
– vertebral arch defect (spina bifida) 5-034
– vulva 5-716
– wound 5-890
– – abdominal wall 5-545
– – deep 5-890
– – scalp 5-890
– – – with skin graft 5-893
– – superficial 5-890
Repeat
– operation
– – vascular graft 5-394
– prescription 9-130
– previous treatment 9-131
Replacement
– acetabulum 5-816
– – and femoral head 5-815
– battery
– – hearing aid 9-313
– bladder
– – with ileal loop 5-577
– – with sigmoid 5-577
– bladder drainage 8-135
– catheter
– – cerebral ventricle 5-024
– – indwelling
– – – bladder 8-135
– – urethral 8-135
– cord (umbilical) (to assist delivery) 5-739
– cystostomy tube 8-136
– drainage device
– – urinary tract 5-599
– electrode
– – endocardial 8-882
– – myocardial 5-378
– femur 5-786
– – head 5-816
– heart 5-375
– – assist system 5-376
– – valve 5-352
– hip
– – total 5-815
– indwelling catheter
– – bladder 8-135
– intravenous electrode 8-882

Replacement - *continued*
— inverted uterus
— — puerperal (manually) 8-256
— — surgical 5-759
— iris 5-136
— pacemaker 8-882
— — heart 5-378
— — — battery 8-881
— plaster 8-313
— pleural drain 8-155
— prolapsed rectum 8-242
— prosthesis
— — limb 5-855
— pulse generator 8-881
— retroverted gravid uterus 5-759
— stapes 5-191
— testis (in scrotum) 5-624
— — by prosthesis 5-626
— therapy 9-111
— tracheostomy tube 8-700
— umbilical cord (to assist delivery) 5-739
— ureter
— — with ileal segment 5-564
— valve
— — heart 5-352
— — Holter
— — — for hydrocephalus 5-024
— — Spitz-Holter 5-024
— — ventriculostomy 5-024
— vascular graft 5-394
— vitreous 5-157
— — for retinal reattachment 5-154
Reposition (see also Replacement,
   reimplantation) 5-909
— cilia base 5-096
— cord (manually) 8-254
— fetus (manually) 8-253
— pterygium 5-122
— uterus
— — gravid, retroverted 8-252
Rerouting
— nerve 5-045
Resection (see also Excision) 5-909
— aneurysm
— — heart 5-373
— — — with replacement 5-374
— aponeurosis 5-833
— — hand 5-823
— artery 5-385
— — with reanastomosis 5-382
— — with replacement 5-383
— bladder (urinary) 5-575
— — endoscopic 5-573
— — neck 5-573
— — segmental 5-575
— — transurethral 5-573
— bone 5-784

Resection - *continued*
— bone 5-784 - *continued*
— — jaw (lower) 5-773
— — — upper 5-772
— breast 5-860
— — with graft reconstruction 5-869
— bronchus 5-321
— bursa 5-834
— caecum 5-455
— chest wall
— — lesion 5-343
— colon
— — partial 5-455
— conjunctiva for pterygium 5-112
— esophagus 5-423
— exteriorized intestine 5-460
— fascia 5-833
— — hand 5-823
— gallbladder 5-511
— infundibular
— — heart 5-351
— intestine NEC 5-455
— — for interposition 5-453
— — large 5-455
— — small 5-454
— kidney 5-553
— ligament (joint) 5-809
— lip 5-884
— lung 5-323
— Meckel's diverticulum 5-451
— mesentery 5-543
— muscle 5-833
— — hand 5-823
— — ocular 5-101
— — — levator palpebrae 5-094
— — — oblique 5-101
— — — orbicularis 5-096
— — — rectus 5-101
— — — with recession 5-101
— nose 5-213
— ovary (partial) 5-651
— palate 5-272
— pancreas 5-524
— — radical 5-526
— — total 5-525
— pancreatico-duodenal (radical) 5-526
— pelvic viscera, en masse
— — female 5-687
— — male 5-576
— pharynx 5-292
— prostate - see Prostatectomy
— rectosigmoid
— — pull-through 5-483
— rectum (see also Excision, rectum) 5-485
— rib 5-784
— — drainage of chest 5-340
— sclera 5-132

Resection - *continued*
- sclera 5-132 - *continued*
- - for anterior chamber drainage 5-132
- - with implant 5-132
- scrotum 5-612
- septum
- - nasal 5-214
- sigmoid 5-455
- sternum 5-784
- stomach - see Gastrectomy
- submucous 5-214
- - larynx 5-302
- - nasal septum 5-214
- - vocal cords 5-302
- synovial membrane
- - joint 5-805
- tendon 5-833
- - hand 5-823
- tongue 5-251
- trachea
- - with reanastomosis 5-314
- ureter 5-563
- vocal cords (submucous) 5-302
Reserve
- alkaline 2-122
Resettlement
- vocational 9-538
Residual urinary volume
- determination 1-331
Respiration, respiratory
- artificial 8-722
- assistance
- - endotracheal 8-711
- function test 1-719
- intensive care unit 9-151
- postmortem bacteriology 2-561
- quotient 1-762
Response
- to carbon dioxide 1-716
Restoration
- cardio-esophageal angle 5-537
- extremities (see reattachment) NEC
  5-859
- eye socket 5-167
- orbital 5-167
- tooth
- - amalgam 5-232
- - by filling 5-232
- - by inlay 5-233
- - other 5-234
Restraint
- by appliance 8-359
Resuscitation 8-729
- closed cardiac massage 8-520
- hyperbaric oxygen 8-762
- manual 8-720
- mechanical ventilator 8-710

Resuscitation 8-729 - *continued*
- mouth to mouth 8-721
- operative 8-724
- pulmonary 8-710
Resuture (see also Suture) 5-890
- abdominal wall 5-545
Reticulocyte count 2-804
Retinaculotomy
- carpal 5-821
- - for nerve decompression 5-043
- phalangeal 5-821
- tarsal 5-831
- - for nerve decompression 5-043
Retinopexy 5-154
- photocoagulation 8-622
Retraining
- work oriented 9-533
Retroversion
- gravid uterus
- - repositioning
- - - manually 8-252
Revascularization
- arterial
- - endarterectomy 5-381
- cardiac
- - arterial implant 5-362
- - bypass graft 5-361
- - direct 5-361
- - endarterectomy 5-360
- - indirect 5-362
- femoral artery
- - bypass 5-392
- myocardium (see also Revascularization,
  cardiac) 5-363
Reversion to sinus rhythm 8-642
Revision
- amputation stump 5-850
- anastomosis
- - artery 5-394
- - intestinal 5-469
- - stomach 5-444
- bladder neck 5-578
- colostomy 5-464
- enterostomy 5-464
- fenestration
- - inner ear 5-206
- ileostomy 5-464
- laryngostomy 5-315
- mastoid antrum 5-209
- mastoidectomy 5-209
- palatoplasty 5-275
- pedicle graft 5-897
- prosthesis 5-566
- salivary duct
- - scar 5-263
- scar tissue 5-891
- spectacles 9-322

Revision - *continued*
— stapedectomy 5-192
— stoma, artificial, intestine 5-464
— tracheostomy 5-316
— tympanoplasty 5-196
— ureteroenterostomy 5-567
— valve
— — cardiac 5-353
— ventricular shunt 5-024
Rhesus
— antibodies 2-823
— negative mothers
— — postpartum protection 4-440
— protection 4-440
Rhinocheiloplasty 5-898
Rhinoplasty 5-217
Rhinorrhaphy 5-217
Rhinoscopy 1-243
— foreign body
— — removal 8-104
Rhinotomy 5-211
Rhizotomy
— acoustic 5-040
— spinal (roots) 5-031
— trigeminal 5-040
Rhytidectomy
— eyelids 5-096
— facial 5-900

Rhytidoplasty 5-900
Ring biopsy
— cervix 1-474
Ring's operation 5-815
Ringing
— hemorrhoids 8-341
Root canal therapy 5-237
Rorschach test 1-934
Rose bengal test 2-324
Rose-Waaler test 2-664
Rosette inhibition test, lymphocytes 2-874
Rotation
— fetal head
— — by forceps 5-724
— — manually 8-253
Rotation tests
— vestibular function 1-235
Roux-Herzen-Judine operation 5-425
Rubin's operation 5-667
Rupture
— membranes
— — artificial 5-730
— ovarian cyst
— — manually 5-650
Rush' operation 5-787
Rutger drawing test 1-939

S

Sabourauds medium 2-701
Saccharose
– blood 2-139
Sacculotomy 5-207
Sacrectomy
– partial 5-784
Sacropromontory fixation of rectum 5-486
Saemisch's operation 5-121
Salicylate
– blood assay 2-163
Saliva
– examination 2-288
Salpingectomy 5-665
– bilateral 5-662
– for sterilization 5-980
– partial 5-665
– unilateral 5-661
Salpingo-oophorectomy
– bilateral 5-655
– for sterilization 5-980
– unilateral 5-653
Salpingo-oophoroplasty 5-656
Salpingo-oophororrhaphy 5-656
Salpingo-oophorostomy 5-666
Salpingo-oophorotomy 5-650
Salpingo-uterostomy 5-666
Salpingocolpostomy 5-666
Salpingohysterostomy 5-666
Salpingoplasty 5-666
Salpingorrhaphy 5-666
Salpingosalpingostomy 5-666
Salpingostomy 5-666
Salpingotomy 5-660
Salt
– loading test 1-740
Salting (intrauterine)
– for termination of pregnancy 5-750
Samaritans advisory service 9-651
Sampling
– blood 1-914
– – continuous (monitoring) 8-945
– – fetus, intrauterine 5-755
– coronary artery 1-276
– selective
– – organ
– – – venous catheterization 1-860
– – venous 1-860
– – – adrenal 1-862
– – – renal 1-861
Santonin

Santonin - continued
– excretion 2-322
Saturation analysis
– thyroxine 2-402
Saucerization
– bone 5-783
– jaw 5-771
– skull 5-015
Scalenotomy 5-831
Scalp suction delivery 5-728
Scapulopexy 5-789
Scarification
– conjunctiva 5-112
Schanz operation
– osteotomy 5-781
Schauta-Amreich operation 5-686
Scheie's operation 5-132
Schilling
– blood count 2-881
– hemogram 2-881
Schlatter's operation 5-439
School child
– care by other personnel 4-788
– – first attention 4-788
– – home visit 4-793
– – subsequent 4-789
– interview with nurse 4-737
– medical examination 4-730
– – primary school 4-730
– – – entrance 4-730
– – – other 4-731
– – secondary school 4-732
– – – entrance 4-732
– – – other 4-733
– nurse home visit 4-738
– parent interview with nurse 4-736
Schuknecht's operation 5-191
Sclera 5-153
Sclerectomy 5-132
– with retinal reattachment 5-153
Scleroplasty 5-137
Sclerosis, induction
– vein 5-970
– veins
– – leg 5-971
Sclerostomy 5-132
Sclerotomy 5-132
– exploratory 5-139
Scotch tape
– collection of perianal parasites 1-911

Scraping
 – conjunctiva 5-112
 – cornea 5-123
 – rectal mucosa 1-911
 – skin
 – – fungus 2-700
 – skin lesion
 – – virology 1-911
 – trachoma follicles 5-112
Screening 4-279
 – adult 4-249
 – anticancer 4-259
 – battered baby suspect 4-221
 – biochemical 4-260
 – – disorders 4-260
 – – neonatal 4-215
 – chest x-ray 4-240
 – childhood 4-239
 – congenital hip disease 4-211
 – cot death liability 4-220
 – deafness
 – – childhood 4-230
 – feto-placental products 4-202
 – for prematurity 4-210
 – galactosemia 4-214
 – hemoglobinopathy 4-213
 – infant examination NEC 4-229
 – infectious conditions
 – – childhood 4-233
 – multiphasic 4-270
 – phenylketonuria 4-212
 – physical disability
 – – childhood 4-231
 – prenatal 4-209
 – psychological
 – – childhood 4-232
 – sicklemia 4-213
 – sickling 4-213
 – thalassemia 4-213
Scrotectomy 5-612
Scrotoplasty 5-613
Scrototomy 5-610
Sculpturing
 – valve
 – – cardiac 5-351
 – – heart 5-351
Secretin
 – production 2-314
 – response 2-333
Section (surgical)
 – brain (fibres) NEC 5-012
 – – prefrontal 5-012
 – – thalamus 5-013
 – cauda equina 5-031
 – cingulate gyrus 5-012
 – cornea 5-121
 – corneoscleral 5-132

Section - continued
 – corpus callosum 5-012
 – ganglion
 – – sympathetic 5-050
 – – trigeminal tract 5-040
 – globus pallidus 5-013
 – hypophyseal stalk 5-075
 – ligament
 – – spinal 5-801
 – medulla oblongata 5-012
 – mesencephalon 5-012
 – nerve
 – – acoustic 5-040
 – – cranial 5-040
 – – in skull 5-040
 – – peripheral (sensory root) 5-040
 – – spinal (root) 5-031
 – – sympathetic 5-050
 – – trigeminal tract 5-040
 – – – within skull 5-040
 – spinal
 – – cord 5-032
 – – ligament 5-030
 – – nerve (root) 5-031
 – tendon
 – – Achilles 5-831
 – thalamus 5-013
 – thyroglossal tract 5-060
 – tooth 5-231
 – whole organ (for examination) 2-950
Sedimentation rate (erythrocytes) 2-810
Selective organ sampling by venous
  catheterization 1-860
Semen specimen
 – collection 1-341
Seminal stains
 – forensic examination 2-942
 – identification 2-942
Sengstaken's operation 5-428
Sensitized tanned red cell agglutination
  2-631
Sensory mapping 1-200
Separation
 – choroid 5-156
 – conjoined twins 5-859
 – fused labia 5-719
 – sutured layers
 – – abdominal wall 5-545
Septectomy (nasal) 5-214
Septoplasty (nasal) 5-217
Septostomy
 – atrial 5-355
Septotomy
 – heart
 – – balloon catheter 5-355
 – – open operation nos 5-355
 – – transvenous 5-355

Septotomy - *continued*
− nasal 5-211
Sequestrectomy 5-780
− jaw 5-770
− nose 5-211
− skull 5-011
Serial plasma CEA
− assay 2-662
Serological diagnosis 2-629
− conditions NEC 2-669
− fungi 2-702
− infectious disease NEC 2-619
− non-infectious diseases 2-669
− parasites 2-759
− syphilis 2-609
− treponemal disease 2-609
− treponemal diseases 2-609
− virus 2-558
− with micro-organism 2-619
Seromucoid
− blood 2-134
Serum (see also Blood and Plasma)
− acute phase protein 2-107
− alanine
− − identification 2-100
− − transaminase 2-460
− amylase 2-470
− anti-alpha fetoprotein 2-667
− antiamebic
− − fluorescent antibody test 2-753
− antileucocytic 2-640
− antitrypsin activity 2-659
− cholecystokinin pancreatozymin 2-335
− complement level (hemolytic) 2-655
− gastrin 2-334
− glutamic oxaloacetic transaminase 2-460
− glutamic pyruvic transaminase 2-461
− haptoglobins 2-643
− iron 2-835
− lactate dehydrogenase 2-450
− lysozyme 2-484
− neutralizing antibodies 2-624
− phosphate 2-154
− proinsulin 2-339
− protein bound iodine 2-400
− sample 1-914
− − paired 1-914
− thyroid stimulating hormone 2-406
− T-4
− − free 2-404
− − total 2-402
Sex
− chromatin 2-922
SGOT 2-460
SGPT 2-460
Shaving
− burn 5-883

Shaving - *continued*
− scar
− − cornea 5-123
− skin
− − for graft 5-893
Shea's operation 5-191
Sheep cell agglutination test 2-664
Shelf operation (hip) 5-816
Sheltered employment 9-537
Shirodkar's suture 5-674
Shock therapy 9-192
Short wave therapy - see Diathermy
Shortening
− bone 5-789
− endopelvic fascia 5-693
− eyelid
− − margin 5-096
− − muscle 5-094
− fixation device
− − internal 5-787
− ligament (joint) 5-819
− − broad 5-693
− − round 5-693
− − sacrouterine 5-693
− − uterus 5-693
− muscle 5-837
− − eye 5-104
− − eyelid 5-094
− − levator palpebrae 5-094
− scleral 5-153
− tendon 5-837
− − hand 5-828
− ureter 5-563
− − with reimplantation 5-563
Shunt (see also Anastomosis and By-pass)
  5-022
− endolymphatic 5-207
− femoropopliteal 5-392
− intestines 5-458
− lumbar subarachnoid peritoneal 5-036
− lymphovenous 5-405
− mesocaval 5-391
− portal to vena cava 5-391
− saccus endolymphaticus 5-207
− salpingothecal 5-036
− semicircular-subarachnoid 5-207
− spinal 5-036
− splenorenal 5-391
− subarachnoid-peritoneal 5-036
− subdural 5-022
− superior mesenteric-caval 5-391
− ureter 5-567
− ventricular
− − formation 5-023
− − irrigation 8-151
− ventriculoatrial 5-023
− ventriculocaval 5-023

Shunt - *continued*
- ventriculocisternal 5-022
- ventriculopleural 5-023
- ventriculosubarachnoid 5-022
Sialoadenectomy 5-262
Sialoadenolithotomy 5-260
Sialoadenotomy 5-260
Sialodochoplasty 5-263
Sialolithotomy 5-260
Sickling (blood red cells) detection 2-840
Sigmoid bladder operation 5-577
Sigmoidectomy 5-455
Sigmoidomyotomy 5-469
Sigmoidopexy 5-466
Sigmoidoproctostomy 5-459
Sigmoidorectostomy 5-459
Sigmoidoscopy 1-642
- biopsy 1-451
- destruction of lesion 5-452
- foreign body removal 8-113
Sigmoidosigmoidostomy 5-459
- end to end 5-455
Sigmoidostomy 5-461
Sigmoidotomy 5-450
Sigmoidoureterostomy 5-566
Silver nitrate
- application 5-950
Single breath
- CO diffusing capacity 1-715
- expiration test 1-713
Single ureter
- urine sampling 1-654
Sinusectomy 5-225
- ethmoid 5-225
- frontal 5-223
- sphenoid 5-225
Sinusotomy
- combined 5-224
- ethmoidal 5-224
- frontal 5-223
- maxillary
- - aspiration 5-221
- - external 5-222
- - intranasal 5-221
- - radical 5-222
- - simple 5-221
- sphenoid 5-224
Size-reduction 5-901
- abdominal wall 5-901
- breast 5-874
Skeletal traction 8-471
Skin
- examination
- - for parasites 2-732
- fold thickness (measurement) 1-952
- heavy metal 2-940
- reaction

Skin - *continued*
- reaction - *continued*
- - to fungi 2-703
- snip
- - bacterial investigation 1-911
- - helminthic search 1-911
- - histology - see Biopsy, surgical, skin
- specimen for examination 1-911
- temperature
- - measurement 1-370
- test 1-700
- - allergy 1-702
- - bacterial antigen 1-704
- - hydatid 1-704
- - hypersensitivity 1-702
- - pollen 1-702
- - provocation 1-704
- - susceptibility 1-701
- - tuberculin 1-703
- traction 8-420
Sleeve resection
- bronchus
- - wide 5-321
- stomach 5-438
Slide
- agglutination test (bacterial) (microscopic) 2-612
- stained (see also Stain) 2-503
- unstained (for microscope) 2-500
Sling
- application 8-301
- - fracture 8-303
- - pelvic 8-302
- fascial
- - for facial weakness 5-900
Sling operation
- eyelid 5-094
- fascial 5-837
- - uterus 5-693
- levator muscle 5-593
- orbicularis muscle 5-093
- rectum (puborectalis) 5-486
- retropubic 5-595
- suprapubic 5-594
- tongue 5-254
- urethral 5-594
Slitting
- canaliculus for
- - passage of probe 5-084
- cornea 5-121
- lens 5-143
Slocum's operation 5-848
Smear
- cytology 4-250
- - cervix (uteri) 4-251
- superficial
- - biopsy - see Biopsy, non surgical

Smith's operation 5-493
Snaring
− polypus
− − aural 5-204
− − cervix 5-672
− − nasal 5-212
Snellen test type 1-211
Social case work 9-719
Social worker intervention 9-719
Socioeconomic care 9-762
Sociopsychological care 9-769
Sodium
− balance 2-351
− plasma 2-150
Somatotyping 1-950
Somogyi units 2-470
Somogyi-Nelson test 2-130
Sondage
− esophagus 5-428
Sondergaard's operation 5-357
Sounding
− urethra 5-585
Special bed 8-373
Special school
− for handicapped children 9-512
Special transport 9-800
Specific conductance
− lung 1-712
Spectacles
− for aphakia 9-325
Spectrophotometry 2-491
Spectrum
− antibiotic 2-530
Speech
− therapy 9-410
− training 9-411
− − esophageal 9-414
− − for defect correction 9-415
Sperm
− count 2-915
− mobility 2-915
− stains, forensic examination 2-942
Spermatic fluid
− chemistry 2-285
− examination 2-915
Spermatocelectomy 5-631
Spermatocystectomy 5-606
Spermatocystostomy 5-606
Spermatocystotomy 5-606
Spermiogram 2-915
− amniotic fluid 2-917
Sphenoidectomy 5-225
− approach to brain stem 5-029
Sphenoidotomy 5-224
Sphincter saving
− operation
− − rectum 5-485

Sphincterectomy
− anal 5-494
Sphincteroplasty
− anal 5-496
− − postpartum 5-758
− bladder (neck) 5-578
Sphincterorrhaphy
− anal 5-496
− − postpartum 5-758
Sphincterotomy
− anal 5-494
− cardia 5-426
− iris 5-135
− pancreatic 5-518
− transduodenal ampullary 5-518
− Oddi 5-518
Sphingolipids
− blood 2-145
Spinal
− brace 9-343
− carriage 9-800
− frame 8-371
− stabilization 5-810
− support 9-343
− traction 8-410
Spinelli's operation 5-759
Spirography 1-710
− basic 1-710
Spirometry 1-710
− basic 1-710
− dynamic 1-711
Spitz-Holter valve 5-023
− replacement 5-024
Spivack's operation
− gastrostomy 5-432
Splanchnicectomy 5-051
Splanchnicotomy 5-050
Spleen, splenic
− blood pool 2-814
− pulp smear 2-800
Splenectomy (partial) (total) 5-413
Splenolysis 5-544
Splenopexy 5-419
Splenoplasty 5-419
Splenopneumopexy 5-419
Splenorrhaphy 5-419
Splenotomy 5-412
Splint, splinting
− dental
− − external 8-335
− dislocation
− − hip 8-322
− finger 8-321
− fracture 8-324
− hand 8-320
− knee 8-323
− limb 8-309

Splint - *continued*
- periodontal 5-246
- pneumatic 8-351
- teeth 8-335
- ureter 5-562
- urethral 8-360
Split thickness graft 5-893
Splitting
- lacrimal papilla 5-084
- larynx 5-313
- spinal cord 5-032
- sternum 5-781
- tendon sheath 5-830
- - hand 5-820
- trachea 5-313
Spondylosyndesis 5-810
Sputum
- collection 1-912
- parasite examination 2-731
Ssabanejev-Frank operation 5-432
Stabilization
- ankle 5-811
- bone 5-789
- foot 5-811
- hip 5-812
- joint (see also Arthrodesis) 5-812
- shoulder 5-812
- teeth, fractured mandible 5-762
Stain, staining
- bacteria slide 2-503
- bipolar 2-503
- fluorescent antibodies 2-646
- for abnormal morphology
- - red blood cells 2-805
- for eosinophils 2-882
- giemsa 2-805
- gram 2-503
- hematoxylin and eosin, for histology
  2-902
- indirect for leucocytes 2-883
- papanicolaou (uterine cervix) 2-916
- quinacrine mustard 2-925
- reticulum, for histology 2-902
- vital 2-804
- Ziehl-Neelsen 2-504
Stamm-Kader operation 5-432
Stanmore's operation, hip 5-815
Stapedectomy, stapectomy 5-191
- revision 5-192
- with
- - fenestration of footplate 5-191
- - graft 5-191
- - wire prosthesis 5-191
Stapedial reflex response 1-231
Stapediolysis 5-190
Stapes mobilization
- with stapedectomy 5-191

Stapling
- diaphysis 5-787
- epiphyseal plate 5-787
Starr-Edwards valve 5-352
Static compliance 1-712
Stationary bicycle 9-453
Steinberg's operation 5-444
Step test 1-724
Stereoscopic vision
- testing 1-216
Stereotaxis
- globus pallidus 5-013
- pituitary 5-075
- spinal 5-032
- thalamus 5-013
Sterilization
- female 5-980
- - culdoscopic 5-980
- - endoscopic 5-980
- - laparoscopic 5-980
- - ligation of fallopian tubes 5-980
- - peritoneoscopic 5-980
- - permanent 5-980
- - salpingectomy 5-980
- - surgical 5-980
- male
- - orchidectomy 5-981
- - surgical 5-981
- - vasectomy 5-981
Sternotomy 5-781
- for bone marrow biopsy 5-418
Steroid
- blood NEC 2-143
- - by caval sampling 2-439
- prophylaxis 4-450
- supression test 2-425
- urine NEC 2-449
Stimulation, stimulator
- ACTH 2-420
- adrenocorticotrophic 2-420
- atrial 8-657
- - overdrive suppression 8-655
- electrical 8-669
- urethral testing 1-330
- venous flow 8-544
Stomach
- contents
- - chemical analysis
- - - forensic 2-943
- - macroscopic examination 2-951
- emptying time 2-305
Stomal calibration 1-322
Stomatoplasty 5-274
Stomatorrhaphy 5-274
Stools - see Feces
Strayer's operation 5-831
Strength

Strength - *continued*
- of grip 1-751
Stress tests
- pregnancy 4-201
Stretching
- eyelid (and elongation) 5-096
- fascia 8-216
- foreskin 8-227
- muscle 8-215
- nerve (peripheral) 5-049
- phimosis 8-227
- tendon 8-215
Stripping
- artery 5-381
- larynx 5-300
- nerve
- - peripheral 5-043
- saphenous vein, varicose 5-384
- subdural membrane 5-014
- sympathetic, periarterial 5-397
- - carotid 5-397
- - nerve 5-051
- varicose veins 5-384
- vocal cords 5-300
Stromeyer-Little operation 5-500
Study
- temperature gradient 1-736
Subcutaneous
- filler 5-880
- tunnel
- - for esophageal substitute 5-427
Sublingual test
- allergy 1-708
Substitute mothering 9-751
Suction
- clearance
- - middle ear 8-172
- drainage
- - continuous 8-179
- - stomach 8-122
- urethral catheter 8-133
Sulfhemoglobin 2-832
Sulkowitch test 2-230
Summerskill's operation 5-087
Support
- bodily 8-370
- - fracture 8-303
Suppression
- sinoatrial node 8-655
- steroid, test 2-425
- tri-iodothyronine, test 2-407
Suprapubic
- catheterization 5-571
- cystostomy 5-572
Surveillance 4-319
- infectious disease 4-319
- - carrier 4-311

Surveillance 4-319 - *continued*
- infectious disease 4-319 - *continued*
- - contact 4-310
- - search
- - - carrier 4-314
- - - contact 4-313
- - - new cases 4-312
- local disease 4-501
Suspension
- balanced 8-430
- - for traction 8-430
- Buck's 8-430
- diverticulum, pharynx 5-294
- kidney 5-556
- ovary 5-656
- periurethral 5-596
- pharyngeal diverticulum 5-294
- thyroid 5-069
- urethra 5-597
- urethrovesical 5-597
- - gracilis 5-597
- - junction 5-596
- - levator muscle 5-593
- - pubococcygeus muscle 5-593
- - retropubic 5-595
- - suprapubic 5-594
- uterus 5-693
- vagina 5-706
- vesical, retropubic 5-597
Suture (see also Repair and Ligation) 5-890
- abdominal wall 5-545
- - delayed 5-545
- - secondary 5-545
- aneurysm NEC 5-395
- - arteriovenous 5-395
- - endoaneurysmorrhaphy 5-395
- anus 5-496
- - postpartum 5-758
- artery 5-393
- - ligation 5-387
- bile duct 5-516
- bladder 5-578
- blood vessel 5-393
- - ligation 5-387
- bowel 5-467
- breast (skin) 5-875
- bronchus 5-334
- canaliculus, lacrimal 5-086
- capsule of joint 5-819
- cervix 5-675
- - encirclement 5-674
- - obstetric trauma 5-757
- - postpartum 5-757
- - supporting
- - - pregnancy 5-674
- cleft palate 5-275
- conjunctiva 5-115

Suture - *continued*
- cornea 5-124
- cul-de-sac 5-707
- dehiscent wound
- - abdominal 5-545
- delayed 5-890
- diverticulum, intestinal 5-467
- ear, external 5-183
- esophagus 5-427
- eye, socket 5-167
- eyeball 5-169
- eyebrow 5-890
- eyelid 5-095
- - ptosis repair 5-094
- - repair 5-095
- face 5-890
- fascia 5-835
- - hand 5-824
- - to skeletal attachment 5-837
- - - hand 5-828
- gallbladder 5-519
- gum 5-242
- heart NEC 5-374
- - septum 5-357
- hemostatic
- - liver 5-505
- - stomach 5-443
- hepatic duct 5-516
- hymen 5-706
- intestine 5-467
- kidney 5-557
- lacerations 5-890
- larynx 5-315
- ligament (joint) 5-819
- - broad 5-693
- - gastrocolic 5-546
- - knee 5-819
- - - cruciate 5-814
- - sacrouterine 5-693
- lip 5-898
- liver 5-505
- meninges 5-021
- - cerebral 5-021
- - spinal 5-034
- mesentery 5-546
- mouth 5-274
- - external 5-898
- - internal 5-274
- muscle 5-835
- - hand 5-824
- nerve
- - cranial 5-042
- - peripheral 5-042
- - sympathetic 5-053
- nose 5-217
- - external 5-890
- - internal 5-217

Suture - *continued*
- omentum 5-546
- ovary 5-656
- palate 5-275
- palpebral fissure 5-092
- pancreas 5-529
- paraurethral tissues
- - to symphysis 5-595
- peptic ulcer, perforated NEC 5-443
- - duodenal 5-443
- - gastric 5-443
- perforation intestine 5-467
- pericardium 5-374
- perineum
- - female 5-716
- - - postpartum 5-758
- - male 5-890
- periosteum 5-789
- pharynx 5-294
- rectum 5-486
- retina for reattachment 5-154
- ruptured chordae tendinae 5-354
- salivary duct 5-263
- salivary gland 5-263
- sclera 5-137
- scrotum 5-613
- secondary 5-890
- - abdominal wall 5-545
- - peritoneum 5-545
- Shirodkar 5-674
- skin 5-890
- - breast 5-875
- - ear 5-183
- - eyelid 5-095
- - nose 5-890
- - penis 5-643
- - scrotum 5-613
- - vulva 5-716
- spermatic cord 5-634
- spinal meninges 5-034
- spleen 5-419
- stomach 5-445
- sympathetic
- - nerve or ganglion 5-053
- tendon 5-835
- - hand 5-824
- - to skeletal attachment 5-837
- - - hand 5-828
- testis 5-625
- tongue 5-254
- trachea 5-316
- tunica vaginalis 5-613
- ureter 5-568
- urethra 5-583
- uterus 5-695
- - nonobstetric 5-695
- - obstetric 5-757

Suture - *continued*
- uvula 5-276
- vagina 5-706
- - postpartum 5-758
- valve 5-354
- - heart 5-354
- vas deferens 5-637
- vault 5-707
- vein 5-393
- - cranial sinus 5-021
- - injuries
- - - cava, inferior 5-393
- - - peripheral 5-393
- - ligation 5-387
- vulva 5-716
- - postpartum 5-758
- wound 5-890
Swab
- conjunctival 1-910
- from wound 1-917
- nasal 1-910
- oral lesion 1-910
- throat 1-910
- urethral 1-916
- vaginal 1-916
Swallowing defect
- amelioration 9-421
Sweat
- chemistry 2-284
- sodium chloride 2-284
- test 2-339
Swenson's operation 5-483
- cystoplasty 5-577

Syme's operation 5-847
Sympathectomy 5-051
- lumbar 5-051
- periarterial 5-397
- - adrenal 5-073
- preganglionic 5-051
- tympanic 5-209
Sympatheticotripsy 5-050
Symphysiotomy
- kidney 5-557
- nonobstetric 5-801
- obstetric 5-739
Symphysis
- pleural 5-345
Synchondrotomy 5-801
- temporomandibular 5-774
Syndesis (see also Arthrodesis) 5-812
Syndesmotomy 5-801
Synechotomy (iris) 5-136
Synovectomy
- joint 5-805
- - jaw 5-774
- tendon sheath 5-833
- - hand 5-823
Synovial fluid
- examination 2-288
Syringing 8-179
- ear 8-171
- lacrimal duct 8-170
- lacrimal sac 8-170
- middle ear 8-172
Syringotomy (anal) 5-491

T

T-3 suppression test 2-407
Takata-Ara reaction or test 2-321
Taking down
– gastric anastomosis 5-444
– shunt
– – ventricular 5-024
Tamponade
– esophageal 5-428
– intrauterine
– – following delivery or abortion 5-759
– – to assist delivery 5-739
– obstetric 5-759
– uterus
– – obstetric 5-759
– vaginal
– – following delivery or abortion 5-759
Tap, tapping
– hydrocele 8-163
– subdural 5-010
Tape
– perianal
– – sample, ova 1-911
Tarsal rotation operation, eyelid 5-096
Tarsectomy (eyelid) 5-091
Tarsoplasty 5-096
Tarsorrhaphy 5-095
Tartrate resistance
– acid phosphate
– – tissue 2-904
Taste threshhold 1-200
Tattooing
– cornea 5-129
– skin defect 5-880
Tautening eyelid for entropion 5-093
Temperament
– assessment 1-931
– gradient study 1-736
Tendon
– loop operation, hand 5-825
– pulley reconstruction 5-827
– – hand 5-827
– reflex 1-201
– – timing 1-202
Tenectomy 5-833
– hand 5-823
– ocular 5-101
– – levator palpebrae 5-094
Tenodesis 5-837
– hand 5-828
Tenolysis 5-839

Tenolysis 5-839 - *continued*
– fingers 5-829
– hand 5-829
Tenoplasty 5-837
– hand 5-828
– thumb 5-827
Tenorrhaphy (see also Suture, tendon) 5-835
Tenosuture (see also Suture, tendon) 5-835
Tenosynovectomy 5-833
– hand 5-823
Tenosynovotomy 5-830
– hand 5-820
Tenotomy 5-831
– Achilles 5-831
– – elongation 5-837
– adductor 5-831
– eye muscles 5-100
– hand 5-820
– levator palpebrae 5-094
– ossicles 5-193
– scalenus muscle 5-831
– stapedius 5-190
Tensing
– orbicularis oculi 5-096
Terminal care 9-191
Termination of pregnancy 5-752
– amniotic injection 5-750
– by
– – hysterectomy 5-744
– – hysterotomy 5-744
– – intra-amniotic injection 5-750
– dilatation and curettage 5-752
– hysterotomy 5-744
– specified technique NEC 5-752
– vacuum aspiration 5-751
Test, testing (of) (see also Reaction)
– absorption
– – xylose 2-312
– adrenal function 2-354
– agar gel diffusion
– – viral precipitation 2-614
– antiglobulin
– – indirect 2-824
– antihuman globulin 2-824
– attitudes 1-933
– biliary obstruction 2-320
– capillary resistance 2-860
– cardiovascular stress 1-732
– complement fixation

Test - *continued*
- complement fixation - *continued*
- - syphilis
- - - blood 2-600
- - - cerebrospinal fluid 2-603
- deficiency
- - vitamin 1-953
- detrusor reflex 1-330
- drawing (rutger) 1-939
- eye muscle balance 1-216
- fluorescent antibody
- - antiamebic serum 2-753
- function - see Function tests
- hemagglutination
- - indirect
- - - malaria 2-754
- hemostasis 2-869
- hepatic protein dysfunction 2-321
- histamine (augmented) 2-302
- intelligence 1-930
- intestinal function 2-319
- latex fixation 2-663
- LE cells 2-872
- LSAR 2-286
- lymphocyte
- - rosette inhibition 2-874
- - transformation 2-873
- muscle
- - power 1-205
- nerve conduction 1-203
- nitro blue tetrazolium 2-885
- personality 1-932
- phenylketonuria 2-240
- pituitary response
- - to antidiuretic hormone 2-411
- - to metyrapone 2-410
- plaque reduction neutralization 2-620
- projective 1-934
- prothrombin 2-862
- psychological 1-930
- - specified NEC 1-939
- psychometric 1-930
- reflexes 1-201
- - time recording 1-202
- renal function (see also Specific chemical procedure) 2-349
- rose bengal 2-324
- sensibility, topographical 1-200
- sheep cell agglutination 2-664
- sweat 2-339
- taste 1-200
- thyroid function (see also Specific chemical procedure) 2-409
- VDRL
- - qualitative 2-601
- - quantitative 2-602
- vision - see Vision testing

Test
- Ascheim-Zondek 2-444
- Benedict 2-223
- Bernheim 2-115
- Coombs 2-824
- Fehling 2-223
- Folin-Wu 2-130
- Fouchet 2-115
- Frei 1-704
- Friedman 2-444
- Gerhardt
- - acetoacetic acid 2-240
- Guarinii 2-106
- Guthrie 2-100
- Hagedorn 2-130
- Hanger 2-321
- Hay 2-214
- Herzfeld 2-115
- Khan 2-602
- Kleihauer 2-843
- Lange 2-274
- McLean 2-130
- Millon
- - urine 2-200
- Napier 2-629
- Nonne-Apelt 2-274
- Pandy 2-274
- Paul-Bunnell 2-651
- Rorschach 1-934
- Rose-Waaler 2-664
- Somogyi-Nelson 2-130
- Sulkowitch 2-230
- Takata-Ara 2-321
- van den Bergh 2-115
- van Slyke 2-121
- Wight 2-654
Testape
- glucose in urine 2-220
Tetanus
- immunization 4-335
- - with pertussis and diphtheria 4-336
Tetraethyl lead
- blood 2-164
Thalamectomy 5-013
Thalamotomy 5-013
Theleplasty 5-872
Therapeutic pool 8-551
Therapy
- dietetic (see also Diet) 9-149
- diversional 9-501
- domestic tasks 9-521
- drug - see Drug
- educational 9-510
- electroconvulsive 8-630
- family group 9-610
- - residential 9-610
- not elsewhere classified 9-199

Therapy - *continued*
- shock (insulin) 9-192
- short wave - see Diathermy
- specialized NEC 9-299
- whirlpool 8-553
Thermal test
- vestibular function 1-234
Thermocautery (see also Cauterization) 5-914
- brain 5-014
Thermography
- skin 1-736
Thompson's operation, hip 5-816
Thoracocentesis 8-155
Thoracolysis 5-333
Thoracoplasty 5-332
Thoracoscopy
- foreign body removal 8-108
- transpleural 1-691
Thoracostomy
- without lung collapse 5-340
Thoracotomy 5-340
Three-segment balloon intra-aortic assist 5-376
Three-snip operation on punctum 5-084
Three-wheeler 9-805
- invalid 9-806
- - powered (motor) 9-805
Thrombectomy 5-380
Thrombin
- clotting time 2-861
Thromboelastogram 2-864
Thromboendarterectomy (see also Endarterectomy) 5-381
- coronary 5-360
Thrombokinetic studies 2-856
Thromboplastin
- generation time 2-865
Thrombosis
- venous
- - production 5-970
- - - leg 5-971
Thymectomy 5-077
Thymol flocculation 2-321
Thymopexy 5-079
Thyrochondrotomy 5-313
Thyrocricoidectomy 5-302
Thyrocricotomy 5-313
Thyroglobulin
- antibody 2-631
Thyroid function
- chemical tests 2-407
- other tests 2-409
Thyroid hormones
- release 2-405
Thyroidectomy 5-062
- complete 5-063

Thyroidectomy 5-062 - *continued*
- complete 5-063 - *continued*
- - by transsternal route 5-064
- partial 5-062
- subtotal 5-062
- total 5-063
- - by transsternal route 5-064
- transsternal 5-064
- with radical neck dissection 5-063
Thyroidotomy 5-060
Thyroparathyroidectomy 5-063
Thyropexy 5-069
Thyrotomy 5-313
- with (tantalum) plate 5-315
Thyrotrophic release factor 2-416
Thyroxine
- assay 2-401
Thyroxine-binding globulin 2-401
Timing
- tendon reflex 1-202
Tissue
- chemical analysis 2-952
- culture 2-930
- digestion for parasites 2-954
- examination 2-939
- immunofluorescence 2-953
Toe-to-thumb transfer 5-826
Toilet
- compound fracture, by surgery 5-795
- middle ear 5-204
- wound 8-191
- - by surgery 5-883
Tongs
- caliper 8-411
- Crutchfield 8-411
Tonometry
- cornea 1-225
Tonsillectomy 5-281
- by dissection 5-281
- by guillotine 5-281
- with adenoidectomy 5-282
- - by guillotine 5-282
Tonsillotomy 5-280
Topectomy, brain 5-014
Topical
- caustic application
- - endoscopic 5-951
Torek's operation 5-624
Torkildsen's operation 5-022
Total
- body water 2-352
- flow resistance 1-712
- leucocyte count 2-880
- lung capacity 1-710
Toti's operation 5-087
Toxocaria
- detection of antigen 2-750

Toxoplasma
– detection of antigen 2-750
Trabeculectomy
– retrocorneal 5-133
Trabeculotomy
– retrocorneal 5-133
Trace elements
– blood 2-156
Trachelectomy 5-673
– with colporrhaphy 5-673
Trachelopexy 5-693
Tracheloplasty 5-675
Trachelorrhaphy 5-675
– obstetric 5-757
Trachelotomy 5-680
– obstetric 5-739
Tracheocricotomy 5-313
Tracheofissure 5-313
Tracheolaryngotomy 5-313
– emergency 5-311
– permanent opening 5-312
Tracheoplasty 5-316
– with substitute voice box 5-316
Tracheorrhaphy 5-316
Tracheoscopy 1-621
– by tracheotomy 1-690
Tracheostomy 5-311
– emergency 5-311
– permanent 5-312
– tube
– – removal 8-109
Tracheotomy (emergency) 5-311
– permanent opening 5-312
Tracing
– carotid artery 1-252
– infectious disease 4-319
– – carrier 4-314
– – contact 4-313
Traction 8-479
– abduction 8-476
– adhesive tape 8-420
– balanced skeletal 8-402
– balanced suspension 8-430
– bone 8-471
– boot 8-421
– by extension 8-470
– cervical 8-412
– for dislocation 8-474
– forceps obstetric - see Delivery, forceps
– fracture
– – closed 8-472
– – jaw 8-473
– gallows 8-423
– hinged 8-475
– infixed pin
– – bone 8-400
– intermittent 8-477

Traction 8-479 - continued
– intermittent 8-477 - continued
– – skeletal 8-403
– joint 8-479
– Kirschner wire 8-401
– lumbar 8-413
– pelvic 8-430
– plaster cast 8-424
– skin 8-420
– skull caliper 8-411
– spinal 8-410
– Thomas splint 8-422
– vacuum
– – fetal scalp 5-728
– 90-90 8-402
Tractotomy
– brain 5-012
– spinal cord 5-032
Training
– after delivery 9-476
– blind person 9-550
– – lead dog 9-551
– co-ordination 9-432
– deaf persons 9-417
– during pregnancy 9-475
– dyslexia 9-412
– dysphasia 9-413
– esophageal speech 9-414
– finger reading 9-416
– gait 9-440
– joint movement 9-463
– – passive 9-463
– lip reading 9-416
– masticatory 9-420
– muscular endurance 9-454
– muscular strength 9-453
– speech defect correction 9-415
– use of lower limb prosthesis 9-441
Transaminase
– serum 2-460
Transection
– bone 5-781
– – femur 5-781
– – foot and toes 5-781
– – jaw 5-779
– fallopian tube
– – bilateral 5-664
– – remaining tube 5-664
– – unilateral 5-669
– muscle 5-831
– – hand 5-821
– – ocular 5-100
– nerve
– – sympathetic 5-050
– – vagus (transabdominal) 5-440
– nerve tract
– – spinal cord 5-032

Transection - *continued*
- pylorus 5-433
- tendon
- - hand 5-821
- thyroid isthmus 5-069
- uvula 5-276
- vein 5-387
- - varicose
- - - intra-abdominal 5-387
- - - peripheral 5-387
Transfer
- digital 5-826
- - to thumb 5-826
- muscle
- - hand 5-825
- - origin 5-836
- - with bone division 5-781
- skin flap 5-896
- tendon 5-836
- - hand 5-825
- - patellar 5-836
- - with bone division 5-781
- tibial tuberosity 5-781
- toe to thumb 5-826
Transfer factor
- extraction 2-932
Transferase 2-469
Transferrin
- estimation 2-835
Transfixion
- iris 5-135
Transformation
- sex
- - operation 5-644
- sexual
- - by surgery 5-644
Transfusion 8-809
- antihemophilic factor 8-814
- blood 8-801
- - cut-down 8-802
- - expander 8-812
- - intravenous 8-801
- bone marrow 8-804
- cut-down 8-802
- dextran 8-812
- dried plasma 8-813
- exchange 8-803
- - exsanguination 8-803
- - in utero 5-754
- - intraperitoneal 5-754
- - with hysterotomy 5-754
- intraperitoneal, fetal 5-754
- intrauterine 5-754
- intravenous 8-800
- - blood 8-801
- packed cells 8-805
- plasma 8-810

Transfusion 8-809 - *continued*
- plasma 8-810 - *continued*
- - dried 8-813
- platelets 8-806
- replacement 8-803
- serum 8-811
Transillumination 1-962
- antrum 1-244
- sclera 1-229
- skull 1-209
Transplantation
- aorta, thoracic 5-392
- bone
- - jaw (lower) 5-773
- - - upper 5-775
- - marrow 5-410
- - with metallic fixation 5-786
- colon 5-453
- - for esophagus 5-424
- conjunctiva 5-122
- - for pterygium 5-122
- corneal 5-125
- dura 5-021
- eye muscle 5-103
- - levator palpebrae 5-094
- hair follicles 5-902
- heart 5-375
- ileal stoma to new site 5-462
- kidney 5-555
- - cadaver 5-555
- - donor 5-555
- - heterotopic 5-555
- liver 5-504
- lung 5-335
- lymphatic 5-409
- mammary artery to myocardium 5-362
- mucous membrane
- - to eyelid 5-096
- muscle 5-836
- - hand 5-825
- nerve 5-044
- nipple 5-872
- ocular muscle 5-103
- - levator palpebrae 5-094
- ovary 5-659
- - autograft 5-656
- - homograft 5-659
- pancreas 5-528
- pterygium 5-122
- salivary duct
- - opening 5-263
- salivary gland 5-263
- skin (see also Graft, skin) 5-893
- spermatic cord 5-634
- spleen 5-419
- stomach
- - into chest 5-424

Transplantation - *continued*
- stomach - *continued*
- - - to esophagus 5-424
- temporalis muscle to orbit 5-167
- tendon 5-836
- - hand 5-825
- test 2-646
- testis 5-625
- thymus 5-078
- thyroid tissue 5-069
- tooth 5-235
- ureter 5-567
- - isolated loop 5-564
- - to
- - - bladder 5-567
- - - colon 5-566
- - - ileal conduit 5-564
- - - ileum
- - - - external diversion 5-564
- - - intestines 5-566
- - - skin 5-565
- vein
- - for bypass 5-392
- - for portal shunt 5-391
- - replacement 5-383
- vitreous 5-157
Transposition
- eyelash, flaps 5-096
- muscle 5-836
- - eye for ptosis 5-094
- - hand 5-825
- - ocular
- - - intrinsic 5-103
- nerve 5-045
- - peripheral 5-045
- - radial 5-045
- - ulnar 5-045
- nipple 5-872
- pterygium 5-122
- tendon 5-836
- - hand 5-825
- vocal cords 5-315
Transsection
- cervix
- - inverted uterus 5-759
- vagus 5-440
Transsphenoid surgical approach to brain
  stem 5-029
Transversostomy 5-461
Trapping
- cavernous sinus fistula 5-021
Tray splint 8-323
Treatment
- specialized 9-779
Trendelenburg's operation
- pulmonary embolism 5-380
- varicose veins 5-384

Trephine
- bone sequestrum 5-780
- corneal 5-121
- corneoscleral 5-132
- cranial 5-011
- - with removal of hematoma
- - - extradural 5-011
- dura 5-011
- pupil 5-135
- sclera 5-132
- skull 5-011
Treponema
- fluorescent antibody absorption test
  2-605
- hemagglutination absorption test 2-605
- immobilization 2-604
Trial forceps
- failed 5-733
Trial labor 8-960
- monitoring 8-960
Tricycle
- hand powered 9-804
- invalid 9-804
- - powered (motor) 9-805
Trigonectomy 5-575
Trigonostomy 5-561
Trimming
- alveolus (dental) 5-244
- amputation stump 5-850
- colostomy 5-452
Tripolar catheter electrode (heart) 1-265
Tubbs pyloric dilator 5-430
Tubeless gastric analysis 2-303
Tuberculin testing 1-703
Tubular (renal) reabsorption capacity 2-344
Tucking
- ocular muscle 5-104
Tumbling E test 1-212
Tumor antibodies 2-661
Tuning fork tests (for hearing) 1-232
Tunnel, subcutaneous, antethorax 5-427
Turbidity
- plasma 2-146
- thymol 2-321
- zinc 2-321
Turbinectomy 5-215
- electrocoagulation 5-215
- with ethmoidectomy 5-225
Turbinotomy 5-211
Tympanectomy 5-204
Tympanogram 1-231
Tympanoplasty
- epitympanic 5-194
- revision 5-196
- type 1 5-194
- type 2, 3, 4, 5 5-195
- with fenestration 5-205

Tympanostapediopexy 5-195
Tympanosympathectomy 5-209
Tympanotomy 5-200
Typewriter
− electrically controlled, for handicapped
   9-241
Typing
− bacteria
− − by bacteriophage 2-524

Typing - *continued*
− bacteria - *continued*
− − by phagocytosis 2-524
Tyrosinase 2-452
Tyrosine
− serum identification 2-100
TAB
− immunization 4-322

U

Ultrafiltration
- blood 8-857
- - removal of microfilaria 8-857
Ultraviolet
- irradiation 8-621
- radiation 8-621
- therapy 8-621
Ultraviolet light
- examination for fungi 2-704
Umbilectomy 5-542
Uncapping
- ureterocele 5-561
Undercutting
- cortical (brain) 5-012
- hair follicle 5-882
- perianal
- - denervation 5-490
- skin 5-882
Underwater seal
- pleural drainage 8-740
Unification
- double uteri 5-695
Units (of)
- King-Armstrong 2-472
- - acid phosphatase 2-473
- Maclagan 2-321
- Somogyi 2-470
Unroofing
- cranial abscess 5-011
- pancreatic duct 5-523
Unsaturated fat diet
- prophylactic 4-464
Uptake
- iodine (by thyroid) 2-403
Uranoplasty 5-275
Uranorrhaphy 5-275
Urban's operation 5-864
Urea
- clearance 2-341
- excretion 2-341
- nitrogen, serum 2-112
- urinary 2-215
Ureteral catheterization 1-654
Ureterectomy 5-563
- with ureteroureterostomy 5-563
Ureterocecostomy 5-566
Ureterocolostomy 5-566
Ureterocystostomy 5-567
Ureteroenterostomy 5-566
Ureteroileocutaneostomy 5-564

Ureteroileostomy 5-566
- external diversion 5-564
- internal diversion 5-566
Ureterolithotomy 5-562
Ureterolysis 5-568
Ureteroneocystostomy 5-567
Ureteropexy 5-568
Ureteroplasty 5-568
Ureteroplication 5-568
Ureteroproctostomy 5-566
- closure 5-568
Ureteropyelostomy 5-557
Ureterorrhaphy 5-568
Ureteroscopy 1-650
- operative 1-695
Ureterosigmoidostomy 5-566
- with colostomy 5-566
Ureterostomy 5-565
- cutaneous 5-565
- external 5-565
- in situ 5-565
Ureterotomy 5-562
- with calculus removal 5-562
Ureteroureterostomy 5-567
Urethral pressure measurement 1-335
Urethrocystopexy 5-597
Urethrocystoscopy 1-652
Urethrolithotomy 5-580
Urethrolysis 5-584
Urethropexy 5-597
- with colporrhaphy 5-704
Urethroplasty 5-583
Urethrorrhaphy 5-583
Urethroscopy 1-655
Urethrostomy 5-580
Urethrotomy
- external 5-580
- internal 5-584
Urethrovesicopexy 5-597
Uric acid
- blood 2-113
- urinary 2-216
Urine, urinary
- acetoacetic acid 2-240
- acetone 2-240
- acidity 2-250
- alanine 2-201
- albumin
- - estimation 2-204
- alcohol 2-243

Urine - *continued*
- aldosterone 2-442
- aminoacids 2-200
- — detection 2-200
- — estimation 2-201
- ammonia 2-210
- amylase 2-470
- arsenic 2-234
- ascorbic acid 2-241
- Bence-Jones protein 2-670
- bile pigments 2-212
- bile salts 2-214
- bilirubin 2-212
- biochemistry 2-259
- blood detection 2-253
- boric acid 2-236
- bradykinin 2-206
- bromide 2-236
- calcium 2-230
- calculus analysis 2-251
- carbohydrate 2-229
- — constituents 2-229
- catecholamines 2-442
- chloride 2-231
- chorionic gonadotrophin 2-444
- chromium 2-234
- citric acid 2-242
- collection from single ureter 1-654
- concentration test 1-741
- copper 2-234
- creatine 2-211
- creatinine 2-211
- cystine 2-201
- d-aminolevulinic acid 2-201
- density 2-258
- depression of freezing point 2-252
- drug detection 2-244
- electrolyte
- — constituents 2-239
- — other 2-239
- estrogens 2-443
- examination
- — for parasites 2-733
- exogenous organic constituents 2-248
- fluoride 2-235
- fructose 2-229
- function test 1-749
- galactose 2-221
- glucose 2-220
- glycine 2-201
- gonadotropin 2-444
- heavy chain protein 2-671
- heavy metals 2-234
- hemoglobin 2-205
- — detection 2-205
- hemosiderin 2-839
- histidine 2-201

Urine - *continued*
- homogentisic acid 2-201
- hormone NEC 2-449
- hydrogen ion concentration 2-250
- hydroxyproline 2-201
- inorganic constituents 2-239
- iron 2-234
- kallidin 2-206
- ketoglutarte 2-229
- ketones 2-240
- lactose 2-229
- lead 2-234
- leucine 2-201
- light chain protein 2-670
- magnesium 2-235
- mandelic acid 2-242
- manganese 2-234
- mercury 2-234
- microscopic examination 2-346
- — crystals 2-254
- mucopolysaccharides 2-222
- myoglobin
- — detection 2-205
- nickel 2-234
- oestrogens 2-443
- organic acid 2-242
- osmolality 2-252
- other nitrogenous compounds 2-219
- other organic constituents 2-249
- oxalic acid 2-242
- pentose 2-229
- pH 2-250
- phenylpyruvic acid 2-240
- phosphate 2-239
- physicochemical test 2-258
- pituitary hormones 2-440
- placental lactogen 2-444
- plasma peptid products 2-206
- porphyrins 2-213
- potassium 2-232
- pregnancy hormone 2-444
- progesterone 2-444
- protein
- — clinical detection 2-202
- — estimation 2-203
- — product NEC 2-209
- rejection products (incompatibility) 2-645
- renin 2-206
- routine clinical examination 2-255
- saccharometry 2-224
- salicylic acid 2-242
- salicylsulphonic acid 2-242
- sediment
- — microscopic examination 2-254
- sodium 2-233
- specimen 1-915

Urine - *continued*
— steroids 2-441
— sugar 2-229
— thallium 2-235
— thyroid excretion 2-405
— trace elements 2-235
— tyrosine 2-201
— urea 2-215
— — concentration 2-215
— — total 2-215
— urea-creatinine ratio 2-341
— uric acid 2-216
— urobilinogen 2-212
— uroporphyrin 2-213
— vanillyl mandelic acid 2-201

Urine - *continued*
— vanillylmandelic acid 2-242
— xylose 2-229
— 5-hydroxyindole acetic acid 2-219
— 17-hydroxycorticosteroids 2-441
— 17-oxocorticosteroid 2-441
Urinometer
— refractive 2-258
Urobilinogen
— blood 2-115
Urobilistix 2-212
Uteropexy 5-693
Uvulectomy 5-276
Uvulotomy 5-276

V

V-Y operation
– eyelid 5-096
V-Y plasty
– bladder sphincter 5-578
– rectal prolapse 5-486
– renal pelvis 5-557
– skin 5-890
– thoracic artery 5-395
– tongue 5-254
Vaccination (see also Immunization) 4-359
– smallpox 4-340
Vaccine (see also Immunization)
– antirabies
– – therapeutic administration 9-222
– autogenous 9-221
– typhus 4-344
Vacuum aspiration
– termination of pregnancy 5-751
Vagectomy
– subdiaphragmatic 5-440
Vagina, vaginal
– aspirate, for cytology 1-476
– contraceptive device 4-658
– cytology 2-916
– secretion
– – examination
– – – for parasites 2-734
– smear, for hormone study 1-476
Vaginectomy
– see colpectomy 5-702
Vaginofixation 5-706
Vaginoperineotomy 5-701
Vaginopexy 5-706
Vaginoplasty 5-705
Vaginorrhaphy 5-706
Vaginoscopy 1-663
Vaginotomy 5-701
– for pelvic abscess 5-701
Vagotomy 5-440
– abdominal 5-440
– parietal cell 5-440
– superselective 5-440
– truncal 5-440
– with
– – gastroenterostomy 5-442
– – other gastric operation 5-445
– – partial gastrectomy 5-438
Valine
– serum identification 2-100
Valve

Valve - *continued*
– Bjork-Shiley 5-352
– Braunwald-Cutter 5-352
– Cutter-Smeloff 5-352
– Harken 5-352
– Holter - see Holter valve
– Kay-Shiley 5-352
– Lillehei-Kaster 5-352
– Spitz-Holter - see Spitz-Holter valve
– Starr-Edwards 5-352
Valvotomy
– cardiac
– – closed 5-350
– – open 5-351
Valvulectomy 5-352
Valvuloplasty
– cusp 5-353
– gastric 5-537
– with graft or prosthesis 5-352
Van den Berg test 2-115
Van Slike test 2-121
Varicocelectomy 5-630
Varicotomy 5-380
Vasectomy 5-981
– bilateral 5-981
– for excision of lesion 5-636
– sterilization 5-981
– unilateral 5-636
Vasoligation
– gastric 5-387
– varicocele 5-630
Vasopressin
– concentration test 1-741
Vasorrhaphy 5-637
Vasotomy 5-635
Vasovasotomy 5-637
VDRL slide test 2-601
Vector cardiography 1-263
Vena cava sieve 5-386
Venectomy 5-385
– varicose 5-384
– – with reanastomosis 5-382
– – with replacement 5-383
Venesection, venisection 8-820
Venipuncture 8-846
– base of brain 5-010
– diagnostic 1-869
– intracranial 5-010
Venotomy 5-380
Venovenostomy 5-392

Venovenostomy 5-392 - *continued*
− intra-abdominal 5-391
− portacaval 5-391
− splenorenal 5-391
Ventilation
− minute 1-711
− standardized exercise 1-724
Ventilatory
− control test 1-716
− function test NEC 1-719
− regional function 1-713
Ventouse
− assisted delivery 5-728
− traction
− − fetal head 5-728
Ventricular outflow tract pressure gradient 1-720
Ventriculocisternostomy 5-022
Ventriculocordectomy 5-302
Ventriculopuncture 5-010
Ventriculoseptopexy
− with prosthetic device 5-356
Ventriculoseptoplasty 5-357
− with prosthetic device 5-356
Ventriculostomy (cerebral) 5-022
Ventriculotomy (heart) 5-371
− septum 5-355
Ventrofixation (uterus) 5-693
Ventrosuspension (uterus) 5-693
Verification
− spectacles 9-322
Version
− bipolar 8-251
− cephalic (obstetric) 5-732
− combined (obstetric) 5-732
− external 8-251
− internal (obstetric) 5-732
− Wigand 8-251
− with breech extraction 5-725
Vesicle fluid
− micro-organisms 1-911
− virology 1-911
Vesicolithotomy (suprapubic) 5-571
Vesicostomy 5-572
Vesicourethroplasty 5-578
Vesiculectomy 5-606
Vesiculotomy 5-606
Vestibular
− tests
− − clinical 1-234
− − function 1-239
− − − clinical 1-234
− − − rotation 1-235
− − with specialized equipment 1-234
Vestibuloplasty 5-244
− buccal 5-244
− dental 5-244

Vestibulotomy 5-207
Vibration
− cervix 8-543
Vickers chamber 8-772
Vidianectomy 5-051
Villusectomy 5-805
Vineberg's operation 5-362
Virus
− animal passage 2-544
− culture 2-549
− − chick embryo 2-545
− − organ 2-542
− − tissue 2-543
− cytophatic effect 2-540
− demonstration
− − electron microscopy 2-541
− − light microscopy 2-540
− detection 2-549
− identification 2-559
− − complement fixation 2-554
− − counterimmunoelectrophoresis 2-553
− − extraction of antigen 2-556
− − hemadsorption inhibition test 2-550
− − hemagglutination 2-550
− − immunodiffusion 2-552
− − neuraminidase 2-551
− − phage typing 2-555
− − serological 2-558
− − varieties 2-559
− immunofluorescent reaction 2-615
− isolation 2-549
− neutralization 2-620
Viscometry
− blood 2-183
Vision testing 1-211
− binocular 1-216
− illiterates 1-212
− infants 1-212
Visual fields
− testing 1-210
Vital capacity 1-710
− forced 1-711
Vital staining 2-804
Vitamin
− supplement 4-473
Vitamin B 12 assay 2-570
Vitamin deficiency
− test 1-953
Vitamin A
− blood 2-160
Vitamin C
− blood 2-161
Vitamin D
− metabolism 2-365
− supplement 4-472
Vitrectomy (anterior) 5-157
Vocational

Vocational - *continued*
- assessment 9-531
- retraining 9-530
- schooling 9-513
- training
- - general 9-532
Voice training 9-415
Volume
- corpuscular, mean 2-813
- packed cell 2-811
- red cell 2-813

Volume implant
- with radiotherapy
- - tongue (requires radiology code) 5-259
Voluntary agency 9-729
Vomit
- retrieval for analysis 1-312
Von Kraske's operation 5-485
Vulvectomy 5-715
- complete 5-715
- partial 5-715
- radical 5-714

W

Waiting list 9-183
Walking frame 9-333
− loan 9-812

Warm immune antibodies 2-627
Wash-out
− antrum
− − with puncture 5-220
− bladder 8-132

Wassermann reaction 2-600
Water
− loading test 2-429
− retention test 1-740
Water bed 8-374
Waterston's operation 5-390
Wedge resection
− bladder 5-575
− − neck, transurethral 5-573
− bone 5-784
− breast 5-860
− cervix 5-672
− − with trachelorrhaphy 5-674
− kidney 5-553
− liver 5-501
− lung 5-323
− nail 8-186
− ovary 5-651
− − for biopsy 1-570
− stomach 5-434
− tongue 5-251
Wedging
− plaster 8-230
Weight reduction diet 4-461
Weil-Felix reaction 2-613
Weir's operation 5-479
Well baby care
− by nurse 4-716
− − conference (with parent) 4-716
− − − first 4-715
− − − subsequent 4-716
− − home visit 4-718
− − − first 4-717
− − − subsequent 4-718
− by other health personnel 4-785
− − first attention 4-784
− − home visit 4-791
− − subsequent attentions 4-785
− − medical 4-712
− − initial 4-710
− − subsequent 4-712
Wertheim's operation 5-685

West's operation 5-087
Westergren method 2-810
Wet colostomy 5-566
Wharton-Jones operation 5-096
Wheeled chair 9-803
− powered (motor) 9-802
− supply 9-803
Wheeler's operation 5-093
Whipple's operation 5-526
Whirling
− acupuncture (for anesthesia) 8-541
− − with moxa 8-606
− bath 8-583
− brush 8-183
Whirlpool therapy 8-553
Whispered speech test (for hearing) 1-232
White cell (see also Blood, white cell) 2-880
− count 2-801
− − differential 2-881
− − total 2-880
Whitehead's operation 5-493
Wigand's version 8-251
Wight test 2-654
Window operation
− antrum (maxillary) 5-221
− aortic 5-395
− bone cortex 5-780
− pericardial 5-371
Wiring
− anal 5-496
− aneurysm 5-395
− − aorta 5-395
− bone
− − fractured
− − − open reduction 5-792
− cervix 5-674
− dental 8-334
− − fractured jaw 5-762
− − − open operation 5-763
− − orthodontic 5-246
− jaw
− − external 8-334
− − open operation 5-763
− olecranon 5-792
− rectal 5-486
− teeth 8-334
Wirsungojejunostomy 5-527
Withdrawal
− blood
− − for donation 8-821
− − for examination - see Sampling, blood

X

Xenobiochemistry 2-289
Xenodiagnosis 2-563
− protozoa 2-745
Xenon

Xenon - *continued*
− wash-out
− − kidney 2-343
Xylose absorption test 2-312

Y

Y-ostectomy
− jaw (upper) 5-772

Yount's operation 5-831

Z

Z-plasty
− canthus 5-092
− eyelid 5-096
− face 5-891
− relaxing 5-891
− − scar 5-891
− skin 5-891
− thoracic artery 5-395
− wrinkled scar 5-891

Z-suture
− esophagus 5-427
Ziegler's operation 5-135
Ziehl-Neelsen (strain) 2-504
Zinc
− blood 2-156
− turbidity 2-321
Zonulolysis, zonulysis (lens) 5-144